FIT FOR THE FUTURE

Report of the Committee on Child Health Services

Chairman: Emeritus Professor S D M Court, CBE, MD, FRCP, FCST

VOLUME 1

Presented to Parliament by the Secretary of State for Social Services, the Secretary of State for Education and Science and the Secretary of State for Wales by Command of Her Majesty
December 1976

LONDON
HER MAJESTY'S STATIONERY OFFICE
£6.50 net

Cmnd. 6684

ISBN 0 10 166840 6

MEMBERS OF THE COMMITTEE

Emeritus Professor S D M Court, CBE, MD, FRCP, FCST (Chairman)

Mrs M Bannister (resigned June 1976)

Miss B M Barchard, SRN, RSCN

Mrs G Gorell Barnes, MA, MSC (appointed August 1974)

Mrs B Barnett (resigned July 1974)

Mrs M Best, SRN, SCM (resigned November 1973)

Mrs M Bickerton, SRN, HV

Professor P H Burke, MDS

Mrs G Carter

Miss E M Davies, BA (appointed November 1974)

Mrs J Davies, MA

Dr R Harvard Davis, MA, DM, FRCGP

Miss F Drake, MA

Dr H McC Giles, MB, FRCP, DCH

Dr A Parry Jones, MB, BCH, DPH, FFCM

Professor C R Lowe, MD, PhD, FRCP

Mr A G McPherson, BA, MB, MChir, FRCS

Dr S R W Moore, MD, MFCM, DPH

Professor T E Oppé, MB, BS, FRCP, DCH

Dr M G H Rogers, MA, MB, BChir, DPH, DCH

Professor M L Rutter, MD, FRCP, FRCPsych, DPM

Professor J Tizard, CBE, PhD

Mr J R G Tomlinson, MA, FRSA

Mr J E Knight (to January 1976)

Mrs M Palmer (from March 1976) } Joint Secretaries

Dr T K Whitmore, MRCS, LRCP, DPH

iii

To:

The Rt Hon. DAVID ENNALS, MP
Secretary of State for Social Services

The Rt Hon. SHIRLEY WILLIAMS, MP
Secretary of State for Education and Science

The Rt Hon. JOHN MORRIS, QC, MP
Secretary of State for Wales

Dear Secretaries of State,

I am glad to submit to you the Report of the Committee on Child Health Services.

When Sir Keith Joseph called us together we were left in no doubt of his concern to improve the child health services and his belief that the reorganisation of the National Health Service and the transfer of the School Health Service provided an unrivalled opportunity to achieve this improvement. Your predecessor Mrs Castle shared this view and encouraged us by saying that she considered health services for children a potent investment in the country's future. It is with this sense of need and opportunity that our work has been done. Three years is not long for a far reaching inquiry of this kind, touching some of the most significant and sensitive aspects of family and public life. And there was no guiding precedent since such a review has not been carried out in this country before.

We are sorry that our report will not fit comfortably into one volume. With so wide and serious a review, it seemed essential to set down in full the evidence and the judgements which led to our recommendations. Our convictions that a sound service must be epidemiologically based led to the collection of a rich store of statistical data which we felt should be made available in the report. We were also conscious of other possible groups of readers beyond Parliament and Government—professional groups of doctors, dentists, nurses, therapists, social workers, teachers and psychologists, in this country and in comparable countries in Europe and beyond; older children; parent associations; members of Community Health Councils; and the interested public. The design of the Report has this potential readership in mind.

The Introduction, complete in itself, speaks of needs and values in a changing society and of our response. Part I examines continuity and change in children and their families, in the picture of health and disease and in the available services; how other countries are facing similar needs and opportunities; and ends with a description of the objectives and structure of an integrated child health service which could meet contemporary needs more effectively. Part II examines the needs of defined areas of child development and childhood illness more closely, to establish whether these particular needs could be met by the type of service put forward at the end of Part I. Part III describes the professional and administrative structure required for this integrated service for all children. Our conclusions and recommendations are shown in italic in each chapter and given in summary in Part IV which concludes the Report.

To suggest that we were agreed in every detail would be foolish. We started from our traditional positions and grew, at times painfully, to the unity and conviction which I believe can be seen and felt in the report. We are also aware of the severe social and economic demands which this country is facing and which for some time will be the setting in which our proposals would be implemented, but we believe the investment in the future set out in this report is a part of that wider investment on which our national wellbeing depends. We know that Reports in themselves do not solve problems. We can only hope that our recommendations, drawn from the experience of so many, will prove as sensible in practice as they seemed in committee.

Three years of unremitting enquiry is a major addition for men and women already committed to full time professional responsibilities. As chairman I am very grateful that their critical attention and collective loyalty has been maintained throughout. Such a quality of public service is necessary and should be highly valued in a democratic society. In turn the Committee thank our "observers" from the Departments for providing necessary information at the right time and helping us to see how the desirable can become the possible. We also thank the Office of Population Censuses and Surveys for work so efficiently carried out on our behalf. And we have come to regard Mr Frank Whitehead, the statistical master-builder of the Report, as an indispensable support to the committee. We have left our warmest thanks till last. The efficiency of a committee like ours depends on the skill, patience and tenacity of the secretaries. We are deeply grateful to Mr Jeremy Knight, Mrs Mary Palmer, Dr Kingsley Whitmore and to other members of the secretarial team, particularly Mrs Joan Dickson, Mr Bryan Harrison, Mr Michael Brown and Miss Karen Higgs. Without their sustained efforts, especially in the final stages, the Report would not have been completed in good time.

Yours sincerely,

DONALD COURT

CONTENTS

VOLUME 1

PART II

PARTICULAR NEEDS AND REMEDIES

CHAPTER 13: THE PATH TO DENTAL HEALTH

PART III

THE WAY FORWARD: THE MACHINERY OF CHANGE

PART IV

SUMMARY OF MAJOR RECOMMENDATIONS

APPENDICES

VOLUME 2
STATISTICAL APPENDIX

INTRODUCTION

"By health, I mean the power to live a full, adult, living breathing life in close contact with what I love—I want to be all that I am capable of becoming."—Katherine Mansfield†

Our task has been to review the existing health services for children, judge how effective they are for the child and his parents, and to propose what the new, integrated child health service should try to achieve and how it should, therefore, be organised and staffed.

The purpose of this opening chapter is to give a simple account of what we discovered about the existing services, to sketch the philosophy we developed of the most helpful relationship between the professionals, the children, and others caring for the children, and thus to reveal the deeper purposes lying beneath the recommendations we make.

---

† Quoted by permission of the Society of Authors as the literary representative of the Estate of Katherine Mansfield.

Surveying the Scene

Children and Childhood

Over the last twelve years in Britain there has been a marked decline in the birthrate and the small natural decrease in the year ending March 1976 was the first occasion in peacetime since central records were first instituted 140 years ago that deaths exceeded births in any 12 month period. Between 1974 and 1981 the number of children aged under 15 in England is expected to fall by 9%—1,000,000 fewer children. Moreover, over the rest of the century the number of children under age 15 is likely to remain lower than that of 1974. There is, therefore, a very practical reason for reviewing at this time the health care we give our children since there will be fewer of them growing up in our society, parents will have even higher expectations, and improvements could be made without an increase in expenditure. While all that is true, and we take account of it in the detail of our recommendations, we wish to assert beyond any possibility of misunderstanding, that we have tried to base our arguments on the nature and needs of children and their families, on knowledge and insight which reach to the ground of our being as the human species.

In the last two or three generations we have come to realise how precious is our inheritance of children and also to recognise their needs as being different from those of adults. At one time children were dressed in adult clothes, scaled down to size, which seemed to reflect an attitude that they were in a sense retarded adults. Childhood was thought of as an inadequate and incomplete form of the adult state. By contrast we have become increasingly aware of childhood as a separate state, as a period of human experience in its own right. And more important still, we have come to realise the extent to which experience in childhood determines the adult outcome.

It is the mark of the human species that our young are born incomparably more "immature" than the young of other species. Man is the only species which has gone all-out for general immaturity and open mindness: they are his particular strategies for development. The human baby and child faces a long period of development and dependence during which he develops the fundamental human attributes of speech, thought, self consciousness and reflection. During these stages the child is a biological organism with biological propensities which needs constant inter-action with his environment, especially the adults around him so that he can learn in innumerable ways and emerge a social as well as an individual being. As the human child grows he is in many important ways literally being created by the slowly forming imprint of experience, the essential tension between the biological and the social, hereditary and environmental influences. That is why the rearing of the young is the fundamental issue in a human society—and why the quality and philosophy of health, education and other care available to the child and his family are so important.

We have found no better way to raise a child than to reinforce the ability of his parent(s), whether natural or substitute, to do so. Almost all parents want the best opportunities for their children but too many still set low expectations and assume that their child's life will be governed by

2

innate ability and maturation, as though mental, physical and emotional development were things that simply happened up to a determined level by an automatic process. One conviction that informs this report is that parents need to be made more aware of the learning (in the widest sense) that goes on day by day through experience, and of their part in it. Future improvements in the health of children will depend as much on the beliefs and behaviour of parents as on the services provided.

Another of our convictions is that the disadvantages of birth and early life cast long shadows forward. Many parents have to contend with circumstances which grossly hamper their natural and acquired ability to be good parents and many children are crippled by circumstance. It should be an objective of a civilised community to ameliorate the condition of those affected in this way and always to strive to remove the causes so far as future generations are concerned. We now know that the effects of early disadvantage can be much diluted by the environmental circumstances the child encounters during the middle and later years of childhood; and that it is especially worth making this corrective effort because early disadvantage tends to lead to later disadvantage, so that, unless there is intervention, there develops a compounding of difficulties. It is this train of events which is influential rather than the critical effect of particular circumstances in early life considered in their own right.

It is striking how many separate but parallel movements in different fields have recently contributed to our understanding of child development. The history of children's literature records the awakening of the artistic and intuitive consciousness of the special state and needs of childhood, and work in education and psychology has mapped the stages and needs of intellectual and emotional growth. Social and industrial legislation has reduced our economic inhumanity to our children, and leaders in social work have tried to enhance the concept of care for children. And in medicine, paediatrics has become established as the specialty dealing with the care and treatment of dependent and developing human beings. It seems possible that our generation will prove to be the one which first tried to apprehend and provide for the needs of the child as a whole. The stage appears set for a concerted effort—if we have the will to make it.

Child Health and Child Health Services

A recognition that children are different from adults and yet the world has been made to suit adults, has two separate and essential consequences for the development of health and welfare services for children. On the one hand we recognise that some different skills are needed: taking blood from a baby for analysis demands different skills from those required for dealing with an adult, and micro methods have to be learnt. Parallel with these special skills is the need to understand the importance to the child's health of his immediate environment. Care for the total needs of the child may be as important as the cure of an immediate problem. If an adult goes into hospital the separation from home, the change of routine, the boredom, the food, may all be factors of secondary importance. For the child, living completely in the present, unable to conceive of the day after tomorrow, the position is quite different. One five-year old wrote about hospital: "I would not like my Mummy and Daddy to leave me

3

there because they might forget me and leave me there for ever—and they might be out the day I come home".[1]

We believe that the training of anyone in professional contact with children should further their understanding of a child's emotional, educational, social, psychological and physical needs; that is, their understanding of the essence of being a child.

What is required from the health services by the child, his parents and others caring for him is by now well known: safe and courteous conduct through pregnancy; skilled attention for mother and child at the point of birth; supervision and advice about the development of the child, especially if there is any kind of handicap; prompt care at home or in hospital during illness or after an accident; and the knowledge that the child's progress at school will be watched, discussed with parents and that educational failure will be recognised, diagnosed and as far as possible remedied. Most of all, doctors must have the skill and make the time to listen to parents' observations and try to understand their anxieties and fears, recognising the great strain that raising children involves and that only the parents can contribute an essential dimension to understanding a child.

On the credit side

The improvements in the health of children during this century have been spectacular and heartening. Most of the killing or crippling diseases of the nineteenth century have been eradicated or brought under control. Between 1948 and 1973 the infant mortality rate fell from 34 to 17 per 1,000 and mortality within the age group 1–14 years fell by more than half. Local studies suggest that the mean height of children entering school is 7.5cm greater and their weight 2,270g heavier than forty years ago.[2] This improvement is maintained throughout childhood and adolescence so that the majority are taller and heavier on leaving school than any generation of their predecessors.

Most of the improvements have resulted from a reduction in overcrowding, better nutrition, smaller and more "spaced" families; others are due to a variety of specific measures such as immunisation or new, effective treatments. Further improvements have resulted from higher standards of medical and nursing care and a recognition of the educative rôle of these services in the care of mother and child.

Shortcomings

And yet in many crucial respects our findings have given us profound anxiety about the present state of child health in this country, about the shortcomings of the services and those working in them, and about the prospects for new generations if they are to grow up in the same deprived physical and emotional circumstances as many children today contend with.

Twenty years ago this country had one of the lowest rates of infant mortality but since then we have fallen behind other countries, Sweden, the Netherlands, France, Switzerland and Japan among them. In 1960 for example, the rates in England and Wales were the same as in Finland,

---

[1] Hales—Tooke, A (1975). *Children in Hospital—The Parents' View.* Priority Press.
[2] Court, S D M (1971). Child Health in a Changing Community. *Brit. Med. Jour.* 2, 125-131.

4

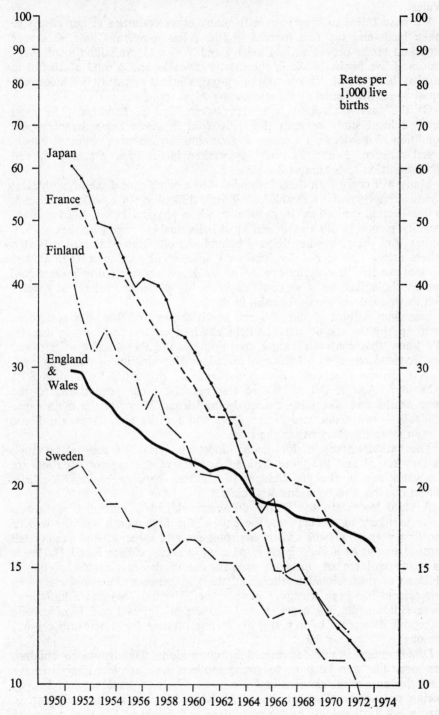

Infant mortality rates in selected countries 1950-1974

Rates per 1,000 live births

Japan

France

Finland

England & Wales

Sweden

but by 1972 the Finnish rate was about one-third below that in England and Wales.

We have failed to keep pace with many other countries in our efforts to make birth and the first months of life a less dangerous time. Of every thousand births occurring in England and Wales 11 are stillborn; of every thousand live births 11 die in the first four weeks and a total of 16 fail to survive the first year. In contemporary terms infant mortality is a holocaust, equal to all the deaths of the succeeding 24 years of life.

Of the survivors, many will suffer some kind of handicap. The most detailed local study suggests that one child in seven has a handicapping condition of moderate or severe degree sufficient to be a cause of educational concern. A parallel study undertaken in an inner city area showed the proportion to be almost double.

Many will carry with them into adult life a significant disability: physical handicap, recurrent or established illness, difficulties in emotional control, or intellectual limitation. In particular, while physical health has improved steadily, mental health and the ability of individuals to cope with the ordinary demands of their lives have lagged behind. As one kind of hazard is beaten others arise. This is not forgivable on account of our ignorance. As one witness put it: "If only we applied all we know about children's emotional and psychological needs we could make as big advances in the next generation as we made in physical health in the last".

Less than a third of our children reach the age of five with decay-free teeth and by the age of seven half the children are affected by gum disease. We know that control of sugar consumption and the practice of personal oral hygiene could go a long way to reduce this amount of dental disease; it is a disease that could be almost entirely prevented by a change in behaviour. And if dental disease has reached gross proportions so too have deaths and disabilities caused by accidents. They are the main cause of death between one and fifteen years and for the under-fives, the home is even more dangerous than the roads.

The national statistics for death, illness and disability conceal as much as they reveal and the more striking features of the present situation are the variations in the life chances of children between regions, localities within regions, and between social classes.

A child born into the family of a semi-skilled or unskilled worker is twice as likely to die between the end of the first month and the end of the first year of his life (when environment and other related factors tell most strongly) as a child born to parents in social classes I and II. Twice as many children of unskilled workers die in the first month of life as children of professional workers and the gap between the social classes in this respect has been widening steadily for 25 years. Two and a half times more children die in classes IV and V than in classes I and II of certain infectious diseases. Children still die in our lifetime for nineteenth century reasons.

Disadvantage is not determined by class alone. Disadvantaged children are more likely to be born to young mothers who are less likely to have used the ante-natal services and are more likely to have smoked heavily during pregnancy. They are more likely to be born prematurely and to have a low birthweight. In the early days and weeks of life they are more exposed to the risk of infection and death. Evidence to this Committee suggests that it is largely possible for this group to be identified.[3]

Children who live in urban conditions are more likely to suffer from ill-health than those who do not and children in inner London areas are twice as likely to be psychologically disturbed as their counterparts in rural areas. The physical health of inner-city children is likely to be poorer and yet the services in urban areas, especially in the North and Midlands, are likely to be less numerous and of a poorer quality. More money is spent on health services in those areas where there are more well-off people in the population. Despite recent efforts to bring about more equality, the variations in regional provision of service are still much the same as they were in 1948 when the National Health Service began.

Environmental Handicap

One result is that children already suffering disadvantage for social or geographical reasons often suffer double disadvantage on account of poor services. We believe that in the long run only a combined approach from housing, health, education and social services can even begin to eradicate the causes of the initial disadvantage, but meanwhile the health services must respond to the needs of these children and their families by providing more, better and in some respects, different health care. In the first place the service must seek out and reach out to those in need. It must not only provide health care but also assist in the growth of self-confidence and knowledge that will enable such families in the future to do more for themselves.

It is most likely in a population such as Britain's that people have essentially the same potentialities; and that, therefore, the wide divergencies between region and class that we have found, and that health services have to try to cope with, are largely caused by the different conditions in which people live—in which we include their attitude to each other and to their children. Our contention is that a society that wanted to remove these differences would not only provide remedial health services but would also concentrate on preventive health services and on environmental improvement.

Physically and Mentally Handicapped Children

The standard of diagnosis, assessment, treatment and care for children suffering from physical, mental or multiple handicaps whether in the hospital or the community does not reach that largely achieved by the NHS for the treatment of acute illness. It is also evident that families often get little relief from the economic and social difficulties that arise because they care for a handicapped child. In this respect they are often worse off than families with children with acute disease, although their burdens are often more severe and last much longer. Health, education and social services for handicapped children and their families are the product of the historical development of

---

[3] Emery J, *et al*. Unexpected death in infancy: child development team, Sheffield. Evidence submitted to the Commitee.

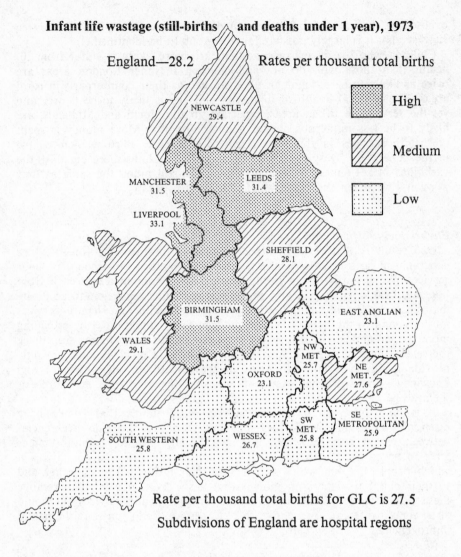

Infant life wastage (still-births and deaths under 1 year), 1973

England—28.2   Rates per thousand total births

High

Medium

Low

NEWCASTLE
29.4

MANCHESTER
31.5

LEEDS
31.4

LIVERPOOL
33.1

SHEFFIELD
28.1

BIRMINGHAM
31.5

EAST ANGLIAN
23.1

WALES
29.1

NW
MET
25.7

NE
MET.
27.6

OXFORD
23.1

SE
METROPOLITAN
25.9

SOUTH WESTERN
25.8

WESSEX
26.7

SW
MET.
25.8

Rate per thousand total births for GLC is 27.5

Subdivisions of England are hospital regions

services which have grown in an uncoordinated manner; they are consequently patchy and vary both in quality and coverage.

Some of the most depressing evidence we have received concerned handicapped children both at home and in hospital.

The mother of a handicapped child talks about her early experiences: [4] she felt from the start that B, her second child, would be abnormal in some way. He was a quiet, good baby . . . so good, he never moved. When she compared him to her first, the health visitor reassured her; he's just backward, it'll be all right. She took him to the local clinic but "as soon as the weight is o.k. they don't think any more"—and she just had to keep to herself her knowledge, now more than a fear, that she had a backward

[4] Fox, M (1975). *They get this training but they don't really know how you feel.* National Fund for Research into Crippling Diseases.

8

**Areas of above-average expenditure on community-health
services and above-average socioeconomic status.**

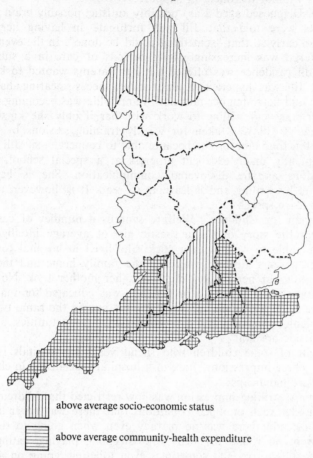

☐ above average socio-economic status

☐ above average community-health expenditure

J Noyce, A H Snaith, A J Trickey, (1974) Lancet Vol 1. No 7857. p. 556.

child. When he was nearly three he had a fit. The local hospital said this
was due to teething but she knew he wasn't teething when he had the fit
and she insisted on going to a children's hospital. "I had to put up a fight,
but I got there". She saw "the greatest expert in the country", and after an
EEG was told there was nothing the matter, no need to see B again. "Oh
yes, they said he was backward", but seemed to imply that there was nothing
to be done about it. She spent two years waiting and wondering, B made
little or no progress. This mother's and child's experiences with two schools
before finally the child was found a place at a suitable training centre for the
severely mentally handicapped indicate a depressing lack of communication
between services or understanding of the family's needs.

A research worker's notes[5] about another child indicate the uselessness of diagnosis without treatment or support:

JILL, 10. Diagnosed aged 2 as "possibly autistic, possibly brain damaged". Her parents were told that Jill was fortunate in having her condition diagnosed so early so that "something could be done". In the event, the only support offered was increasingly long periods of care in a sub-normality hospital. Full residence was offered but her parents wanted to keep her in the family. Jill was hyperactive, destructive, faeces-smearing, had no span of attention and fierce temper tantrums. Family life was becoming impossible. Her mother was very willing to work with her if only she knew where to start. At age 8 Jill was taken for weekly training sessions by a research centre. Within four months she became able to cooperate, sit still and attend and subsequently made excellent progress at a special school, controlling her obsessions as she discovered communication. She is beginning to communicate by writing and is learning to read. It is, however, too late for her ever to learn speech.

The Council for Children's Welfare sent us a number of case histories among them the story of CJ, a spastic girl of average intelligence, independent and able to walk with a stick. She lived in hospital for ten years because her parents' divorce broke up the family home and there was no accommodation for her in the "digs" that her mother took. No residential special school could be found for her. She was educated for that ten years in the same room adjoining her ward, always having the same two teachers. She was denied virtually all the educational opportunities available to children outside hospital.

The plight of some children who spend years in hospitals is especially disturbing. These impressions[6] are of a hospital specialising in children with chronic severe handicaps:

"The most striking impression was how restricted the children were; they lived under such cramped conditions that there was never a chance to be alone, and there was no privacy even when going to the lavatory. Life went on round the beds with sleeping, playing, eating, washing, treatments, visitors and sometimes even toileting, going on at the same time in one room. A child such as Tony (aged 8 spina bifida, who had been there for two years) who was not ill but was an in-patient because he needed schooling, physiotherapy and a home, had to sit on a bed-pan in his bed just as if he was a sick patient recovering from an operation; this was simply because there was no room in the bathroom and it was quicker to put him on a bed-pan. Because the ward was upstairs there was no access to the outside, and even on the brightest of days the children remained indoors. This was particularly shocking when one realised that the children did not live in the ward for just a few weeks, but that this was their home for several years".

"Elsewhere in . . . hospital a ground floor ward accommodated 24 mentally able children aged from 4 to 6, who were physically handicapped by spina bifida or thalidomide. Although this ward had a day-room and access to a small paved courtyard, life there was as

(5) Newson, E Unpublished notes.
(6) Oswin, M (1971). *The Empty Hours.* Allen Lane, Penguin. pp 77-8 and 80-81.

restricted as in the upstairs ward . . . it was not unusual for naked and half-naked limbless four year olds to sit on their little yellow plastic pots, tight together, in a row against the bare wall, for an hour or an hour and a half, whilst bathing routines went on above and around them. The going to bed routine for these little children started at 3.30 p.m. . . . because these small, mentally alert children had no opportunities to satisfy their normal craving for play, they inevitably derived bizarre play habits from their environment. . . ."

Many handicapped children who live in hospital are vulnerable to various forms of deprivation which may eventually create additional handicaps for them . . . further intellectual retardation, social incompetence and deep-seated unhappiness. Their initial disadvantage is compounded by the provision we make or fail to make for them.

Educational failure

The connection between health and education is one of the most important aspects of paediatrics. Educational failure should be recognised early and requires precise diagnosis just as much as physical disease, for many difficulties at school could be anticipated before school begins. The connection between low birthweight, nutrition and the development of intelligence has been investigated. So also has the connection between attainment and the size of the family to which the child belongs. Yet in general our understanding of disorders of learning is still rudimentary and the problems of intellectual limitation, defective speech, inadequate reading ability, excessive clumsiness, disturbed behaviour, truancy, school phobia and delinquency create a formidable array of disability. These problems will yield only to the combined efforts of doctors, teachers, psychologists and psychiatrists, social workers and others. Yet we found a good deal of evidence that as yet services were not disposed so as to cooperate in the interests of the child.

Non-accidental injury

The failure of services becomes most stark and tragic when it contributes to the death of a child at the hands of those who should care for him. While we were working as a Committee the results were published of investigations into the deaths at the hands of their parents of six young children, among them Maria Colwell. They were the children whose names became known to the public. Many others died whose cases received no such publicity. The exact size of the problem has not yet been determined; figures quoted on a national basis are generally extrapolated from local studies. These suggest that more than 5,000 children are affected in this way every year of whom 1,000 will be seriously injured and nearly 100 die.

The failure to prevent this suffering is of two kinds. Health, social and education services do not react well enough individually or collectively to signs of need; and too little is known and done about the reasons which cause individuals to lose control and injure their children.

Such omissions and failures of insight by professionals must be remedied by a determined effort of those responsible for giving the services and for training new generations of doctors, teachers and social workers.

The implications for society as a whole of "non-accidental injury" to

11

children are very disturbing because the cases which come to light are almost certainly only the tip of the iceberg. It is likely to occur among parents who are hard pressed by life, burdened by their children, and especially their young children, from whom they cannot get the physical relief of removing themselves or the psychological relief of sharing their burdens with others. It is not only a matter of individual behaviour since one could expect that in a healthy society child battering would happen only in rare pathological cases.

Trends and Innovations

The changing pattern of family and social life

An effective health service, and especially an effective child health service, must be knowledgeable about the social and economic circumstances of those it serves and have developed a philosophy of how its expertise and facilities can best be made available to those in need of them. It was part of our remit to examine the use made of existing services and although there is regrettably little statistical evidence so that we have had to rely a good deal on anecdote, it is none the less clear that health services in the future will have to take much more account of the realities of life and its constraints for most families with children if the services are to reach them more satisfactorily.

The average age of marriage in the 1960s and first half of the 1970s has been lower than at any time since civil registration began in 1836 and more than 90% of women have married at least once by the time they reach the end of child-bearing age. In 1974 spinsters were marrying $2\frac{1}{2}$–3 years younger than their counterparts 40 years ago (at an average age of 22.7 instead of 25.5); and whereas in 1931 17% of women aged 45–49 had never married, in 1974 the proportion was only 7%. Thus marriage is becoming more popular and is being undertaken younger, although the trend seems to have levelled off in recent years.

Divorce, too, is getting more popular. There has been a long term upward trend in the divorce rate ever since civil divorce first became available in 1857. But up to 1940 the number each year never exceeded 10,000. After the second world war a much steeper upward trend began and the 1970 figure (58,000) was double that of 1960. Since the new legislation of 1970 there has been a further doubling of the annual rate: 120,000 divorces in 1975. Not only has the divorce rate risen steadily but there is also a growing tendency for husbands and wives to divorce at younger ages and after shorter durations of marriage. Marriages where the bride was under 20 are twice as likely to end in divorce as those where she was 20–24 years old. Yet the divorced frequently remarry very soon and there is an upsurge in this trend also. In 1965 11% of marriages involved a divorced bride or groom—by 1972 it was 22% and in 1974 25%.

Yet though marriage is more popular and entered into younger there has been no consistent increase in the number of children. A general picture of declining annual births and earlier marriage reflects the way in which getting married and starting a family are no longer so closely connected as they were even a few years ago. Moreover, recent trends in births have, in particular, shown a fall in the number of births to married women who

12

already have two or more children and in the number of first births—that is, a decline in the number of large families and a delay in the start of childbearing. Since two of the major causes of these trends—the changed social position of women and more satisfactory methods of family planning—are likely to be of continuing significance it may be assumed that these new patterns of family-building and life are likely to be with us for some time.

Two other aspects of this theme are of special significance for child health services: the rise in the illegitimacy ratio and in the number of abortions, especially to teenage girls. In 1973 67% of all live births to women under 20 were conceived extra-maritally and 30% were illegitimate at the time of birth.

Family planning and the consequent decline in family size result in women being involved in child-bearing for a much shorter period of time, and related to this, there has been a rapid increase, which is still continuing, in the numbers of women with young children who go out to work. In Britain the proportion of women with children under the age of five who are doing paid work outside the home increased by more than 70% during the 1960s. By 1971 nearly 600,000 mothers with young children (that is, children under five) were in paid employment. Of these, 30% worked more than 30 hours a week. This implies that more than a quarter of a million children under the age of 5 had mothers who worked full-time.

There is still a tendency in Britain to regard the employment of mothers of young children as something that will decrease rather than increase during the next few years. There is no evidence that this is the case and all the indications are that we share with all other industrial countries a developing trend towards women beginning work when their children are under school age. Nor is it true that mothers who go out to work when their children are young are the ignorant ones who do not know what is good for their children. Evidence from countries as different as France, Sweden, Germany, Hungary, New Zealand and the USA supports the British experience that better educated women of higher social class are more not less likely to seek employment while their children are very young. Moreover there is evidence that the mothers who behave in this way are less likely to suffer from depression, loneliness, anxiety and feelings of low self-esteem. The sad truth is that our society has in no way come to terms with this social fact nor tried to use the opportunity it could afford through day care and education to improve the quality of services for children. Most countries in Western Europe make very much more provision for young children than we do. And, once again, when a move is made, through nursery education, it is based on the concept of 'priority groups' where all the evidence points to the need for a high general level of service. The present deplorable and serious situation of young children put into inadequate day care has been well documented.

Enquiries into the prevalence of psychiatric disorder among the parents of young children have yielded dismaying results. Little is known about fathers but something is known about mothers from local surveys undertaken in urban areas. These indicate that probably 16% (one in every six) of the mothers of young children suffer from a definite psychiatric disorder. But, once again, social class and circumstance are the most telling factors. Recent

13

surveys have shown that feelings of severe depression are part of the common experience of a large minority—possibly more than 40%—of working class mothers with young children. The circumstances connected with this were, as might be expected, chronic difficulties in housing, with money, with children, health or marriage; and traumatic recent events such as a husband losing his job or going to prison, the threat of eviction, older children being in trouble with the police and so on. There is evidence that a trusting and confiding relationship with another adult helped to protect women from the impact of such circumstances and yet these mothers have to accept the very conditions of life which least help marriage or friendship.

Since about 26% of working men in Britain are semi-skilled or unskilled manual workers living in an environment in which many adverse characteristics are to be found, the magnitude of the problem of psychiatric disorder in mothers and its effects on children are very obvious indeed.

More than one million children (1 in 15) are being looked after by a single parent; 920,000 of them by 520,000 lone mothers. We found no evidence that health services have tried to adjust to the routines and special needs of this group of children and parents. Contrary to common belief only 15% of "single parents" are unmarried mothers and unmarried mothers account for only 11% of all the children. The majority are deserted wives and husbands, or those whose partner has died. To provide single handed for all the needs of children must be physically and mentally exhausting. The Finer Committee spoke of the sense of loss and suffering to be found among these parents; the sense of social isolation, the burden of coping alone with unfamiliar household tasks and the emotional and material needs of children. The child suffers the risk of having a lonely or depressed mother or father, the grief of loss and the sense of being different from other children. The results for some children will be poor performance at school or disturbed or delinquent behaviour.

In the last generation our society has become more multi-racial, as ethnic minority groups from almost all parts of the world have made a permanent home in this country. Although a small proportion of the total population, they represent a significant element in certain areas. The health problems of immigrant communities are largely related to two aspects of their life within our society: the cultural differences and the environmental conditions. The contrast in mores, habits of family rearing and dietary laws and traditions can cause stresses which need sensitive understanding by caring outsiders. The environmental health problems arise because the areas in which ethnic minority groups settle tend to be those already suffering environmental disadvantage; such health problems are largely preventible and more needs to be done.

Although there have been marked improvements in the real standard of living in this country, poverty remains. Moreover, considerable inequalities of income and wealth, among them regional disparities, persist in spite of improvements over many years. The quality of housing has continued to rise, yet still one child in four is reared in a home which is overcrowded or lacking in basic amenities. The proportion of the population in each social class has remained roughly the same during this century although there has been a long term tendency to a reduction of the proportion of semi-skilled and unskilled workers. However, the gap between social classes with respect to infant mortality, educational progress, working conditions and ill-health remains almost as wide as it has ever been.

What general conclusions may be drawn from this brief survey of our national life style so far as it has consequences for the life experiences of children, those who are bringing them up and for the health services?

The majority have exchanged stability for prosperity. The minority remain as disadvantaged as ever. The proportion of children who are likely to be in a family that breaks up or contains children from a previous marriage has very much increased. Whether the amount of marital discord has also increased cannot be proved on statistics now available but many believe it has. Without doubt, there is evidence of a marked degree of depression among women who have young children under 5. The proportion of children being brought up by one parent has probably increased; the proportion of illegitimate children has certainly increased; and the proportion of young children whose mothers go out to work has also increased.

Our society does not seem adequately to have adjusted to its basic condition as industrial, urban, multi-racial and undergoing continual change. Material standards of living measured by conventional indicators of domestic consumption, car ownership, paid holidays, income and so on have about doubled in the last twenty years.[7] We believe that many of the regrettable aspects of our findings are the results in part of the unacknowledged consequences of these material changes in life style. For example, increased job opportunities and improvements in housing have both led to much greater geographical mobility: one third of all families move house every five years, often to places very far away from their kin. And families with young children are especially likely to move. So the older style of three-generation family is broken up and young parents get much less support from relatives and long-established neighbours. At the same time urban planning provides fewer opportunities for places in which children can play and traffic makes streets too dangerous for the younger ones to go out alone. The tower blocks which have replaced terraced houses all over England deny access to play space or garden for children; and provide no substitute for the back yard or front steps on which adults meet regularly and gossip casually. From 1911–1966 the population of this country increased by less than one third but the number of households nearly doubled. Between 1961 and 1971 alone the proportion of households containing two or more families declined from 2.7% to 1.4%. Thus the overwhelming majority of households are composed of "nuclear" families and live in independent dwellings. In consequence mothers and their young children probably spend far more time alone together today than ever they did in the past, and very large numbers of young women live lonely and unhappy lives.

The total picture which emerges is one of fundamental change in the pattern of family life, and from this several important consequences follow:

> To talk about the family as the basis of child-rearing is not sufficient; we must clarify what we mean by the family and its essential contribution.
>
> If our services are to be based on working with and through the

---

[7] Eversley, D (1974). *New Society*. 29.616.

family then the professionals concerned must understand and respond appropriately to the new conditions.

If families can now no longer do everything that they were formerly supposed to do, and services have to provide instead, they must do so in a way that supports rather than denigrates the family.

Titmuss argued as long ago as 1948 that while we have always assumed as a society that the family was fundamental to our social structure, we have never really acted as though we believed this and have allowed its importance and effectiveness to be eroded, not wilfully, but by neglect.[8]

In any case the family is not always the ideal environment for child-rearing. Arguably it is only in recent, post-industrial society, that we have expected the family to be the centre and mediator of the child's experience of sociability. The density of social life in earlier times left little room for the family. Once asked to carry this weight and narrowed to the "nuclear" family of our days it can for some become oppressive and restrictive. It is an irony that we have "discovered childhood" and its special needs for sociability and richness of real experience just when our social forms were draining these very characteristics away from the family upon which the responsibility for providing them was mainly placed. Perhaps that is why we have become so conscious of these issues. Auden remarked in 1938 that "The breakdown of the old village or small-town community left the family as the only real social unit, and the parent-child relationship as the only real social bond . . . The problem for the modern poet, as for everyone else today, is how to find or form a genuine community, in which he has his valued place and can feel at home . . . Virtues which were once nursed unconsciously by the forces of nature must now be recovered and fostered by a deliberate effort of the will and the intelligence."[9] It has been made clear to us how fragmented and often irrelevant our transfer from one generation to the next of knowledge about child-bearing has become, so that each mother (and father) has to develop her own ways of coming to terms with her child. Seldom are the ways of infants learnt at first hand before one's own need of them and we must appreciate how dependent this makes parents on the sometimes contradictory advice of professionals. Professionals' wisdom has changed several times this century and seems often to have reflected our moral concerns about children rather than any science.

If we wish to redress this we must create a total system. Our Committee can only point to the need and try to show the health services' part in it.

The changing pattern of disease

The child health services not only have to take account of the changing pattern of family life, but also of the changing pattern of illness, disease and treatment.

As congenital and hereditary conditions become more significant in the totality of illness and as more children survive with handicapping conditions, new demands are made on services. Families with a chronically sick or

---

(8) Titmuss, R M (1948). Parenthood and Social Change. *Lancet*. 2 797.

(9) *Oxford Book of Light Verse* (1938). Introduction pp xviii-xix. Reprinted by permission of the Clarendon Press.

16

handicapped child need to be in a continuing relationship with health workers and this relationship demands new sensitivities. In short-term acute illness, the parents, child and health workers can direct their attention to the minimising of time spent in treatment. The treat-and-cure model, which is the traditional medical one, is also familiar to parents, and one in which doctors, nurses and patients can identify common objectives. Efforts can be directed towards ending the patient's need for professional help as soon as possible.

The care of the handicapped, however, demands on-going support and specialised knowledge at a level immediately, easily and continually available to parents; the support and knowledge will not be purely medical—nurses, teachers, therapists, social workers all have a part to play. Most important of all, services for the handicapped child must include the parent as part of the assessment, decision-making and management team. Good support services for families with handicapped children depend on the professionals' ability to work as a team reinforcing the parents' ability to cope; and where parents cannot cope, the services must try to provide what a good home would offer.

The development of new drugs and new procedures have made it increasingly possible to reduce the length of time children have to spend in hospital; much recurrent and chronic illness can be managed at home and children can often be treated on a day-care basis when they do need hospital services. At the same time, we are becoming increasingly aware of the importance of a child's environment to his whole development, and this also has contributed to the shift of emphasis from hospital to home care. The integration of health services since 1974 provides new opportunities to encourage this trend towards care in the home and makes it increasingly possible for the hospital to be seen as a locality where children can be cared for, nursed and treated, and as part of the general community health services, not the only place where expertise is available. The greater emphasis on home care means that the nursing, medical and therapy services must be more flexible, more able to respond immediately to patients' and families' needs.

Despite the increasing control of infectious illness, some serious infections do remain; 2,000 children die from respiratory infections every year, 3 out of 4 are infants and half the deaths occur at home. These and other infections depend for their early diagnosis and successful treatment on better trained doctors and greater parental awareness. The position with many illnesses of childhood is that the knowledge to prevent and cure does exist, but the gap between the knowledge and its application is a wide one. This is as true of psychological and emotional disorders as of physical illness. Families at present do not always have easy direct access to the specialist knowledge they need when their children are ill; sometimes the knowledge is not available locally, at other times they do not know where and when they should seek it.

Nevertheless even if specialist knowledge is increased at primary level and in the district, some conditions remain which will demand further resources which cannot be spread throughout the country but will have to be concentrated at regional level. In such cases it is more than ever important to give the family the support it needs to allow a parent to stay with the child and other members of the family to visit frequently.

Many diseases and health problems which affect a large part of our adult population have their origin in life-style. Those affected eat, smoke or drink too much, take too little exercise, fail to keep teeth and gums in good condition. The earlier in life good patterns of health-related behaviour can be established, the healthier we are likely to be. An integrated child health service has therefore to include the practice of preventive medicine in its widest sense, covering not only procedures, but also advice and the provision of information, and has a responsibility to consider how best it can influence the behaviour of families and children.

The recognition that many future improvements in health depend on changes in behaviour has far-reaching implications for the whole health service. In preventive medicine, more even than in acute medicine, the need of the users of the service at different stages of their lives must dictate the form in which the services are delivered, and unless services are able to respond in the terms required by the users, the gaps between provision and use, knowledge and its application will remain.

Parents for example do not always welcome professional advice about the care of a well child and professionals may not always have found the best way of giving their help. Some parents see no advantage in visiting a child health clinic. "They worry you too much, the baby is not heavy enough, not doing this and that. It makes you think your baby is backward. I got upset." "It's not easy to get down there. You have to wait in a queue and you have to meet the other children from school; there isn't always time". "We don't go to the welfare, they tell you one thing and you believe in another." Families learn about keeping healthy from a variety of sources, from friends, relations, neighbours, books, newspapers, television, and it is against this background that health professionals have to work, and have to seek for a shared framework of understanding. Every contact with the health services is an opportunity for education in health and all health workers should use such opportunities to make children and parents better able to take care of their own health.

On-going health support services for children, more appreciation of emotional and psychological problems, earlier and more accurate diagnosis of illness and handicap, the shift from hospital to home care . . . all these aspects of the care of children make substantially the same demands on health workers: that they must be more willing to share knowledge and share responsibilities with both colleagues and parents.

The changing pattern of health care

Health services for children have not developed consistently in response to what children and families actually require in the way of medical advice, diagnosis and treatment, and the boundaries between community services, general practice and hospital have been clearer to the professionals than they ever have been to the users of the services.

The child health clinics, health visiting and school health services, which developed from the 19th century community services, are continuing a tradition of providing advice and health surveillance, both for families who seek, and for families neither willing nor able to seek, health care. The allocation of duties and responsibilities at the start of the National Health

Service in 1948 perpetuated the division between the preventive services based largely on the Local Health Authority Services and the acute services provided by the general practitioner in time of illness. This division has often been wasteful of resources and confusing to families. In neither of these services, however, has there ever been any requirement that the doctors have any specialist training in the care of children. The medical specialty of paediatrics developed during the 1920s in the hospital setting and there it has remained.

The reorganisation of 1974 offered fresh opportunities for providing an integrated service and our proposals aim at a child-centred service which looks at the needs of children and their parents in the family and educational setting, which takes into account the changing pattern of child illness, combines all aspects of medicine and offers access through a single door.

Several trends in general practice have affected our thinking about future patterns of care. The increasing numbers of group practices and the creation of health centres, the attachment of health visitors and district nurses to general practice, the idea of the primary care team are all developments which point to the possible integration of preventive and curative medicine. The proposed vocational training for general practitioners and the concept of special interest within group practice are two other developments which we have taken into account in making our proposals.

We have also recognised a change of attitude in general practice and the most effective developments indicate a desire on the part of general practitioners to acknowledge agreed objectives and work jointly to provide a public service as well as individually with individual patients. Among paediatricians too we have noted a desire to marry their traditional clinical skills with more concern and skill in dealing with populations and groups of children.

One trend which we think is against the interests of children can be discerned since the attachment of health visitors to general practice. Our impression is that, since attachment, families with young children have had less than their previous share of the health visitor's time, and this is a development we should like to see reversed.

Training

Apart from the obvious need for more doctors and nurses to have a specialised knowledge of the illnesses of childhood and the normal development of children, a service directed towards prevention of disease and the reinforcement of personal responsibility for health will make new demands on professionals' abilities to communicate.

Studies indicate that patients generally are diffident about asking for information, that anyhow they forget a proportion of what is told to them, and that they are more likely to forget advice than other statements.

On the other hand doctors and nurses are not always aware of what patients are trying to tell them. A study of 800 mothers and children in an American hospital walk-in clinic[10] showed that the interviews with paediatricians brought to light only 24% of the mothers' main worries about their children. The paediatricians often failed to realise how much the

---

(10) Korsch, B M, Gozzi, E K, Francis, V (1968). Gaps in Doctor-Patient Communication: 1. Doctor-patient interaction and patient satisfaction. *Paediatrics*. 42 855-71.

19

mothers blamed themselves for their children's illnesses, and questions asked by the mother were frequently ignored. This unresponsiveness on the part of the doctors led, in some cases, to mothers ceasing to try to give further information and lapsing into silence.

Nearer home, only three years ago, a doctor, forewarned about possible child abuse, failed to interpret a child's silence as a possible sign of distress.

The national picture and national planning

Child health in this country, therefore, emerges as a story of contrasts and contradictions; much that is commendable and much also which must be unacceptable in a civilised society and yet is either not appreciated as creating an imperative or else ignored by those who should be taking action.

This led us to ask how far successive governments since the inception of the National Health Service have consciously planned Child Health Services —and, if they have, upon what criteria and priorities. What we discovered provides, we believe, one key to the present unsatisfactory situation and to a better future. It is a remarkable fact that from 1948–1972 children's services were never identified separately in the finances or planning of the NHS. Expenditure was largely planned and recorded according to the type of service (hospitals, GPs, health visitors, health centres etc.) not according to specific groups in need of a service. Such a system of planning for and monitoring expenditure on a nation's health services over the period of a generation reveals assumptions about the relative unimportance of thinking about the recipients of these services and their total effectiveness for them which are very far removed in philosophy from those we are advocating in this report. We recommend that planning should begin with the needs of the child and his family and proceed from there to the provision of appropriate services according to agreed priorities. It is also clear that a fundamental change from "service" to "client" orientation is necessary not only in the interests of children or any other "client group" but because the NHS now has responsibility for preventive as well as curative medicine. It is a nice paradox that although curative medicine would appear to be concerned with individuals its growth historically has led to organisational concern mainly with services; whereas preventive medicine though working more in the public arena and concerned with whole populations has developed an organisational concern for the individual and his special needs, circumstances and private actions. Hence the unification of the NHS creates an imperative that the service should be organised so as to be able to consider the needs of specific groups and accept at least the same degree of accountability as was required of the former public health services. The weakness of national planning for children is brought out starkly in the light of details of expenditure that are available for 1972–73 when DHSS attempted for the first time a "grouped planning statement" for children's health services. This statement estimated (no doubt very approximately) the total expenditure on children's health services to be £220 million†—or about 9% of the total. At that time children constituted approximately 24% of the total population. Without wishing to suggest that health services should be apportioned simply on a pro rata basis, this does raise a question

---

† Excluding the cost of family practitioner services.

of whether children are receiving an appropriate share. If these patterns of expenditure on children's services under the previous system of planning were intentional they call for explanation. If they were not intentional they would appear, a priori, to be unjustifiable. Those with the responsibility of facing this will also have to face the unresolved question whether children should have only a commensurate share of the total resources or more than would be directly proportional to their numerical strength in the population because their future is our future. If it is accepted that health care for children is first and foremost a basic human right and also extremely cost-effective because conditions are better prevented or cured early than managed for a life time, then the lack for so long of any national thought or purpose in this field becomes even more apparent and unacceptable.

We, therefore, welcome the moves made in the DHSS recently to create administrative arrangements for considering children's health services. Chief among these is the creation of a "Children's Division" at DHSS. The division does not have responsibility for all services affecting children (which would lead to divided responsibilities in other respects and also no doubt the danger of becoming unwieldy) but has the potentially more valuable duty to ensure that health and personal social services are as effective as possible in meeting the needs of all children. It is exactly this holistic view, of the child and his world, which we believe necessary. Supporting this approach is the Department's planning cycle based on an annual grouped planning statement which is the method by which objectives are translated into targets expressed in terms of resources. We particularly welcome the recent initiative to reallocate health service resources so as to create a more even balance between regions. At Area and District level the proposed District Planning Teams for Children should prove a valuable innovation though it is too early for us to be able to judge their effectiveness. At the level of district management where there are no medical or nursing staff with specific responsibility for children's services, it remains to be seen whether there will be sufficient attention to children's needs.

Looking to the Future
Who speaks for Children?
There are, therefore, grounds for believing that the dispositions of the NHS could lead to appropriate attention being paid to children's health services. We appreciate that the appointment of our own Committee is of a piece with this. The 1960s and 70s saw a welcome upsurge in political concern for children and especially disadvantaged children—the National Children's Bureau (1964), Child Poverty Action Group (1965), the Plowden Report (1967), the Children and Young Persons Act (1969), the Education Act (1970), the White Paper on Education (1972) and the Children Act (1975) for example. Our work as a Committee has convinced us, however, of the need for a small, powerful national group of both lay and professionals who can speak for children. We propose that this could readily be achieved within the existing framework of advisory committees by the formation of a Joint Children's Committee of the Central Health Services and Personal Social Services Councils.

The beginnings of this proposal arose in our minds from two sources. On the one hand we asked ourselves "Whose job will it be to see that any of

21

our recommendations that are accepted are actually carried out? Not just as elegantly worded circulars of advice and direction but actually in surgeries and clinics, hospitals, schools and homes. And in the spirit we intended?" There seemed to be no group we could ask to take this on.

Secondly, we realised that our work was frequently made more complete and our conclusions deeper because our membership included representatives not only of the relevant branches of medicine and nursing but also of social work and education and of parents themselves. We were enabled to think of the child as a whole. We were also aware that this kind of approach was becoming more frequent on a local and small scale but we could see little evidence of similar developments nationally where they are, we acknowledge, harder to envisage and realise. We were drawn to the idea of a council of wise people who would meet from time to time to think about the needs of children and how far they were being met.

To be effective the council must be concerned with a wider field than child health services. It should already be clear that health as it must be understood in our kind of society depends on more variables than the quality and availability of health services. Services for very young children and their parents for example need to be organised corporately by health, education and social services. The needs of the single parent family, the handicapped and the homeless all reach beyond the competence of any single government department, and across the boundaries of central and local government and voluntary organisations.

The Joint Committee for CHILDREN would constitute a unique bringing together of figures of national standing, politicians, professionals and voluntary workers, from the range of services and organisations now separately provided for children with the purpose of providing a national forum in which the quality and development of services for children would be kept under continuing review. The proposal is rooted in the belief that children have special needs which they cannot articulate for themselves and that society must, therefore, act on their behalf.

There are also other bodies we feel can keep up pressure on behalf of children. Voluntary bodies have a distinguished record and much of the improvement in the care of children results from the monitoring, research and efforts of caring, dedicated and largely unpaid people. We feel there should be continued government and other support for this valuable work.

At district level the recent creation of Community Health Councils indicates that the government accepts the importance of considering the views of the users of health services and we hope that these councils will feel that they have a responsibility to represent the needs of children as well as of more articulate members of the community. Rationalisation of resources and the implementation of some of our proposals will result in a restriction of the consumers' areas of choice and it is important therefore that Community Health Councils press continually for excellence in their local services.

Because we recognise that it is neither possible nor desirable that the consumer representation should be sufficient to maintain standards of service for children we are asking that DHSS assume responsibility for monitoring the acceptance or otherwise within the service of those of our recommendations that are "implemented" by government. We regard this as paramount and urge that the service should aim to be its own most effective critic; it should be acknowledged as part of the duty of everyone within the service never to be satisfied that what is being achieved could not be improved from within the same resources.

Children's Rights

Finally in thinking about ways in which society can act on behalf of children we must confront the fact that there are times when the rights of children (as enunciated for example in Geneva in 1923 and in the Declaration of the Rights of the Child in 1959) must override those of their parents. Anyone going into a long-stay hospital (for example) must become aware that not all children have loving and caring parents and that, even if they have, parental concern alone will not ensure good care for every child in this country.

Our Committee have had to consider whether children should have access to health services whether or not their parents wish it or are able and willing to ensure it. We believe more should be done in this direction and many of our recommendations have the objectives of ensuring that at certain stages all children receive medical surveillance and that at any time a professional who feels concern about a child's wellbeing can require a medical examination, if necessary without parental consent. Above all, we believe that our proposals for better training of the professionals and a new and purposeful style of cooperation between them should prove the greatest safeguard the service can offer.

The Lay and the Professional

The growth in the number and variety of professions connected with child-rearing, however necessary in our kind of society, has in some measure undermined the self-confidence of parents. There is properly a yearning to improve the quality of parenting in our society. Yet it must be remembered that many of the controversial issues—styles of discipline, separation from mother, breast-feeding, weening etc—have less importance than the quality of the relationships within the family since it is these that create or deny a sense of security and give or withhold the experience of love. Those parents who felt confused by the noise of experts might have been better served by a supportive training of the commonsense. The rôle and importance of the professional must not be undermined; the issue is how professionalism should be delivered to and, on occasions, shared with the layman.

Professions tend to gather a mystique to themselves which can be predatory on the proper rôle of the layman. Illness above all things makes us believe in magic as much as in science and perhaps even more, in magicians. Since faith can move mountains such feelings have their value. But outside the realm of illness we feel there is a case to be made at this stage in the development of our society for stating the true relationship that should exist on behalf of children between their parents and the other caring adults who affect the child and the family. Besides doctors and nurses this applies to teachers, especially as nursery education develops, and to social workers. We feel especially keenly that services for the very young child must not be allowed to become over professionalised; instead they should seek to work through the family encouraging its strengths and helping in its shortcomings. There is overwhelming evidence that measures that do not involve parents achieve only short-term gains.

The Way Ahead

The 1970's may come to be seen as the decade in which the industrialised world tried to provide for all children the same range and quality of services as they had already created for some children.

Confronting the health services are, therefore, not only the questions of how to integrate general and specialist care, public and personal medicine, clinical autonomy and public accountability (as though they were not difficult enough) but also how to integrate the health service contribution with the whole range of "pre-school", education and welfare services. For our work has convinced us that the most effective and acceptable services are those that place the child and family at the centre of their thinking and have found ways to make a coherent whole of what they have to offer.

The necessary coordination, cooperation and understanding will not be achieved solely by the pursuit of administrative procedures. It is necessary for the professionals working in these fields to hold certain beliefs and objectives in common; and for there to be a common conviction about how they should relate to and work with the "laity"—in this case the parents of the children, their families and others working voluntarily with young children and families. This leads us inexorably to the belief that there should be common elements in both the initial and in-service training of those professions.

We believe this to be a fundamental issue for the NHS not only because something new needs to be created to body out these new services, not only because the early years of life are so formative, but also because the relationships created with the child, family and other professionals will also largely determine the effectiveness of the Health Service given to all other age groups in our society.

We urge therefore that now is the moment to consider carefully how health and welfare services for children ought to be provided since they must be seen as coherent by those receiving them and must accept that a young child cannot be regarded in isolation from his parents who must therefore share as full partners in the giving of the services. Such an approach we believe would have many advantages. It accepts the philosophy that social provision should wherever possible enhance the capacities of the adult to cope with his responsibilities. It creates a good and we would say proper relationship between the professional and the recipient of his services so that, as far as may be possible, the client becomes the agent of his own improved health. It offers the only way of meeting the ever-growing demand for manpower since the social services cannot indefinitely increase their call upon the nation's human resources and yet, as we shall amply demonstrate, the child health services are still unsatisfactory in many respects and must enlarge their provision. The energies and interest of parents and other involved adults must be harnessed. The pre-school playgroup movement and comparable organisations have shown the power such movements can generate and this is enhanced not diminished once a proper relationship has been formed with the experts working in the same field. The benefits accrue not only to the child and his parents but to the community at large.

We are impressed by the way in which the relationship between "provided services" and the recipients of those services has metamorphosed in the 200 years of our industrial society. In the beginning the expert and the privileged few tried to provide for the needs of the mass of underprivileged. Then the state began to provide a wider and wider range of services, not only in health but in education and welfare leading to an array of professional organisations some of which through their sophistication were in danger of alienating those they sought to serve. Professionalism can potentially be a conspiracy against the laity. We believe that in our generation there is the opportunity to make the next essential step and to move to shared responsibility. The laity are no longer the abject poor but the political nation who by their decisions and taxes create and sustain the services they require.

Hence in much of what we recommend there is the prior need for a change in attitude: a greater concern for the child and the family; a recognition that families could be better at bringing up their children if they were given the right information, support and relationships with the caring professions when it was needed and in a more acceptable way; and an acceptance that the welfare services of this country must now bring into partnership the better educated and more concerned society that a hundred years of social amelioration has created.

PART I

CHILDREN, HEALTH, AND SERVICES: TODAY AND TOMORROW

CHAPTER I

CHILDREN AND FAMILIES

The Child Population

1.1 It is the health and wellbeing of children up to and through the school years, with which we are concerned. These children number 12¾ million and constitute 26% of the population.

CHILDREN IN ENGLAND AND WALES 1974, 000s

Infants	Pre-school	School Children		Total	Total
(under 1 yr.)	1–4 yrs.	5–15 yrs.	16–19 yrs.	0–19 yrs.	All ages
641	2,942	8,641	533	12,757	49,201

1.2 Numbers define the frontiers of our territory but tell us nothing of the countryside or the people who live there: these comprise unborn children, the newborn, babies, young children, school children, adolescents. They have widely differing health needs but the thread that connects is that they are growing and developing—moving from complete dependence towards increasing independence. At each stage, and in each child, needs and achievements differ as constitution and environment shape personality and determine performance. It is development, with the potential for improvement and susceptibility to damage, that makes childhood such a special period of life, a time when changing needs call for individual response and relevant services. With every child at every age a person, our aim is a *child and family centred health service for children.*

The Family

1.3 The majority of children belong to families; they are born and grow in the light and shadows of family life. We cannot use the word "family" as though it had a single, self-evident and accepted meaning; but in considering the needs of children we must start with the families in which they live. The family is a social arrangement for the protection and rearing of children; a commitment by man and woman, together or alone, to care as well as they can and for as long as is needed for the children born to them or chosen by adoption. It is a special example of the bonding that is biologically natural between men and women, adults and children. Although child-rearing patterns are changing and may change further the pattern we have described is still the central one in our society.

26

1.4 The functions of the family include provision of the security and stimulus needed by dependent and growing children and the opportunity of education and enjoyment for children and parents alike, relationships for their protection and nurture, education for responsibility, and mutual enjoyment. Although somewhat simplified this conception of the family can guide us in a necessary examination of family function and dysfunction today and of the direction of change.

1.5 Much of our information about families in England and Wales comes from the Census and other national surveys. National statistics make a distinction between *households,* and *families.* A household includes all those who live at the same address, having meals prepared together and with common housekeeping. A family is defined as a married couple alone, or with their never-married child or children of any age or a lone parent with his/her never-married child or children. Of most interest to us were the households and families containing dependent children.*

1.6 There are some 16½ million households in England and Wales but less than 40% contain a family with dependent children. In 1971 there were some 6½ million families of whom the majority were typical two-parent families. Of these over 90% lived as separate households with no other people and 92% of the children lived in households with their parents alone. The remaining 8% of children lived in households where there were other relatives such as grand-parents or aunts or boarders and a smaller proportion lived in households containing more than one family. There was understandably perhaps, a slightly smaller probability that parents with only one dependent child would be living in an entirely separate household.

1.7 The presence of other relatives within a household has both advantages and disadvantages for the wellbeing of developing children and their parents. On the one hand relatives can provide much needed additional help and companionship for parents and children alike, and the opportunity for parents to enjoy relaxation away from the immediate surroundings to which they are often tied, particularly by very young children. But this is not always so and a shared household can be divisive of family life and lead to neglect of children's welfare. Official statistics provide no comment on this aspect of family life nor indeed on those families living entirely alone for whom some extra presence would be a positive advantage.

1.8 Not all children live in two-parent families. An estimate was made for the Committee on One-Parent Families(1) that in 1971 there were in Great Britain 620,000 one-parent families with 1,080,000 children. Of these, 920,000 children were in 520,000 fatherless families and 160,000 in motherless families.

---

* The Census defines a dependent child as one below the minimum school leaving age or one above this age but receiving full-time education; however, children over the age of 25 are not classified as dependent children even if still receiving full-time education.

(1) *Report of the Committee on One Parent Families* (Chairman: Hon Sir Morris Finer) (1974). HMSO, London.

Marriage and Child-bearing

1.9 Changes are taking place in the age of marriage and child-bearing. Men and women are marrying at younger ages: in England and Wales the average age at first marriage declined from 26.8 for men and 24.4 for women in 1951 to 24.9 for men and 22.7 for women in 1974. In 1973 in England and Wales, nearly 60% of women aged 20-24 and nearly 9% of girls aged 15-19 were already married. At the same time there has been a steep decline in the birth rate which in England and Wales fell in 1973 to 72 per 1000 women aged 15-44, from 93 per 1000 in 1964.

1.10 Younger marriages have thus not brought about an increase in family size. On the contrary, average family size which began to decline from the middle of the 19th century has fallen again in recent years. The lowest point, with an average of 2.0 live births per marriage, was in the 1930s; fertility was higher in the period after the second world war and the average completed family size for marriage in the later 1950s will be 2.4. But for marriages in the late 1960s and the 1970s a lower average is forecast. The interval between marriage and the birth of the first child has fluctuated over the past twenty years; of couples aged 20-24 marrying in 1961, 48% had not had a child after two years and in 1971 this had risen to 65%. A similar pattern can be seen in all age groups. In fact over half of all couples married in 1971 were still childless after two years—compared with just over 40% for couples married in 1961.

1.11 Today technology and society permit highly effective and generally acceptable methods of family planning*, which are becoming available to all; these have undoubtedly helped many families to have the number of children they want at the desired intervals. Thus a study of "family intentions "[2] suggests that " women marrying after 1959 expected to have slightly smaller families than those who married in the 1950s." A further study of the same families five years later showed that these mothers had on average had fewer children than they had anticipated. We can therefore hope for stability of the child population at present levels for the remainder of this century. The trend is of the greatest importance for the planning of services.

1.12 A smaller family size combined with earlier marriage and the concentration of child bearing into a shorter span has profoundly affected the family cycle. The period of family making and the nurture of small children has shortened. Yet although there are fewer children to care for, the increasing time given to education has prolonged the period during which an individual child remains financially dependent on its parents.

1.13 These trends have coincided with an increase in the proportion of married women who work. We shall return to the question of child care facilities later but here it should be pointed out that while women

(2) Woolf, M (1971). *Family Intentions*. Office of Population Censuses and Surveys: Social Survey Division, HMSO, London.
* See also Chapter 8.

have always constituted a sizeable proportion of the country's work force the increase in the prevalence of marriage, the reduction of family size, the concentration of child bearing into a shorter period for most mothers have resulted in, or perhaps been partly dictated by, an increase in the proportion of *mothers* working, particularly part-time. For married women 25–34 the proportion working increased from 25% in 1951 to 39% in 1971 and is expected to rise to over 40%. The need for this may have been financial to increase the family income, or social—to obtain relief from the isolation and monotony of being at home full-time. Whatever the reason it has encouraged the development of what Young and Willmott[3] have termed the symmetrical family where both parents work and share more equally the traditional rôle of the mother in caring for children in the home.

One-Parent Families

1.14 We have already drawn attention to the existence of single parent families. While it is difficult to project the size of this group into the future it seems certain that the number of children who experience this type of family at some stage in their development will increase. The increase in the popularity of marriage, the decline in the average age of marriage and the passage of the Divorce Reform Act in 1969 have all increased not only the number of divorces—from 25,000 in 1961 to 114,000 in 1974—but the number of children whose parents have been divorced.

1.15 Divorce, a critical but often late event in a process of family breakdown, has been widely studied but there has been only limited attention to the long term effects on children. Nor has there been much study of the damaging effects upon children of living in households in which there is excessive tension, quarrelling or violence or in households in which there is separation, if not divorce of parents. The problem of violence in marriage has however become more widely recognised in the last few years, and the Report of the Select Committee on Violence in Marriage drew attention to the effects of violence in the home on children. That both types of family dysfunction are disadvantageous to the well-being of children is plain and the medical, nursing and personal social services have special responsibilities towards such children.

Unmarried mothers

1.16 Another vulnerable group of single parents are unmarried mothers, who care for about 10% of the children in single parent families and who face complex problems. The majority are young when pregnancy occurs, receive late and insufficient ante-natal care, and have a higher rate of stillbirth, premature birth and low birthweight babies with all the physical disadvantages these imply. With competent family planning services provided by the NHS and with abortion more readily available the number should fall. But from conception onwards a complex network of disadvantage begins to affect the illegitimate child and it is clear that poverty and isolation are important and often connected threads. In fact

---

[3] Young, M, and Willmott, P (1973). *The Symmetrical Family: A Study of Work and Leisure in the London Region*. London: Routledge and Kegan Paul for the Institute of Community Studies.

although the incidence of illegitimate births has fallen somewhat since 1964 the proportion of all births that are illegitimate has risen slightly as the overall birth rate has declined. It is perhaps significant that the illegitimate birth rate among girls aged 15–19 has tended to increase since 1964 while that for other age groups has markedly declined. These births, especially those to girls under 16, are of particular concern to us.

Children's Children

1.17 Often the saddest within the complex of illegitimacy are the children who are having children. In 1951 the total births to girls in England and Wales aged under 16 was 196, in 1972 the number was 1,618. (In addition 2,804 abortions were carried out on girls under the age of 16.) While not all the children of these girls may have been unplanned or unwanted, a proportion of them will face special difficulties resulting from upbringing in a single parent family. Fortunately however, as the Finer Report[1] pointed out, some will be brought up in stable unions, some will be legitimated, and others adopted, so that "the number who remain dependent upon their lone, unmarried mothers is only a small proportion of the total".

Social Class

1.18 The context of family and child life differs widely within communities and over the country as a whole; and the differences in children's needs, parents' attitudes, family circumstances and the social setting in large part determine a community's local—and changing—needs. Much of our best information nationally about differences in the life changes and needs of children is derived from data describing the families or households in which they live and, in particular, data on the occupation of the head or principal wage earner in the household or family. Knowledge of a person's occupation permits an analysis by social class.

1.19 A grouping of occupations into social classes was first introduced by the Registrar General in 1911; its purpose was to emphasise the great variation in death rates between occupational groups, which persist to this day, even for children. Subsequently its use has revealed "significant and persisting differences in a wide range of social and economic attributes." The classification of the working population by occupational status divides it into six groups or social classes, each of which is relatively homogeneous in respect of the general standing within the community of the occupations concerned, taking into account the skills required to carry out the occupation and the educational qualifications leading to it. These groups are known generally as I professional, etc, II intermediate, III skilled, separating manual and non-manual, IV partly skilled and V unskilled. A sample based on the 1971 census showed 38% of children aged 0–19 in England and Wales in households headed by a skilled manual worker, 16% in households headed by a partly skilled worker and 6.5% in households headed by an unskilled worker.

1.20 There are important differences in what happens to children growing up in households that differ by social class, some of which we outline below. Of especial concern are the children of unskilled workers in social class V. They include many who are disadvantaged socially and economically and who pose important problems for our health and social services.

1.21 There are social class differences in the age of marriage and in fertility—the two are closely linked. A special analysis of legitimate births in 1970-72 taking account of the social class of fathers revealed that the average age of mother, in respect of first births, was considerably lower for the wives of social class V husbands (21.9) than for others.

Average age of Mother at first live birth within Marriage: Social Class of Husband

Social Class of Husband	Average Age of Mother
I	26.3
II	25.8
III N	24.9
III M	23.4
IV	22.9
V	21.9
Not classified	22.8
Total	24.0

Great Britain

1.22 Among married couples where the husband is in a non-manual occupation over 60% of all births are to women over the age of 25, whereas among the manual group over 50% occur before the wife is aged 25. In all social groups however the number of births to women over the age of 40 is small, and their number and proportion are declining—a fact of importance to the child health services since older women are statistically at somewhat higher risk of producing malformed children than younger ones. Women who marry manual workers do so at a younger age than do women marrying non-manual workers; they start their families younger and they have on average more children. However, fertility is now falling in all social classes.

1.23 Social class differences underline the importance of preventive medicine. Social class V contains a higher proportion than other classes of those families where the adverse circumstances e.g. low income, bad housing and poor education, combine to place the children at great risk of ill health or accident. These are the very families who it is most important to ensure get the full benefits of the child health services. Yet there are social class differences in the use households make of various child health services. The report of the National Child Development study "From Birth to Seven"[4] shows that the children of unskilled workers are less likely to have been immunised and to have attended a dentist than other children and their mothers were also less likely in their own childhood to have attended an infant welfare clinic. The 1973 General Household Survey[5] shows that children from social class V consult general practitioners

(4) Davie, R, Butler, N, and Goldstein, H (1972). *From Birth to Seven: A Report of the National Child Development Study*. Longman, London in association with the National Children's Bureau.

(5) Office of Population Censuses and Surveys: Social Survey Division (1976). *General Household Survey* 1973. HMSO, London.

less frequently than other children although there is a great deal of evidence that they suffer more chronic and acute sickness.

Financial Poverty

1.24 It is nearly 100 years since the pioneer studies of modern poverty described the family life cycle in a way that identified the periods and circumstances in which the risk of poverty was greatest. The loss of a father through death or desertion, the loss of his earnings through sickness or unemployment, or his complete absence in the case of illegitimacy, then as now put the mother and her young children in desperate financial straits. Even today, mothers are often compelled to work for low wages, and to live in over-crowded accommodation. And any family whose income is small in relation to basic needs, often dictated by household size, is vulnerable.

1.25 Poverty is a relative term and opinions differ on how best to measure it. One measure is the level of need established for supplementary benefit purposes. On this standard it was estimated in 1974 that 110,000 families containing 260,000 children were living below the supplementary benefit level, while a further 480,000 families containing 1,110,000 children had incomes no more than 20% higher—this includes the 394,000 families with 854,000 children who actually were receiving supplementary benefit in 1974. (Statistical Appendix, Section B.) Nothing is known yet about the distribution of these families and children by social class but many are undoubtedly those of unskilled workers in social class V. Their greater experience of ill health has already been indicated.

Environment

1.26 Poverty is demonstrated not by low income, but by obviously low standards of living, particularly housing. Classical epidemiological studies have shown the connection between poor housing conditions i.e. overcrowding, lack of proper water supply, toilet facilities, and heating, and the incidence of ill health particularly respiratory and infectious disease. Fortunately housing conditions are improving as urban redevelopment replaces the sub-standard housing that has survived from the 19th into the 20th century. Nonetheless in 1973 it was estimated from the General Household Survey that about 400,000 children in England and Wales were living in households with more than 1.5 persons per room. About 750,000 children lived in households lacking exclusive use of a bath and over 1 million children lived in households lacking the exclusive use of an inside wc. Although these numbers are still too large it must be remembered that the proportion of households without the use of basic amenities has declined considerably since 1951 when the first post war census was held.

1.27 Even in 1971 there were particular areas where sub-standard housing conditions prevailed. A special study of the 1971 census data for the 87,500 census enumeration districts showed that, for example, in 5% of such districts the percentage of households living at more than 1.5 persons per room was greater than 10% (compared with the national average of 2.3%);

in 1% of enumeration districts the percentage was greater than 23.5% (i.e. more than ten times the national average). A similar concentration is evident for the proportion of households lacking exclusive use of fixed bath or inside wc. In the worst 1% of enumeration districts 85% or more of households lacked inside wcs—the national average in 1971 was $12\frac{1}{2}\%$. (Statistical Appendix, Table B.24.) It can be inferred that health problems due to or exacerbated by environmental factors are therefore highly concentrated.

1.28 Space and amenities are necessary for family relationships and well-being; they are essential if we are to recommend the increasing management of children's illnesses at home. In 1973, 6% of all households in Great Britain and 23% of large families (3 or more children) were overcrowded by the bedroom standard; this standard is assessed by allowing a bedroom for each married couple and for each other person aged 21 or over and a bedroom for each two members of the household aged under 21 with the proviso that those aged 10 to 20 should share only with someone of the same sex (General Household Survey, 1973 Table 2.12).

1.29 Flats have replaced terraced houses all over the country. Though the physical environment is very much better many housing estates provide a poor social environment for children. Not only are play spaces inside restricted, but in many estates there is no safe playing space out of doors. Large housing estates and high rise flats are worse in these respects, but are not the only culprits.

Transplanted Isolated Families

1.30 In spite of present income restraints, the majority of families in terms of housing, food, clothing, wages, the quality of education and the opportunities for leisure, have never been so prosperous. Much of this improvement represents a real advance in living standards which families are eager to maintain. One sign of this has been the development of better housing in new housing estates on the edge of cities. It would seem self-evident that to change from overcrowded drab houses in the decaying areas to the light and space of a new housing estate must mean that material conditions are very much better. At the same time it should not be forgotten that homelessness has increased, and is a major cause of children being received into care. There can be serious disruptive effects on a child deprived of the security of its own home.

1.31 Many families move either to get nearer to (or further from) a place of work, or to get better accommodation. In 1973 9% of households with children under 16 had moved in the previous 12 months. For many the change is welcome but change of locality can also be a disturbing experience because the move may involve a loss of effective ties with kin and friends. Also there is evidence that the types and arrangements of housing may influence people's behaviour and satisfaction. This illustrates the importance of emotional as well as material geography in plans for rehousing, and the need for services to maintain contact with all families, especially newcomers. Nearly one-third of our children live in the major conurbations of Greater London, West Midlands, Greater Manchester, Merseyside, West Yorkshire and Tyne and Wear and about 75% overall live in urban conditions. The conurbations are gradually losing population and it is likely that somewhat fewer children are now living in the decaying areas of the larger centres than ten years ago; nonetheless, wherever poor housing exists at cheaper than average rents poorer families will be driven by circumstances to live in it until it is replaced.

Immigrants

1.32 It is frequently alleged that immigrant families live predominantly in the worst housing conditions. It is true that the immigrant population tends to be concentrated in particular areas. The special study of the 1971 census enumeration districts showed that although on average the proportion of the population of new commonwealth origin was 3.6%, in 1% of enumeration districts it was 39.4% or higher. And the General Household Survey for 1973, which enabled an analysis to be made of the living conditions and social class of households in which the head of household was "coloured" (as assessed by interviewer assessment), showed that coloured householders are much more likely than other householders to live in overcrowded conditions and/or in a house lacking or sharing basic amenities, like bath or shower and wc. For example 6% of all households were rated as below a bedroom standard, but for "coloured" householders the proportion was 25%; and whereas 5% of all households lacked exclusive use of a wc, for "coloured" households the proportion was 21%.

1.33 It is interesting to note however that the social class distribution of "coloured" heads of household is not markedly different from that of white households. The proportion in the skilled manual category was the same (33%) and also for unskilled (7%) which corresponds to social class V. But "coloured" householders were more likely to be semi-skilled workers and students, and less likely to be employers/managers or junior non-manual workers, than "white" householders. The difference between "West Indian coloured" and "other coloured" was more marked than between "coloured" and "white."

1.34 Many children of these families face problems of adjusting to a culture which differs from the culture of the home. The parents themselves often face discrimination from the indigenous population. Among the Asians, and some of the European immigrants there are serious language difficulties. The reasons for concentration of certain groups in special areas are not hard to understand.

1.35 The pressures on many immigrant families to maintain an income adequate to house themselves and frequently to provide for other dependants not in this country has meant that many mothers have to work and in consequence expose their children to very poor caring conditions. And because a higher proportion of coloured than white people live in poor quality homes, characterised by overcrowding, multiple occupancy and lack

34

of basic household amenities, the children are in consequence, more prone to respiratory infections, accidents and a variety of minor physical disorders. "Nearly all the medical problems of immigrant communities are related to environmental factors. There are many diseases and injuries to which the children of immigrant parents are particularly liable and it is essential that doctors working in these areas should be aware not only of these conditions but also of their aetiologies, for one factor these diseases and injuries have in common is their preventability."[6] The future incidence of physical illness among ethnic minority groups will be greatly influenced by the physical conditions in which they live and bring up their children but the health service and personal social services can assist individuals and families even when they cannot by themselves remedy the material and social conditions that are the primary cause of their problems.

Sick Parents

1.36 The children of sick parents or handicapped parents need particularly careful consideration especially if the illness of one parent is so severe that it requires the constant attention of the other to the neglect of the children—or through lack of income forces a mother into paid employment to boost the family income. Higher rates of disorder in children especially of behaviour and emotion have been shown to be associated with mental and physical illness in their parents.[7]

1.37 The General Household Survey throws some light on the prevalence of limiting long-standing illness among married men and women. In 1973 the rates per 1000 for men were 60 for age groups 15–44 and 180 for men aged 46–64. For women the rates were 60 and 160 respectively. Thus perhaps 6% of parents aged under 45 are likely to be limited in activity as a result of long-standing illness; and rates are higher for both men and women living in semi-skilled or unskilled households. The survey data give no information about the severity of these illnesses. In many cases they will not cause family dysfunction but they are likely to make families more vulnerable to misfortune. Of greater concern are those families where ill health of the father has led to a prolonged absence from work. In Great Britain in 1974 there were about 77,000 fathers receiving invalidity benefit; to qualify for this they had to have been incapable of work for 6 months or more. There were 177,000 dependent children in their families.

1.38 A study "Prolonged Sickness and the Return to Work" was carried out by OPCS in 1972–73.[8] The survey covered men who had been absent for one month, three months, six months and one year. Results showed that prolonged sickness absence of men does not affect employment of wives dramatically at first—but eventually it is more common for a working wife to stop work and look after her husband than for a non-working wife to start work as a result. In all samples there was a much higher

(6) Stroud, C E (1965). The New Environment. *Post. Grad. Med. J.* 41, 599–602.

(7) Rutter, M (1966). *Children of Sick Parents: An Environmental and Psychiatric Study.* Institute of Psychiatry Maudsley Monographs No 16, Oxford University Press.

(8) Martin, J, and Morgan, M (1975). *Prolonged Sickness and the Return to Work.* Office of Population Censuses and Surveys: Social Survey Division, HMSO, London.

proportion of unskilled and semi-skilled men than in the general population —and the proportion of unskilled workers was greatest in the longer term samples.

1.39 In the predominantly working class city of Newcastle, Miller et al.[9] found that in 1962 15% of mothers and 5% of fathers of 15 year old children exhibited mental illness or excessive degrees of depression or fatigue. More detailed surveys have found comparable rates among mothers in London. Brown et al.[10] have made the most intensive inquiries, surveying fairly representative samples of women living in an inner London borough. In the three months prior to interview, 16% of 220 women were judged to have suffered from a definite psychiatric disorder, characterised by depressive mood, and "clusters of symptoms, such as loss of weight, lack of energy, various forms of sleep disturbance, heightened anxiety and other basically unpleasant experiences which distinguish them from other women."[10]

1.40 The prevalence of disturbance in Brown's study varied markedly according to social class and life-stage. Of working-class women, 25% were judged to have had a recent or chronic disturbance as opposed to only 5% of middle-class women. But the group most affected were working-class mothers with a child under five, 42% of whom had been disturbed, compared to 17% with a youngest child of school age and 5% of middle-class mothers with young children. This very high figure for working-class mothers receives confirmation from another study, looking at the health of children under five on a council housing estate in North London: 42% of mothers were assessed as having been clearly psychiatrically disturbed in the previous twelve months, 16% seriously so.[11]

1.41 Moreover, it is not just the case that other mothers, of whatever social class, who are not severely depressed are necessarily problem free. In Brown's total sample, in addition to the many mothers judged to have suffered a recent psychiatric disorder, a further substantial group were rated as "borderline" cases, who had definite symptoms, which were however less severe than those of the most disturbed group. (It should be noted however that this study related to an inner city area.) Taken together these studies show the magnitude of minor psychological disturbance which exists in the general population and which is often presented to the medical services but whose origins are mainly due to social and behaviour factors.

1.42 The pioneer study of 1,000 families in Newcastle[12] showed however that even in adverse circumstances most parents provide adequate care for their children. It is where ill-health—physical or mental—of one or both

[9] Miller, F J W et al (1974). The School Years in Newcastle on Tyne. Oxford University Press, London.

[10] Brown, G et al (1975). Social Class and Psychiatric Disturbance among Women in an Urban Population. Sociology, 9, 225–254. By permission of the Oxford University Press.

[11] Richman, N (1974). The Effects of Housing on Pre-school Children and their Mothers. Develop. Med. Child. Neurol. 16, 53–58.

[12] Spence, J et al (1954). A Thousand Families in Newcastle-on-Tyne. Oxford University Press, London.

parents coincides with a poor environment and the low income to which such families are prey that the health of the children is seriously at risk. In considering children's health therefore there is a need to view the health and circumstances of the family as a whole.

Children unable to live at home

1.43 Where for a variety of reasons natural family care is lacking or seriously inadequate, children may be cared for by local authorities. In 1974 in England and Wales, there were 31,000 children boarded out with foster parents and 45,000 in local authority or voluntary residential care. Some children may have to live away from home because of illness or disability and we are particularly sensitive to the needs of the 8,000 children living in long stay hospitals. The hospital is the only home many of them will ever know. By the end of the century many thousands of children will have completed an entire childhood in a hospital setting.

The Disadvantaged

1.44 Children who grow up in poverty or squalor, whose homes are grossly overcrowded, or who live in decaying inner-city neighbourhoods; children who are neglected or handicapped, or who are discriminated against on grounds of race, language, colour or religion; children whose parents are sick or psychiatrically disordered, who quarrel incessantly—or who are absent; such children are in different ways "disadvantaged". The term has no precise meaning, but the implication is clear enough. Social or personal disadvantage is handicapping and dysfunctional. Of course many children who are disadvantaged personally or socially may develop normally and function adequately. But they face greater odds than other children: they are more likely to suffer from physical illness or psychiatric disorder, or to fail educationally, or to drop out of school or be "early leavers", more likely to truant or become delinquent, or to leave school for unemployment or poorly skilled jobs.

1.45 When we look at the kind of hazards to which some children are exposed, the need for a social policy for children which goes beyond certain kinds of primary health and educative care becomes apparent. A sensitive indicator of government's awareness and concern is the level of financial support given to families though we have noted in this connection that the Chairman of the Supplementary Benefits Commission, Professor Donnison has recently stated that "Despite recent improvements, British standards of family support are still far behind those of the French, the Belgians and other neighbouring countries".[13]

1.46 We have already referred to the increase in the proportion of mothers who work. We expect this to continue and emphasise the need for more day care services for children under 5. In 1974 in England and Wales, there were 26,000 children on local authority day nursery registers, about 4,000 more than in 1970. But there were 10,000 "priority" children on

[13] Reported in *The Daily Telegraph*, 14 June 1976.

waiting lists for places. These would include children with only one parent; those who need temporary day care on account of the mother's illness; those whose mothers are unable to look after them adequately because they are incapable of giving young children the care they need; those for whom day care might prevent the breakdown of the mother or the break-up of the family; those whose home conditions (e.g. because of gross overcrowding) constitute a hazard to their health and welfare; and those whose health and welfare are seriously affected by a lack of opportunity for playing with others.

1.47 The lack of adequate local authority provision has left many working mothers with no alternative but to use childminders, many of whom are not registered. Childminders can, at best, provide excellent substitute care; but childminding is not always of good quality and the child is often moved from minder to minder, sometimes because of the parents' own dissatisfaction. The conditions still existing in some childminding situations are appalling. Overcrowding, lack of play materials and lack of stimulus may be features replicated in children's own homes; but bad childminding situations which include malnutrition, neglect and a high degree of unsanitary care are not features which many working mothers would fail to be concerned about. We see expansion of day care services for young children as an urgent need. At present the health surveillance of some young children in day care is seriously inadequate.

1.48 For children over 5 compulsory schooling provides not only education, but adult supervision and care during school hours. There is however a great shortage of after-school provision, and play centre places during school holidays. Streets are no longer safe places to play in. The mobility of the population weakens community feeling and often also lessens the frequency of contact with relatives. This is particularly important when children are young since, in the absence of services, mothers have fewer opportunities to make local contacts and are thrown more on their own resources.

CHAPTER 2

THE CHANGING PICTURE OF HEALTH AND DISEASE

2.1 The health of its children must be a prime concern of every society. The state of health of any child is a function of many diverse factors: his constitution, growth before birth, quality of parenthood, the effects of environment—material, emotional, educational—of illness and the services available to deal with it and the attitude of society and of government generally to children. Many of these lie outside our terms of reference, but they have inevitably formed the wider framework for our inquiries. Moreover health is not an absolute that can easily be measured. We can only point to increased survival, improved growth and the absence of particular forms of ill-health as indicators of progress. In this chapter we have recorded improvement in this sense and identified those conditions which constitute the major forms of ill-health and intellectual or physical impairment in children today. In doing so, we have asked ourselves what implications such conditions have for the future organisation of health services for children, for their rôle in prevention, in treatment, and where cure is not possible, in minimising the adverse effects of disability.

Improvement in Health

2.2 *There has been an impressive improvement in the health of children in this century.* In the first place, more children are surviving the hazards of infancy and early childhood. Table 1 shows the continuing reduction of mortality in our own life-time and Table 2 the diseases which have been eliminated or reduced in severity to make it possible. The main factor in this saving of child life has been the decline in deaths from the "infectious fevers", and the continuing decline in the prevalence and severity of these illnesses has resulted in a general improvement in the health of children (Statistical Appendix, Tables D4, D5).

2.3 Increased survival has been accompanied by improved growth. Over the last seventy years children in average economic circumstances have gained in height at ages 5 to 7 by 1 to 2cm each decade, and at ages 10 to 14 by 2 to 3cm each decade.[1] For those whose memories go back beyond the second world war this improvement in physique is a pleasure to see. However the factors which have brought about a reduction in infant mortality and morbidity have also resulted in the saving of the lives of more low birthweight babies and those with inherited disease and congenital conditions.

Illness in Children Today

Acute illness

2.4 There is little doubt that increased survival is now followed by less severe illness and even on this limited basis few would challenge the general proposition that the majority of children enjoy better health than ever

---

[1] Tanner, J (1969). Growth of Children in Industrialised Countries. *In Nutrition in Pre-school and School Age*. Symposia of the Swedish Nutrition Foundation, Uppsala, Almquist and Wiksells.

before. In fact immunisation and antibiotics have proved so effective in the control of infective illness that the illusion exists that all childhood illness is diminishing. The facts are otherwise. *There is a large amount of acute illness in children;* some is minor in a medical sense, but much is severe and some life-threatening or fatal. It is natural to begin with consideration of these acute conditions.

2.5 Except in local studies, most of the data on morbidity are related to use of services rather than the incidence of specific disorders. One view of the range and frequency of childhood illness can be gained by examining the reasons for which children are taken to see their general practitioner. (Statistical Appendix Table D15). The commonest reasons for consulting him are respiratory.diseases including asthma (28%), symptoms and ill-defined conditions (12.7%), infectious disease (11.0%), skin diseases (10.1%), preventive procedures (9.9%), and accidents (5.8%).

2.6 Infections form the largest single part of respiratory disease. These cause half of all illness in children under 5, and resulted in 2,000 deaths in 1974; 1,400 of the deaths occurred in the first year of life and nearly half take place at home. These infections are mainly due to viruses which are not susceptible to existing antibiotics, and although understanding of these illnesses is increasing rapidly current research suggests that safe and effective preventive measures are unlikely to be available in the near future. Their prevalence increases as social conditions become less favourable, and bronchitis and pneumonia are found most commonly in families in Social Class IV and V. An important characteristic of respiratory infection is its tendency to recur. The familiar sequence of coughs, colds, sore throats, earache throughout the first 8 years of life is a tiring and worrying experience for both children and parents. At the same time it is essentially part of the normal immunological development of the child and it is important that parents have this explained to them. Most respiratory conditions can be successfully managed at home and only the severe forms require hospital admission, but if parents are to be able to cope successfully then they need ready access to skilled professional help. The condition of a sick child can change rapidly and parents need a better understanding of the significance of symptoms, and to be confident that help from doctors and nurses well trained in the management of children's illness is readily available.

2.7 A view of illness from hospital reflects the severe forms of the common infections and a range of less frequent diseases. These include urinary tract infection, meningitis, congenital heart disease, diabetes, other endocrine and metabolic disorders, intestinal malabsorption, of which coeliac disease is one example, and cancer including leukaemia. There are also a range of conditions requiring surgery: some relatively common such as hernia, others moderately frequent for example appendicitis, and infrequent complaints such as congenital pyloric stenosis and intussusception. Uncommon but serious disorders create problems for doctors. Though a practitioner may only see a condition once in 5 years his initial knowledge of the disease must be precise and his memory refreshed by continuing education if he is to function effectively. Knowledge has increased and is increasing; but

TABLE 1

Deaths in Infancy, Childhood and Adolescence. England and Wales.

Year	Under 1	1–4	5–9	10–14	15–19
		Number	of Deaths		
1911	114,600	54,470	12,668	7,210	9,632
1931	41,939	18,038	7,073	4,740	8,518
1951	20,223	4,133	1,771	1,328	2,061
1961	17,393	2,662	1,320	1,186	2,137
1971	13,720	2,204	1,484	1,109	2,169
1974	10,459	1,922	1,225	1,091	2,212
		Rates per 1,000			
1911	130.1	17.68	3.42	2.05	2.88
1931	66.4	7.55	2.14	1.47	2.50
1951	29.7	1.35	0.55	0.47	0.76
1961	21.4	0.93	0.40	0.32	0.66
1971	17.5	0.70	0.37	0.30	0.65
1974	16.3	0.65	0.31	0.28	0.63

Rates for those under 1 year are per 1,000 live births; those for age 1–19 are per 1,000 population.

TABLE 2

Deaths of Children aged 1–14 years from Certain Causes, 1931–35, 1956–60 and 1970–74. England and Wales.

	1911–15		1931–35		1956–60		1970–74	
	No	Rate per Million	No	Rate per Million	No	Rate per Million	No	Rate per Million
Pneumonia and Bronchitis	76,643	1,464	28,226	635	3,347	70	2,330	43
Tuberculosis	46,459	887	14,544	327	306	6	71	1
Diphtheria	23,380	447	13,820	311	15	0	1	0
Accidents	18,500	353	12,126	273	6,736	140	7,214	133
Measles	48,986	936	10,874	254	210	4	111	2
Whooping Cough	20,182	385	6,071	137	72	1	7	0
Gastro-enteritis	25,560	488	3,485	78	447	9	487	9
Appendicitis	3,997	76	2,992	67	379	8	151	3
Cancer	2,388	46	2,853	64	3,971	83	3,743	69
Diseases of the ear	2,515	48	2,700	61	106	2	59	1
Rheumatic fever*	3,495	67	2,465	55	139	3	6	0
Scarlet fever	9,901	189	2,589	58	7	0	0	0

* The figures for rheumatic fever are not strictly comparable because of revision of the ICD code.

its application depends on those who are at the point of first contact with the patient and responsible for ongoing primary care having sufficient expertise in paediatrics to be able to make a correct diagnosis and arrange early referral for specialist treatment.

2.8 The illnesses reaching University Centres or major children's hospitals are those which call for special technical facilities and the professional skill and experience to use them. They include complex or unusual forms of disease in every system of the body and the range is shown in Table E23 in the Statistical Appendix. These illnesses make special demands on children, parents and hospital staff. There has been increasing publicity about the work of specialist hospitals but many parents are still not aware of the very great technical advances which have been made in the management of diseases which should be treated there. This emphasises the need for greater knowledge of these advances on the part of general practitioners and the communication of it to parents, if affected children are to receive the range of specialist care which is available.

Dental Disease

2.9 Dental caries remains an uncontrolled endemic disease in childhood. It has been estimated that 6 million school children have active caries; 1 in 5 in the early school years and 1 in 10 between 9 and 15 have 5 or more decaying teeth.[2] Extraction is the least desirable form of treatment and yet by the end of school life a third of children have lost one or more permanent teeth. Many children who need dental treatment do not receive it and this applies particularly to those who are physically and mentally handicapped. In addition to widespread dental caries, disordered development of the jaws and teeth leads in more than half of all children to crowding or faulty occlusion. At the same age, between 7 and 15, a similar number will develop inflammation of the gums. Between 12 and 15, 1 in 5 boys and 1 in 10 girls will damage their front teeth in accidents. The full meaning of these figures is considered in Chapter 13.

Accidental Injury

2.10 *Accidents are the principal cause of death between 1 and 15 years and although rates in the younger age groups have declined, for the 15-19s they are significantly higher than they were 20 years ago.* The extent of non-fatal accidents is unknown and the professional time spent in treating them unmeasured. In 1972 141,000 children were admitted to hospital with accidental injuries and 1,800 died. The main facts have been recently described.[3] The home is more dangerous than the roads, especially with limited space and with limited parental understanding. In 1971 burns and scalds were responsible for 4,651 admissions of children aged 0–4 and 2,126 aged 5–14, a hundred children under 5 died, but many more survive with unsightly scarring and with recurrent admission to hospital for skin grafting. Only the children, parents, doctors, nurses and teachers involved know the distress to the child, the strain on the family and the disruption of school and social life which this involves. Deaths from accidental poisoning are lower than we might expect, between 30 and 40 a year; but in 1971, 25,000 children were admitted to hospital, four times the number ten years earlier, and the parental distress and medical and nursing attention is considerable. The management of accidents carries implications for Accident and Emergency Departments, Children's Departments and Specialist Surgery. Since accidents, are, in the main preventable, it is

(2) Todd, J E (1975). *Children's Dental Health in England and Wales,* 1973. HMSO, London.
(3) Jackson, R H, and Wilkinson, A W (1976). Why don't we prevent childhood accidents? *Brit. Med. Jour.* 2, 1258.

depressing to find that they are the main cause of death between the first birthday and leaving school. They are the results of the encounter of developmentally immature children with a dangerous environment, and the risks become greater as social circumstances become less favourable.

Non-accidental Injury

2.11 Consideration of accidental injury leads on to that of the *disturbing phenomenon of non-accidental injury.* Violence to children by parents has been part of human society from the beginning; awareness of it in society today, and the willingness to accept the implications began in the United States.[4] In the past 10 years an increasing number of professional studies and public enquiries have exposed the extent and gravity of the problem. The true prevalence of violence to children is unknown but evidence from limited local studies suggested a figure of not less than 5,000 affected children a year in England.[5] The report (unpublished) of a special inquiry carried out by the British Paediatric Association and the British Association of Paediatric Surgeons indicate that from 7 to 8% die—the fourth commonest cause of death in the first five years—and that of those who survive 11% have residual brain damage and 5% visual impairment of varying degree. The professions concerned (medicine, social work and the law) were at first unable to grasp the tragic plight of the children and the needs of the parents. Continuing study also suggests that non-accidental injury is but a manifestation of a range of child abuse.[6,7] More vividly than any other this problem illustrates the family dimensions of childhood ill-health today.

Chronic Disorders

2.12 There are many conditions affecting children which can be regarded as recurring or persistent disorders. It is not always easy to draw a clear line between these and the developmental conditions referred to in paragraph 2.13 below. They share with them, to a varying extent, a number of characteristics of importance for the development of services. There is a special need for professional help which recognises that management is more than clinical treatment; it must take into account the personal, family and educational implications of growing up with chronic illness and support parents in the none-too-easy task of maintaining the high degree of discipline in behaviour which is often required on the part of children if their disorders are to be successfully controlled. The group includes asthma, epilepsy, urinary tract infections, other forms of renal disease, obesity, diabetes, cystic fibrosis, coeliac disease and other examples of defective absorption of food. The complete list would be a long one. The two most familiar examples are asthma and epilepsy. At the lowest estimated prevalence (2%) there are 170,000 school children with asthma,

(4) Kempe, C H, Silverman, F N, Droegemueller, N, and Silver, H K (1962). The Battered Child Syndrome. *Jour. Am. Med. Ass.* 181, 17–24.

(5) Evidence from National Society for Prevention of Cruelty to Children to Select Committee on Violence in the Family, 1976.

(6) Franklin, A W (ed) (1975). *Concerning Child Abuse.* Churchill Livingstone.

(7) Carter, J (ed) (1974). *The Maltreated Child.* Priory Press.

and in the majority it will have started in the pre-school years.[8] In few conditions has treatment improved so much in the last 10 years, but the application of the more effective preventive and therapeutic substances available requires from the clinician concerned an understanding of the disordered respiratory physiology and how these substances improve it, and the patience to ensure that child and parents understand exactly what is required. The prevalence of epilepsy in the middle school years is about 0.7% and it is estimated that there are some 60,000 school children with epilepsy. Again effective drugs are available, but their use calls for regular administration and the maintenance of satisfactory levels in the blood. In most affected children neither of these conditions should require frequent consultant supervision, but the doctor who is responsible for ongoing management must have an understanding both of the conditions for effective treatment including the need for regular supervision and equally of the important family and educational implications.

Developmental Conditions

2.13 There are a range of conditions which can broadly be called developmental. One study[8] found that the commonest is bedwetting which at 5 can affect 18% of children, at 10, 12%, at 13, 6% and at 15, 2%. Some 7% of children will have one or more seizures in the first 5 years, half associated with infection. In the first 7 years 8% will have impaired vision from errors of refraction, and from 3 to 5%, an established squint. At 5 the speech of 5% of children may be sufficiently abnormal to cause concern to their parents and impair easy adjustment to school. During the school years 1% of children will develop an established stutter. Some 20% of school children may have recurrent headaches and 10% recurrent abdominal pains.[9] These conditions give rise to considerable personal and parental distress; although understanding has increased it has not reached the majority of parents and doctors and in consequence management is often unsatisfactory. Parents and teachers—and indeed the child himself—require professional advice which can set the disorder in the context of normal development and relate treatment to the child's particular experiences at home or at school.

Malformations

2.14 In some 2% of total births (liveborn and stillborn) substantial malformations are evident at birth. (Statistical Appendix, Tables D 1–3.) As children get older latent conditions develop or are discovered.[10,11] To give one example some 5 children in every 1,000 born alive have malformed hearts, and at present half of them die in the first year. All need specialist assessment, and many continuing observation leading to skilled investigation and corrective surgery. Advances in paediatric cardiology and cardiac surgery are proceeding rapidly with a growing prospect that a majority of

(8) Miller, F J W, Court, S D M, Knox, E G, and Brandon, S (1974). *The School Years in Newcastle on Tyne.* OUP, London.

(9) Apley, J (1975). *The Child with Abdominal Pains.* Blackwell Publications, Oxford.

(10) Vowles, M, Pethybridge, R J, and Brimblecombe, F S W (1975). Congenital malformations in Devon: Their incidence, age and primary source of detection. In *Bridging in Health.* OUP, London.

(11) Carter, C O (1976). Genetics of Common Single Malformations. *Brit. Med. Bulletin.* 32, 1.

defects could be corrected before 5 which would lessen the period of parental anxiety, and enable more children to be normal or improved in health and confidence before they start school. To achieve this demands a high level of specialist skills with the concentration of staff, equipment and patients in a limited number of centres. This principle applies, though in differing degrees, to all malformations and the personal and professional implications are considered in Chapters 12 and 18.

Handicap

2.15 A handicap is a disability which for a substantial period or permanently, retards, distorts or otherwise adversely affects normal growth development or adjustment to life. This covers a wide range of conditions. *The most detailed local study[12] suggests that even in a prosperous area of England a prevalence of one handicapped child in every seven may be found during the childhood years.* The main categories are shown in Table 3.

TABLE 3
Prevalence of Four Handicapping Conditions among 9–11 year old Children in the Isle of Wight

Condition*	Physical Handicap	Intellectual retardation	Educational Backwardness	Psychiatric** Disorder
Total with each handicap per cent	2.7	2.6	7.9	6.8

* moderate and severe cases only   ** estimated

2.16 A child however may have more than one handicap; in the above study 75% had one, 18.8% 2, 4.8% 3, 1.4% 4. And as with growth and illness adverse social factors increase the frequency and intensify the demands arising from the handicap.

2.17 In 1973, 2,151 children under 15 years were registered as blind or partially sighted, and 4,330 as deaf or partially deaf. Since diagnosis and notification are not uniform throughout the country these figures are probably an underestimate. If we include refractive errors and squint more children have defective vision than any other condition apart from dental disease. The above figures also leave out the intermittent deafness associated with recurrent colds, middle ear infections and serious otitis and the classroom backwardness that may result from them. The prevalence of these visual and auditory impairments in children and the variety of causes, make a measure of paediatric specialisation a rational development in each specialty.

2.18 Among the physically handicapped the most familiar group are those with the restricted movement and abnormal posture of cerebral palsy. The severe forms make immense demands on the child, parents, therapists,

---

[12] Rutter, M, Tizard, J, and Whitmore, K (1970). *Education, Health and Behaviour* Longman, London.

doctors, social workers, teachers and eventually on the employment service. With a prevalence of 1 to 2 per 1,000 children, such children are less numerous than those in some other categories, yet they have had a special significance in determining the country's response to all handicapped children. In 1952 a group of parents fighting for help with their spastic children drew public and professional attention to the needs of handicapped children of every kind. Their initiative was the real beginning of the assessment and management services which are now being developed, and of other parent societies who followed their example. *The growth of closer relationships between professionals and such societies has been a major advance in the care of a wide range of disorders and should be encouraged.*

2.19 The demands of school increase the needs of children with known handicaps and bring others to light. For a variety of reasons some children have difficulty in learning to read. This facet of educational failure is primarily the concern of teachers and psychologists. It may be part of a general or specific developmental delay; it may be accompanied by unexplained physical symptoms or disturbed behaviour. The most testing, personal, family and educational handicap arises however from seriously diminished intelligence; approximately 48,000 children (0.4% of children aged 0–16) are severely mentally handicapped, three-quarters of them children of school age requiring special education in some form. Detailed studies of their capacity for development and appropriate methods of education are now taking place, and we consider the implications more fully in Chapter 14.

Psychiatric Disorders

2.20 There is a great deal of disturbed behaviour in children of all ages. Studies[12] suggest that between 5 and 10% of children have disorders of sufficient severity to handicap them considerably in everyday life. In most cases these will have been present for several years when they are first identified and many will persist into adolescence and adult life. The figures available suggest that at a conservative estimate a million of the country's children at some time experience significant episodes of psychiatric illness, and for many the duration and severity of the disturbance leads to prolonged family stress, personal unhappiness and educational under-achievement.

2.21 *Chronic illness, handicap and psychiatric disorders are now at the centre of paediatric care.* They are more common than was once thought and make very great demands on parental understanding and courage and professional judgement and care. We do no more here than indicate the size and complexity of the problems; the detailed implications for services are more fully examined in Part II of our report.

Death

2.22 There are times when death is merciful and right. Nevertheless, it is the strongest challenge to our continuing ignorance, to the deficiencies of services, and, in its social inequality, to the nature of our society.

TABLE 4

The Numbers of Deaths at different ages in Childhood and Adolescence in England and Wales 1974

Still Births	First week	Peri-natal	1 week–1 year	All first year	1–4	5–9	10–14	15–19
7,175	5,994	13,169	4,465	10,459	1,922	1,225	1,091	2,212

2.23 Excluding miscarriage in early pregnancy death is now most frequent in the last stage of pregnancy, during birth, on the first day, in the remainder of the first week and from then until the first birthday. (Table 4.) The number is falling yet more lives are lost in these fifteen months than in the next 25 years. The main reasons are failure of fetal growth, complications, especially insufficient oxygen reaching the brain, during labour and delivery, severe malformations and the immaturity or malnutrition of babies of low birthweight. The causes of many perinatal deaths are not fully understood, and *this loss of life is a continuing test of the quality of antenatal care, the place and management of birth, and the facilities for skilled supervision of every newborn infant.*

2.24 In our attempts to understand and reduce perinatal mortality, two aspects are of central importance. The first is that in 1974 76% of first day deaths and 58% of deaths within the first month occurred in low birthweight babies weighing 2.5 kg or less. The proportion of all live births of 2.5 kg or less (6.5%) has hardly fallen in the last 20 years, but the prospects of these infants have greatly improved as a result of advances in neonatal care. This particularly applies to the smallest infants. Twenty years ago many of those who survived suffered substantial physical and mental impairment; today with centres providing expert "intensive" newborn care, the outlook is much more encouraging. This achievement has implications for the number and siting of such facilities and the place of delivery for mothers at special risk. It also raises the wider issue of the prevention of low birthweight, and here results achieved in some other countries notably Sweden, Finland and Japan is more favourable than our own.[13]

2.25 The second important factor is the social and regional inequalities. Perinatal mortality is significantly higher in Social Classes IV and V and varies within and between different regions of the country.

2.26 Vulnerability continues through the first year. After the first week and even more after the first month the causes of death change; congenital malformations continue to take their toll but they are exceeded by acute respiratory, mainly virus, infections, the sudden unexpected death syndrome, and other infections and disorders.

[13] Pharoah, P O D (1976). International comparisons of perinatal and infant mortality rates. *Proc. Roy. Soc. Med.* 69, 335.

Post neo-natal mortality by cause of death

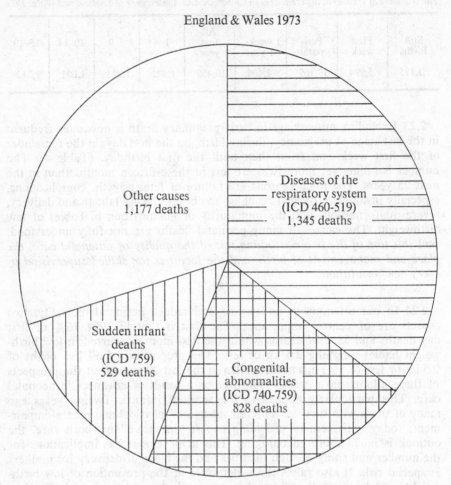

England & Wales 1973

Other causes
1,177 deaths

Diseases of the
respiratory system
(ICD 460-519)
1,345 deaths

Sudden infant
deaths
(ICD 759)
529 deaths

Congenital
abnormalities
(ICD 740-759)
828 deaths

2.27 It is long established practice to consider all deaths in the first year together, and the deaths per 1,000 live births, the infant mortality rate, is a sensitive indicator of child health and attendant services in this period; it allows comparison between countries and within the same country at different times. Table 1 showed that this rate was falling, and we might be content if the fall was comparable with that in other countries. However in both perinatal and infant mortality our improvement has been slower (Statistical Appendix Table C4). *There has been no significant fall in our post-neonatal mortality rate over the past 15 years.*

2.28 More than 70% of deaths between birth and 15 occur in the first year of life. This continuing loss is associated with continuing limitation in our understanding of the causes, and so of prevention, and to a lesser extent is due to our failure to apply known effective treatment. Reduction in deaths from respiratory infection and sudden infant death syndrome (cot death) is proving almost as resistant to present measures as reduction in defective fetal growth, premature birth and congenital malformations. Although not revealed by the national figures, [14] local studies have shown the sudden infant death syndrome as the main cause of post-neonatal infant mortality today.[15]

2.29 The tragedies of sudden infant death have caused widespread public concern. Recent local studies are throwing some light on its aetiology. The condition is not due to a single cause. In a third a known disease capable of explaining the death is present, in a third there are minimal features of disease which, though unlikely by itself to cause, possibly contributes to death; and in the remainder, though recognised disease is absent there is evidence of disturbed growth. The death of a completely well child is a rarity.[16] There is a social pathology too. Epidemiological studies have shown that low socio-economic status is one of the factors commonly present in cases of cot death.[17] In children with recognisable disease, the main factors leading to death lay in "the inability of some parents to recognise the importance of symptoms, or to avail themselves of the health services, the amount of drive and persistence required to obtain general practice services in some areas; and the failure of some practitioners to recognise severely ill children.[18] These findings from the most direct study of its kind in this country, are similar to those of the earlier survey of post-neonatal deaths by the Department of Health in 1970.[15] In this 312 of the 679 deaths occurred at home. Avoidable factors contributing to the death were present in more than a quarter of the cases studied. Over two-thirds of these avoidable factors were described as "social" or were due to parental failure. In one-fifth of the cases an avoidable factor could be attributed to the general practitioner.

2.30 The problem is to decide why one child dies and another in similar circumstances does not. The main factors appear to be limited parental understanding of illness with failure to use the available health services in communities where these are likely to be hard-pressed. Continuing studies in Sheffield of deaths in children aged 1 week to 2 years suggest that it may be possible to identify many of the parents whose children are at potential risk, ideally before the child is born; and that by increased support in the antenatal and infant stage from health visitors who understand exactly what is required, many deaths might be prevented. We believe this approach has clear implications for child health services in the "inner city" and other "disadvantaged areas". *Present knowledge applied through better front line nursing and medical services for children would make a major contribution to reducing infant mortality in this country to levels found in Sweden and Holland.*[19]

[14] Weatherall, J and White, G (1976). *Studies on Medical and Population Subjects,* No. 31. DHSS, HMSO, London.

[15] *Confidential enquiry into post-neonatal deaths* 1964–66. DHSS Reports on Public Health and Medical Subjects, No. 125 (1970). HMSO, London.

[16] Protestos, C D, Carpenter, R G, McWeeney, P M, and Emery, J L (1973). Obstetric and perinatal histories of children who died unexpectedly (cot death). *Arch. Dis. Child.* 48, 835.

[17] Fredrick, J (1974). Sudden Unexpected Deaths in Infants in the Oxford Record Linkage Area. *Brit. J. Prev. Soc. Med.* 28, 164.

[18] McWeeney, P M, and Emery, J L (1975). Unexpected post-neonatal deaths (cot deaths) due to recognisable disease. *Arch. Dis. Child.* 50, 3, 191.

[19] Emery, J (1976). Unexpected Death in Infancy. *Recent Advances in Paediatrics,* No. 5. Churchill, Livingstone.

2.31 Just over a quarter of child deaths occur between one and 15. The main causes are accidents, cancer, respiratory disease, and the continuing effect of congenital malformations. This is the healthiest period of life, and the main cause of death now is accidents, many of which are preventible.

The Social Dimension

2.32 We have already had occasion to refer repeatedly to the correlation between social class and the prevalence of ill-health and disability in children. As we pass from the children of professional families to those of unskilled workers there is a significant increase in bedwetting, squint, stuttering, dental disease and non-infective seizures, and bronchitis and pneumonia and infective diarrhoea are more frequent and more severe. Disease does not occur in a bodily system but in a child, a member of a particular family living in a particular community. Illness in childhood cannot be fully understood without reference to the child's development and social circumstances. Conventional classifications fail to reveal the adverse social factors that may lie behind a diagnostic label and contribute to the form, management and outcome of the illness. Poverty, inadequate housing and unemployment are still with us; and although the majority of parents care for their children faithfully and well, many are hindered from doing so by physical or mental illness, or instability in their personal relationships.

2.33 The effect of environment can also be seen in growth. In one group of urban children at 15 children in social classes I and II were on average 4.5cm taller and 4.4kg heavier than children in social classes IV and V.[8] In a national study,[20] when all adverse factors were compounded, the "social" difference in height was nearly 14cm. In a study[21] of all short children (below the third centile), in a northern city at the age of 10, 82% were normal in terms of freedom from disease. The majority of their families however belonged to social classes IV and V and the children had been brought up in poor conditions. In at least a third of these "normal" children the adverse social conditions were considered the cause of their deficient growth. Short stature can be normal; it can also be a disease of the social environment and an important pointer to a group of socially deprived children.[20] *There is now extensive evidence that an adverse family and social environment can retard physical, emotional and intellectual growth, lead to more frequent and more serious illness and adversely affect educational achievement and personal behaviour.*

TABLE 5

Infant Deaths 1964 England and Wales, Number and Rates per 1,000 Legitimate Live Births

	Social Class	
I & II	III	IV & V
1,714 (12.8)	7,110 (17.2)	4,931 (20.8)

[20] Davie, R, Butler, N, and Goldstein, H (1972). *From Birth to Seven.* Second Report of the National Child Development Study. Longman in association with the National Children's Bureau.

[21] Lacey, K A and Parkin, M J (1974). The Normal Short Child. *Arch. Dis. Child.* 49, 417–424.

TABLE 6

Children 1–14 1959–63 England and Wales([22]), Number of Deaths (and Rates per 100,000 per year)

Age	I		II		Social Class III		IV		V	
1–4	436	(69.0)	1,329	(73.4)	6,147	(88.7)	2,324	(93.3)	1,521	(154.0)
5–9	209	(32.8)	818	(35.1)	3,243	(41.1)	1,234	(41.4)	744	(66.6)
10–14	173	(29.6)	823	(28.8)	2,771	(31.3)	1,091	(30.3)	555	(41.4)

2.34 A special analysis of the 1959–63 child deaths shows that the death rate for children aged 1–4 and 5–9 in Social Class V was approximately twice that in Social Classes I and II and more than 50% higher than that for Social Class IV. The differences for children aged 10–14 are less striking, but nevertheless the death rate in Social Class V was a third higher than that for Social Class IV. The difference in deaths from respiratory diseases is particularly noticeable. For children aged 1–4 the death rate from pneumonia in Social Class V was 25.2 per 100,000 compared with 13.9 for Social Class IV and 10.0 for Social Class I. Children in Social Class V experienced considerably higher death rates from accidents, poisonings and violence. Although these figures relate to a period 15 years ago and the death rate from disease and accident has fallen appreciably since then it is unlikely that the large social class differences have been eliminated. They are a sad commentary on avoidable deaths in childhood.

Prevention

2.35 To what extent have we the knowledge to prevent some of the conditions that most affect children today? The remarkable improvements in children's health which are now taken for granted began with the great improvements in the standard of living of the whole population which had their onset in the changes brought about by the agricultural and industrial revolutions and which are still continuing. Later came critical studies of disease. That dual approach is still valid. We should seek to understand as precisely as possible what we are trying to prevent, if we are to find effective ways of preventing it. Equally we should remember that even incomplete knowledge may be sufficient for effective prevention. Many years elapsed between the discovery of ways of preventing cholera and scurvy and understanding the specific cause of these illnesses.

2.36 If we look back to the previous century it is possible to trace some of the crucial steps that led to the prevention and virtual elimination in some cases of illnesses which were then a common feature of childhood. Increased survival of children began with a decline in mortality from the infectious fevers. As this started well before the application of specific prevention or effective therapy other factors were involved. The first, beginning in the eighteenth century, was improved production and later increased importation of food leading to better nutrition. The second was the concept of "public" as distinct from "personal"

([22]) From: Adelstein, A, *Paedriatrics and the Environment, Fellowship of Postgraduate Medicine*, p 59.

health: the progressive control by the community of water supplies, housing standards, employment and working conditions and environmental hazards. The third was the introduction in 1870 of education for all children. And at the turn of the century came the introduction of the school health service and the maternal and child welfare services, to advise mothers and protect the health of children.

2.37 The 1930's saw the beginning of the rapid increase in the scientific understanding of bodily and mental function which is the basis of modern medical care. The first application of this was preventive: immunization progressively against diphtheria, whooping cough, tetanus, tuberculosis, poliomyelitis, and measles, which not only completed the fall in mortality from these diseases but diminished the costly burden of dangerous, damaging and unpleasant illness. The second was therapeutic: the discovery of antibiotics, specific remedies for the bacterial infections.

2.38 The essential basis of improvement has been an increase in, and wider distribution of national wealth: a rise in the standard of living. Sufficient family income, available food, sound nutrition, safe housing, control of environmental hazards, education, medical and social services, have all played a part in the better health of children in this country today. All are still relevant and will remain the continuing concern of government in the allocation of resources and the choice of priorities.

2.39 We are tempted to plead that causes are now more complex and solutions more difficult than in the past, but to most people the problem of infectious disease seemed "insoluble" before the causes were known and remedies found. The problems for children and adolescents today, the hazards of fetal growth and birth, malformations, unsafe homes, dangerous roads, overeating, smoking, alcohol, family breakdown, parental neglect and abuse are formidable. We are concerned moreover not only with the prevention of children's illness and death but with laying the foundations of health in adulthood. To prevent dangerous heart and lung diseases in adults will call for changes in personal behaviour which should begin in childhood. Many mothers fail to breast-feed yet this provides important protection against infection and death in early infancy, and against obesity in childhood and adult life. We know the dangers of smoking and yet 36% of adolescents aged 16 are already smoking more than one cigarette a week. We accept widespread dental decay when the addition where necessary, of sufficient fluoride to the public water supply to bring the level to one part per million—a policy which we wholeheartedly support— would reduce caries in children to half its present level.

2.40 The solution to many of today's health problems will ask of children and parents a greater understanding of the conditions of health and a willingness to accept the personal responsibility required for their achievement. Government can make an essential contribution through its social policies, support for research, enquiry and public education, and in particular situations by legislation. The impressive fall in smoking and in deaths from lung cancer among doctors, show that they can take the medicine they prescribe for others. *The first responsibility now in professional education and daily practice is to take prevention seriously*. This attitude long established in the community services especially in health visiting, must spread to all the health services for children.

2.41 At the same time, although it raises issues going further than the scope of this report we must recognise that the fetus and child are in many respects specially and uniquely vulnerable to the adverse effects of drugs and to toxic and mutagenic additives and contaminants found in water, food and the atmosphere. Children have the right to be protected from these hazards, and the responsibility for this rests with many bodies and individuals, including Government, manufacturers and distributors and promoters of drugs, foods and all products used by children, as well as parents, guardians and their professional advisers.

Some General Conclusions

2.42 We have attempted a broad picture of the increasing health and continuing ill-health of children in this country today. There has been a remarkable improvement in the survival and growth of children and a decline in the prevalence and danger of infective illness. This has come from increased economic prosperity, improved nutrition, a greater understanding of child health care, specific immunisation against infectious diseases and more rational and effective treatment including the use of antibiotics. A primary aim of today's services must be to promote good health and to prevent disease, in childhood and in adult life. The challenge lies in finding ways of giving health education and advice that will result in parents and young people taking a greater personal responsibility for their health. How best to do this is a matter for research and social action.

2.43 There is still a substantial amount of acute and serious illness in childhood. Disease, injury, stillbirth and death occur more often than is justified with present knowledge, and we are coping with them less successfully than most comparable countries. Of greater significance for the overall development of services is the fact that the emphasis in childhood illness is changing. With the prevention, or more effective treatment of many infective diseases the major health problem affecting children today is no longer acute episodic illness but, increasingly, malformations, chronic illness, physical and mental handicap, psychiatric disorder and ill-health arising from family stress and breakdown. These call for a different approach on the part of professional staff, not least a greater willingness to work together to provide a multi-disciplinary approach which recognises the wider implications of chronic ill-health or handicap.

2.44 Although hospital care, (but not necessarily admission), is still necessary for the treatment of acute and dangerous illness especially in infancy, for the investigation of complex disorders and for the treatment of conditions requiring surgery, more sick or disabled children should be cared for by their parents at home. Parents can however only be expected to carry out this responsibility if they have more opportunity to learn about the care of a sick child, can be sure that professional help will be readily available, and if they have confidence in the ability of the doctor or nurse to deal with their child as well as treat the illness. This has implications both for the accessibility of services and for the level of paediatric knowledge and training required by those involved in professional care.

2.45 Chronic illness and severe handicap have to be lived with. Mumps may mean a fortnight away from school; but asthma can lead to a succession of lost days and interrupted work and leisure, and cerebral palsy to a life very different in its quality from that led by normal brothers, sisters and friends. The ongoing care of a handicapped child calls for a close relationship between parents and professionals, ready availability of specialist skill and judgement, and consistency of professional support, and since the best treatment for handicap is not to have it, for prevention and for the research which can make this possible.

2.46 Finally, although we do not always know how, many illnesses both physical and psychological are caused or intensified by adverse family or environmental factors. Adverse social conditions will doubtless be with us for many years to come. Special efforts are therefore going to be needed to identify those children and families whose health is most at risk, and to provide help and advice in ways which are geared to meet their particular needs. Social as well as developmental and medical knowledge and insight must be acquired if comprehensive diagnosis and management of child, family, and illness are to be achieved. The language of social paediatrics is increasingly used, but the acquisition of real understanding and skills will make strenuous educational demands on all branches of the services for children.

CHAPTER 3

THE ORIGINS AND GROWTH OF SERVICES

3.1 Developments in the provision of health services for children have reflected general attitudes to children at the time. A social interpretation of these changes in the last two centuries is beyond our remit, yet we felt that any review of existing services should be set in historical perspective. Essentially, community health, primary care and hospital services have developed independently and have for the most part separate histories.

Community Health

3.2 Understanding of the especial vulnerability of children came slowly. In the 18th century, when Gibbon, himself the sole survivor of 7 children, could write of the death of an infant "as an unfortunate but highly probable event", half the children born were dead before their 15th birthday. In the middle of the 19th century—a century dominated by increasing industrialisation and devastating epidemics of infectious disease—a third still died before the end of childhood. The first advance in child care came through sanitary reform and control of children's employment. The Factory Act of 1833 established an inspectorate empowered to judge the fitness of children to enter employment and, in the absence of a statutory registration of birth, to estimate their age. By 1867 all children under 16 had to be medically examined when starting or changing employment at the employer's expense, and Edwin Chadwick took a wider approach, convincing government that money spent on sanitation would result in fewer demands on Poor Law Relief, and the addition of at least 13 years to the lives of working people[1].

Health Visiting

3.3 In 1769 George Armstrong established a dispensary for the infant poor in London linked to a scheme for home visiting, commenting that "if you take away a sick child from its parent or nurse you break its heart immediately". An advocate of free medical care for children, he maintained this pioneer service for 12 years[2]. In 1816 J B Davis returned to Armstrong's concept of home visiting but it was not until 1867 that the practice took root. In that year the Manchester and Salford Ladies Sanitary Reform Association supported the employment of "a respectable working woman to go from door to door offering physical help and health advice"[3]. The success of the scheme led to the adoption of similar schemes elsewhere. The health visitor had arrived.

3.4 Florence Nightingale saw this "health missioner" as a new profession for women comparable to "sick nursing", and stressed the need for special training. In 1891 the North Buckinghamshire Technical Committee initiated the first certificated training course: 3 of the 6 who qualified were given wholetime appointments by the Buckinghamshire County Council, the first trained health visitors to be employed by a local authority.

---

[1] General Report on the Sanitary Conditions of the Labouring Population of Great Britain (Chairman: Edwin Chadwick) (1842). HMSO, London.

[2] Neale, A V (1964). *The Advancement of Child Health*. Athlone Press, London.

[3] Hale, R, Loveland, M K, and Owen, G M (1968). *The Principles and Practice of Health Visiting*. Pergamon Press, Oxford.

3.5 The importance of the health visitor in the field of child health was not fully grasped until in 1901 Dr S G Moore, Medical Officer of Health for Huddersfield, decided to use them in his attack on high infant mortality. He arranged a visiting service specifically to help mothers nurse their infants in their own homes and to offer from birth onwards guidance on infant management. Mothers began to use the service but because of delays in notification of births many babies died before a visit could be made. In 1906 a special Act (The Huddersfield Corporation Act) made notification of all births within the city to the Medical Officer of Health compulsory. The following year this was incorporated in the Notification of Births Act, and, though permissive, this allowed local authorities to require the registration within 36 hours of all births after the 28th week of pregnancy. In recognition of the large uptake of these provisions in 1915 they were made compulsory under the Notification of Births (Extension) Act.

3.6 Others were not slow to follow Huddersfield's lead in protecting maternal and child health. In 1899 the first "milk depot" was opened through voluntary effort in St Helens. The model was followed quickly elsewhere. Besides the free distribution of sterilised cow's milk to mothers and infants, some depots offered meals for nursing mothers. Most developed into infant consultation centres, where health visitors gave advice to mothers on hygiene and infant feeding. In Winchester formal courses of instruction were introduced as a "school for mothers". The infant welfare centres of the 20th century had begun.

3.7 By 1916 the extent of development in child welfare services prompted the Local Government Board's report on maternity and child welfare schemes[4]. The guidelines in this report for the numbers of health visitors required (1 : 400 live births) and for proper medical cover for all births were embodied, with other provisions, in the Maternity and Child Welfare Act 1918. This gave recognition to growing practice by empowering local authorities to make arrangements for safeguarding the health of mothers and of children under 5, including the establishment of free ante- and post-natal clinics. (This was, moreover, at a time when only the wage-earner could claim free medical care by right.)

3.8 The expansion of health visiting services led to re-examination of the training and qualifications required for the work. In 1908 an examination leading to certification as a health visitor/school nurse was established by the Royal Sanitary Institute. In 1919 Health Visitors Training Regulations were laid down by the Board of Education and the newly established Ministry of Health. In 1925 the Ministry took responsibility for health visiting and the Royal Sanitary Institute became the central examining body for the health visitor's certificate. And midwifery (but not children's nursing) became a necessary part of a health visitors training.

3.9 The development of health visiting was a reflection both of the growing emphasis on public health and of the concern of some Victorians for the welfare of children—a concern clearly manifest in other fields. The English biologists,

---

[4] Local Government Board, Report on *Maternity and Child Welfare* (1916). HMSO London.

56

men like Darwin and Galton, were pressing the need for a scientific approach to the study of children. Galton himself established an "anthropometric laboratory" where for 3d a child's "form and faculty" could be measured in order to "learn (his) powers or to obtain timely warning of remediable faults in development". By 1896, Sully had opened the first laboratory in Great Britain exclusively devoted to psychology and had also established the British Child Study Association "to encourage teachers to study the individual child and seek advice on their more difficult problems".

Health at School

3.10 In education itself, momentous steps had been taken. The Education Acts of 1870 and 1880 made schooling compulsory and in so doing, exposed for the first time the extent of malnutrition and physical defects among children. The first response by voluntary bodies and local Education Boards was to provide meals for the underfed. This was quickly followed by systematic medical inspection in all grant aided schools and the appointment of school attendance officers. The Medical Officers of Schools Association was founded in 1884 and in 1890 the first full-time School Medical Officer was appointed by the London School Board. Next to malnutrition, physical handicap was now seen as the major problem. Acts in 1893 and 1899 gave local authorities discretionary powers to provide special education for blind, deaf, defective and epileptic children.

3.11 At the turn of the century however many children under 12 were still unable through undernourishment and recurrent illness to benefit from the education provided. Inspection could expose, but not ensure treatment. The arguments echoed the lingering spirit of the last century. Medical services were costly and beyond the reach of large numbers of families, especially those whose children were most in need. The use of public funds was resisted as removing a basic parental responsibility, not least by those defending private medical interests. By 1903 some local authorities began to offer treatment for minor ailments through the appointment of school nurses and by medical officers when conducting inspections.

3.12 The debate was sharpened by the evidence that between 40 and 60% of men enlisting for the South African War were unfit for service. Interdepartmental committee followed interdepartmental committee [5], [6], while the solution, more inspection and more feeding of the malnourished, remained unchanged. In 1907 the Education (Administrative Provisions) Act not only affirmed the duty of all local authorities to inspect but gave them authority to attend to the health of all children in public elementary schools.

3.13 The initial uptake of these powers was slow. Many local authorities were still loth to spend additional money when Poor Law Relief was available as a last resort. Facilities for treatment by general practitioner and hospital were limited and unevenly distributed through the country. Accepting this the Board of Education allowed local authorities to employ doctors for the treatment of

---

(5) Report of the Interdepartmental Committee on Physical Deterioration (1904). HMSO, London.

(6) Report of the Interdepartmental Committee on Medical Inspection and Feeding of Children Attending Public Elementary Schools (1905). HMSO, London.

schoolchildren and the first school clinic opened in Bradford in 1908. The Education Act of 1918 extended this provision to children in secondary schools.

3.14 The original 1907 legislation was directed not only to the physical but also the "mental and moral improvement of coming generations". Compulsory education for all had raised the problem of varying intellectual abilities, necessitating the provision of special schools for children of below normal ability and the consequent refinement of means of assessing intelligence. This clearly pointed to the desirability of a school psychological service. In 1908, the school medical officer for Birmingham wrote[7] "It is perhaps here that one of the most valuable effects of a Medical Department may be found, ie in the close correlation of applied psychology and scientific investigation to the problems which present themselves in adapting the education to the individual needs and capacities of children". First abroad and then in England, stage by stage examinations of children led to the definition of a normative scale of infant development. By 1913 a few authorities had established psychiatric clinics to diagnose those children in need of special education and in the same year Sir Cyril Burt was appointed psychologist to the London County Council to advise on individual problem children, assist in allocating them to school and make surveys of the school population.

The School Dental Service

3.15 In the meantime, the poor state of child dental health became increasingly the subject of attention. A dental surgeon had been appointed to a Poor Law School in 1884 but it was not until 1907 that the first school dental clinic was established at Cambridge: "2 small rooms in a garden, one used as a waiting room supplied with toys for the diversion of the children and the other being the surgery suitably fitted." In the same year the Board of Education recommended that the medical examination of new entrants to public elementary school should include consideration of "teeth and oral sepsis". Local Education Authorities were given powers to make arrangements for the provision of treatment, but only when care for the children could be obtained from no other source. The new powers however allowed LEAs to assist voluntary agencies and by 1909 the first wholetime school dentist had been appointed.

3.16 Surveys demonstrated that the condition of children's teeth was alarming with little evidence of conservative dentistry. In 1910 John Knowles, the school dentist at Bradford, examined 8,657 children and found only 6 fillings. The need for school dental services was now unquestionable, and in 1912 the Board of Education published the first of a series of "Recommendations for the basis of a satisfactory school dental scheme." Dental services were to be under the control of the principal school medical officer and inspections should be carried out by a qualified dentist. Treatment was to be conservative in character, and include preventive measures such as extractions which contributed to the preservation of the dentition as a whole and mechanical devices to regulate the teeth.

Expansion and Development of Community Services

3.17 In the 1920's and 30's, especially after the Local Government Act of

---

(7) Board of Education (1908). Report of the Chief Medical Officer. HMSO, London.

1929, county and county borough councils extended their provision of mid-wifery and public health nursing – a service pioneered by Liverpool in 1866 – maternity and child welfare services, school health and dental services, and domestic help during childbirth and family illness. In response to persisting evidence of large numbers of infant deaths from preventible hazards during the antenatal period and childbirth, the Ministry of Health prompted reforms in medical and midwifery education and obliged local authorities to provide antenatal supervision and a competent obstetric service for every pregnant women. The child welfare centre became the focus for both antenatal and postnatal care, and for the health care of children up to school age. From 1928, all newly-appointed wholetime health visitors were required to hold the Health Visitor's Certificate.

3.18 In 1934, the government introduced its free "milk in schools" scheme, and during that same decade the number of school dentists and clinics increased substantially. Dental attendants began to replace trained nurses and some progressive authorities appointed supervisory dental officers. The school health service extended both its treatment and preventive services. During the '20s the Child Guidance Council under Burt's chairmanship was successfully to promul-gate a new approach to children with behaviour and emotional difficulties. It advocated a nucleus team of psychiatrist, psychologist and social worker who would work together to look beyond the individual child to his family and social setting. Transatlantic exchanges in 1927 led to the publication of a far-sighted report urging the value of preventive work and the need for child guidance clinics to be closely integrated with the school system. Though the first initiatives were exclusively private, by 1935 the provision of child guidance clinics had been accepted as a legitimate addition to the school medical service. In 1932 Leicester became the first local education authority to establish a school especially for nervous and difficult children. In the same year they appointed a psychiatric social worker to assist their psychologist and broadened the scope of their school psychological service to deal with children who had problems not associated with schools.

The Development of General Practice

3.19 Much of what has been described is the preventive aspects of primary care. The complementary curative aspects evolved largely within the general practitioner service. Following the Medical Act of 1858 the concept of the general practitioner service arose because of the necessity for specialisation in medicine which resulted from the growth of medical knowledge and techniques. Specialists in medicine increasingly became dependent upon the facilities of hospitals and the general practitioner came to play a decreasing part in the activities of the large hospital. The National Health Insurance Act of 1911 provided the legislative framework for a general practitioner service for certain groups of compulsorily insured workers, but this Act did not provide for the dependents of these workers, the majority of whom were children. Conse-quently, as we have seen, local authorities began to undertake a measure of personal curative care for these and other needy sections of the population. In this way 3 branches of the health service system, hospital local authority and general practitioner services developed separately. General practice was essen-tially a patient demand service and as such concerned in the main with illness.

Apart from his National Insurance patients a general practitioner had no clearly defined list of patients and hence even if he were interested, was hampered in providing preventive care. A remarkably far-seeing report in 1920[8] advocated the integration of the 3 services to form a comprehensive system of primary and supporting health care but its recommendations were not acted upon.

Hospital, Paediatric and Children's Nursing Services

3.20 Founded in 1722, Guy's Hospital from the beginning admitted children to the womens' wards. A century later St Thomas' Hospital accepted children as in-patients, requiring mothers to enter also "to take them in charge where they were too young to take care of themselves". In 1833 Guy's Hospital again created a precedent by establishing a separate ward for children. The children's hospital movement in this country really began in 1852 with the foundation by Charles West of the Hospital for Sick Children, Great Ormond Street. The example was quickly followed in provincial cities and towns, and many of the original buildings are still in use.

3.21 The Local Government Act of 1929 abolished the Poor Law Authorities, empowered the new County and County Borough Councils to develop work-house wards for the sick as municipal hospitals, and removed the need for those requiring but unable to afford medical treatment to apply for Poor Law Aid. Municipal hospitals were governed by Council representatives. Within medical practice, specialisation was accepted increasingly as a hospital based activity in which general practitioners were becoming less involved. It was however within this hospital setting that the emergence and establishment of paediatrics as the general medicine of children, developed. Hospital-based specialisation provided a focus for research and hence to the development of new forms of therapy. It also led, particularly in the specialist children's hospitals, to a growing understanding and expertise in caring for the sick child not only in terms of providing treatment but of providing it in a setting which took account of his need for personal understanding, play and affection. The professional recognition of this specialty developed more slowly in this country than in Europe and the United States. The British Paediatric Association, founded in 1928 worked steadily to promote recognition of the new discipline and for established training and consultancy posts. By 1928 paediatrics, if not by that name, had been established as a subject for research, teaching and practice in every medical school, but full-time paediatric posts were uncommon outside these centres. It was moreover seen still as essentially a hospital activity. Recognition of the special skills of the sick children's nurse had come earlier, with the establishment of the Register for Sick Children's Nurses in 1919, to be followed in 1928 by the creation of the Association of Sick Children's Hospital Nurses. The hospital service had also provided the basis for specialist work in child psychiatry, starting with Maudsley's observations on "The Insanity of Early Life" in 1867 and leading to the treatment of children both as in-patients and out-patients at the opening in 1923 of the Maudsley Hospital, the first to take only voluntary patients. From this stemmed the development, first of children's clinics, and

---

[8] Ministry of Health, Consultative Council on Medical and Allied Services: Interim Report on the future provision of medical and allied services (Chairman: Lord Dawson of Penn) (1920). HMSO, London.

then of a Children's Department, though this latter initiative was halted by the outbreak of war.

War and the Beginnings of Change

3.22 By 1939 each of these services, the community or local authority based services, the special hospital services for children and the general medical services had developed to a level undreamed of 25 years earlier. The outbreak of war interrupted their growth, but at the same time provided a powerful stimulus for more far-reaching social changes. In particular ways these had an immediate impact on services for children. First the National Milk Scheme was established in 1940 as recognition of the priority in nutritional and welfare policy that should be given to children and expectant mothers. By 1942 the Welfare (Foods) Scheme had been set up, through which every expectant mother and child under 5 was entitled to orange juice, cod liver oil and milk. At the end of the war this was made permanent as the Welfare Foods Service. Second, the voluntary and municipal hospitals were brought together as a nationally organised hospital service with a regional administration. Thirdly, the evacuation of school children forcibly demonstrated the poverty and physical ill-health of many living in the deteriorating centres of large cities, and also the substantial number whose anti-social behaviour made them unacceptable to their temporary foster parents in the reception areas. This last led to demands for more extensive and evenly distributed child guidance facilities, and as a short term solution psychiatric social workers were appointed to work in areas where a full team service could not be implemented.

The Education Act 1944

3.23 Other wartime developments however were to provide a completely new framework for the health and welfare of children. The aim of the Beveridge Report of 1942 was to provide a comprehensive system of social security for all.[9] The legislation it set in train ensured that comprehensive health services would be provided for children (and their families) for the first time as of right. The first steps were taken in the Education Act of 1944. It established two major principles: local authorities were obliged to provide "comprehensive facilities for free medical treatment either under the Education Act or otherwise for pupils in attendance at any school or county college maintained by the authorities", and parents were obliged to submit their children to medical inspection. The School Medical Service was renamed the School Health Service. The new Act extended its functions to cover children in all state schools (from 2 years to 15 years old). Local authorities were to provide school meals and milk; to arrange the free provision through clinics of medical services that included minor ailments, child guidance, orthopaedics, ENT, audiometry, speech therapy, orthoptics, remedial exercises and chiropody, and special investigation for rheumatism, asthma, and enuresis. The Act also required the free provision by local authorities of dental services for the inspection and treatment of all school children; and the School Health Service Regulations 1945 required the appointment of a school dental officer by each authority. Nurses appointed as school nurses were required to have the HV Certificate.

---

[9] Social Insurance and Allied Services: Report by Sir William Beveridge (1942). Cmnd 6404. HMSO, London.

3.24 The Education Act consolidated and expanded the health and education services provided for handicapped children. Local authorities had acquired powers to make provision for the education of handicapped children under the Elementary Education (Blind and Deaf Children) Act 1893, and the Elementary Education (Defective and Epileptic Children) Act 1899, and by 1908 some 17,000 handicapped children were receiving education in 300 special schools. The Mental Deficiency Act 1913 laid on local authorities the duty to ascertain children over 7 who were considered ineducable in special schools and who required supervision or guardianship under the terms of the Act. The need for schools to serve a wider range of needs in the education of "mental deficients" was recommended by the Wood Committee in 1929[10] but only in 1944 was a fundamental reappraisal of special education undertaken. The 1944 Education Act required LEAs to provide schools sufficient in number, character, and equipment to give all pupils opportunities for education according to their different ages, abilities and aptitudes, and gave local authorities for the first time the duty to ascertain and provide for all children over 5, and at the LEA's discretion, for those between 2 and 5 who required special educational treatment.

3.25 Through the Handicapped Pupils and School Health Services Regulations 1945, the types of special educational provision were increased from 5 to 11: delicate, diabetics, educationally subnormal (ESN), epileptic, maladjusted, blind, partially sighted, deaf, partially hearing, physically handicapped, speech defective. In later legislation diabetes ceased to be a qualifying condition. The first state grammar school for the deaf opened in 1945, for the speech defective in 1947, and for the physically handicapped in 1957.

The National Health Service Act 1946
3.26 The central aim of the National Health Service Act 1946 was to provide free health services for everyone at the time of use. The principles on which it was based derived largely from the practices that had evolved up to that time. There was to be no compulsion on either patients or professions; clinical judgments of independent clinicians were not to be questioned; general practitioners were to be free to choose their patients, and vice versa; and GPs and specialists were free to opt for private practice or for NHS work, or both. Although the hospital services were to be organised by regional hospital boards on behalf of the state, general medical and dental services were to be provided for NHS registered patients on the basis of a contract between the general practitioner and the local Executive Council.

3.27 Under the National Health Service Act, it was the duty of the Minister of Health to promote the establishment of "a comprehensive health service designed to secure improvements in the physical and mental health of the people of England and Wales and the prevention, diagnosis and treatment of illness". The need for the service to be comprehensive was thus clearly recognised: that it expressly needed to be coordinated was less apparent at that time. The Act firmly established a tripartite service, comprising separate general practitioner, hospital specialist and local health authority services,

[10] Board of Education and Board of Control (1929). Report of the Committee on Mental Deficiency (Chairman: Arthur Wood). HMSO, London.

each with their own administration. Moreover within the local authority, the health authority's maternity and child welfare service and the education authority's school health service generally retained their separate identities, administration and to a considerable extent staffing. The opportunity to establish a single, comprehensive system of primary and supporting health care was lost once again, as it had been after the publication of the Dawson Report in 1920. Furthermore, this insular approach to the organisation of health services, reinforced as it was by the preoccupation of traditional medical and nursing education with disease and the care of the sick, strengthened the current but unvalidated assumption that prevention could and should be separated from treatment.

3.28 This was the background against which health services for children developed under the impetus of the National Health Service Act and it is essentially with the review of the child health services that have developed within this tripartite administrative structure that we are concerned. We have not been the first committee to concern itself with the implications for children of a tripartite service. In 1967 the Sheldon Committee[11] noted the increasing interest in health, growth and development shown by both general practitioners and paediatricians, and in their report attempted to rationalise the approach to health services outside hospital by recommending a child health service administered then by local health authorities, but provided eventually through general practice. With the NHS still allocating responsibilities between three separately administered branches, such a radical alteration of services was unacceptable; to fulfil their statutory duties, local authorities felt they still needed to employ their own medical staff. In 1973 the NHS Reorganisation Act has sought again to overcome the separation by transferring to autonomous health authorities the responsibility for providing comprehensive medical, dental, nursing, therapist and other necessary professional services for all children. This provided the opportunity for a complete review of child health services, and this report, is our response.

Developments since the creation of the National Health Service

3.29 The tendency in any consideration of services is to concentrate on methods and to overlook the changing attitudes which shape them. These have been more far-reaching than is generally realised, and, as our visits and enquiries have shown, in many areas only now is serious attention beginning to be paid to them. Nowhere is this more evident than in the large and largely undeveloped area between health and welfare, involving medicine, education and social work.

Local Authority Child Care Services

3.30 Developments in social work practice for example, have had, and continue to have an important influence on health services. The focusing of attention on family and "normal" home life in child health care for example since the National Health Service no doubt reflected developments in local

---

(11) Central Health Services Council, Report of a Sub-Committee of the Standing Medical Advisory Committee on Child Welfare Centres (Chairman: Sir Wilfred Sheldon) (1967). HMSO, London.

authority child care stemming from the Curtis Report[12] of 1946 and the enactment of its recommendations. The Children's Act 1948 established, under the overall responsibility of the Home Office, Children's Committees in each local authority to have the duty of care for children deprived of a normal home life. Whilst at first this "care" was restricted to children separated from their families, it became increasingly clear that many children were deprived of the essentials for proper development in their own homes. The effects of both types of deprivation on the physical and emotional health of the child became a recognised health problem that children's officers and the health services together had to contain and prevent. Experience of the problems encountered in trying to help children separated from their parents and the distress and damage which in some instances might have been avoided by earlier intervention led to pressures for increased powers to help children wherever they might be and to spend money on children not "in care".

3.31 The Children and Young Persons Act of 1963 which responded to these pressures greatly extended local authority responsibilities to include the provision of advice, guidance and assistance to prevent children appearing before the courts and being taken into care. Many children whether "in care" or not can only be helped effectively if the whole family situation is modified. The powers given to local authorities to provide preventive and after-care services to children living at home encouraged the development of social work focused upon the family unit as the basis of work with the child. The opportunities afforded by this Act to provide Family Advice Centres, rehabilitation services and day and residential facilities for families have not as yet been fully implemented. The second Children and Young Persons Act in 1969 extended the range of treatment facilities controlled by the present Social Services Department by bringing together the former Approved Schools, Local Authority Children's Homes and some voluntary homes into what is now the Community Homes system and by adding the new "intermediate treatment" provision. It is now possible to plan preventive, care, treatment and rehabilitative social services for children and their families as a rational and integrated whole.

The Local Authority Social Services and Education Acts 1970

3.32 Two other legislative changes in the field of social and educational poiicy since 1946 have also had important implications for the organisation of health services for children. In 1970, following the publication of the Seebohm Report[13] the Local Authority Social Services Act strengthened the concept of a family oriented pattern of social service by bringing the various social service functions of local authorities together in a single social services department. The responsibilities of these departments include the provision of day nurseries, formerly the responsibility of local health authorities. In addition since 1974 they have also been responsible for the provision of social work support to the National Health Service. Also in 1970 the importance of education and training in developing the full potential of every child, whatever his handicap was reflected in the Education Act which transferred to the education service,

---

[12] Report of the Committee on the Care of Children (Chairman: Dame Myra Curtis) (1946). HMSO, London.

[13] Report of the Committee on Local Authority and Allied Personal Social Services (Chairman: Baron Seebohm) (1968). Cmnd 3703. HMSO, London.

from the then local health authorities responsibility for the education of mentally handicapped children of school age. Although these services now lie outside the NHS it is essential that links between them and the health service should be maintained and fostered since many of the most disadvantaged or disabled children will need help from more than one service. Our remit extends only to the provision of health services, but in reviewing them we have endeavoured to keep in the forefront of our thinking the need to provide a health service which can facilitate close working relationships with allied services, and in particular with local authorities' social service and education departments.

65

CHAPTER 4

SERVICES TODAY: THEIR STRENGTHS AND WEAKNESSES

The Tripartite Service

4.1 The NHS Act established a tripartite health service. It recognised and kept separate the community health services provided by local authorities (for children in school, for children under 5 and for expectant mothers), the General Medical Services provided for the listed patients of independently contracted general practitioners, and the specialist health services for all provided by the hospitals. As children of all ages were now entitled to free health services, the duties laid on LEAs to provide comprehensive treatment facilities for school children were relaxed, though the School Health Services retained responsibility for "ascertainment",† child guidance, and speech therapy services, as well as continuing to provide the minor ailments clinics (paragraph 4.31).

4.2 By the Act the permissive provisions of previous Acts were repealed and local health authorities were obliged to arrange for the care of expectant and nursing mothers and of young children and for vaccination and immunisation. Provision of these services was intended to ensure "close integration", on the one hand, with their own midwifery services and the general medical services, and on the other with the hospital and specialist services. Yet because the general practitioners' contract did not explicitly cover preventive services, and local health authorities were debarred from providing treatment services (except in the cases previously mentioned), *the allocation of responsibilities itself helped to create the belief and practice that primary health care, for children could be divided into the separate components of prevention and cure,* with independent services providing for each.

4.3 For the first time, the NHS Act 1946 laid on every authority the duty "to make provision for the visiting of persons in their homes by visitors, to be called 'health visitors' for the purpose of giving advice as to the care of young children, persons suffering from illness and expectant or nursing mothers, and as to the measures necessary to prevent the spread of infection". Under the NHS (Qualifications of Health Visitors and Tuberculosis Visitors) Regulations 1948, all health visitors whether full-time, part-time, or employed by local health authorities through voluntary organisations, were required to have the HV certificate. In the new health service organisation, local authorities generally had responsibility for "community" rather than "patient" oriented services, although the former included "personal" services, such as the specific duty to arrange vaccinations against smallpox and immunisation against diphtheria. In fulfilling this duty and arranging other immunisation programmes the emphasis was on persuasion through the health education and advice offered by clinical medical officers and health visitors.

4.4 The NHS Act also laid on every local health authority the duty to make

---

† The duty placed on local education authorities by Section 34 of the Education Act 1944 to ascertain which children require special educational treatment.

provision, either by direct employment or through arrangements with voluntary organisations, "for securing the attendance of nurses on persons who require nursing in their own homes". This recognised the efforts of the County and District Nursing Associations on which local authorities had hitherto depended for the recruitment and employment of a trained district nursing service which in 1948 was shown to be in reach of 90% of the population.

4.5 It is now nearly 30 years since the NHS Act came into effect and only those who knew the fragmented and variable quality of health care for children which preceded it can appreciate the magnitude of the improvements. It is however our remit to review these services, and "review" must involve critical appraisal aimed at identifying areas for improvement. If therefore in the ensuing analysis we appear to have concentrated unduly on deficiencies, and to have taken much that is excellent for granted, we hope that this will be seen as constructive criticism, aimed at making what is good, even better. We have drawn attention to the significance of parents as the guardians of their children's health, and to some of the implications for the family of the changing pathology of childhood. With this in mind we have in this chapter looked at services not only in terms of functions and administrative structure but also, from the "receiving end", on the grounds that *one of the first criteria for measuring the success of a child health service must be the extent to which it is readily accessible, and comprehensible to those who have to use it.*

4.6 We received considerable evidence on this point. We have been left in little doubt that, while there is still a deep respect for individual doctors and nurses, there is a groundswell of dissatisfaction among parents with many features of the health care of children. Some of this criticism relates to the organisation of the service and its consequences, and we consider this in more detail below. There is also a general feeling of uncertainty and disquiet about the relationships between parents and professionals. Many parents have a strong feeling that they are regarded as passive by-standers rather than active partners in the health care of their children, and expected to accept "what the doctor says", without their opinion being sought. They often find it difficult to talk frankly to doctors and the pressure of time and habit has made some doctors less communicative than they intend. Parents do not always understand what is expected of them but when they need further help they may not reach the same doctor easily, if at all. In view of the increasing importance of parental involvement in prevention and treatment the strength of the comments which we received on these lines has considerable significance for all professional staff involved in the health care of children.

General Practitioner Services

The Responsibilities of General Practice

4.7 Traditionally the general practitioner has been responsible for the provision of a 24 hour service for the treatment of illness. In 1974 there were 21,510 unrestricted principals in general practice in England and Wales. The terms of their contracts with the local Family Practitioner Committee (until 1974 the local Executive Council) are laid down in regulations which require them to provide "all necessary and appropriate personal medical services of the type usually provided by general medical practitioners" to the patients registered with them. These Services include making arrangements for the referral of patients as necessary to any other service provided under the NHS, and advice to enable them to take advantage of local authority services. It is therefore to the general practitioner that most parents are likely to turn in the first instance when their child is ill. Local studies suggest that parents do not seek medical help for 2 out of 5 of all significant illnesses in children under the age of 5[1] but every year approximately 3 out of every 4 children aged 0–14 will see their general practitioner for illness of one kind or another[2], and on average they will have 4 or 5 consultations each. Consultation rates vary both within and between regions, according to factors such as sex, age and social class and the mobility of the families. On average a GP will have between 550 and 600 children under the age of 15 registered with him, although there are considerable geographical variations, and they will occupy 25% to 30% of his time. General practitioners deal with most episodes of illness on their own without seeking further help. 10% of cases might be referred to out patient departments[3] though recent evidence from one community shows that between 1% and 2% may be referred where some of the GPs in the group have increased paediatric experience and regular consultant support is available in the practice.[4]

4.8 The General Medical Services have historically provided an essentially therapeutic service available on request for those children registered with a general practitioner. They are traditionally patient oriented, and although the introduction of the National Health Service brought with it the possibility of general practitioners having a defined population and hence the essential element in the provision of many forms of preventive medicine, there is no defined locality for registration. As noted above parents do not seek help for a substantial minority of illnesses in young children. There are many possible reasons for this and the evidence is conflicting. Clearly a measure of informed self-care by parents is both rational and essential if the health services are not to be overwhelmed but certainly ignorance and the relationship between parents and professionals affects the use of the health services in general and the primary care services in particular. On the one hand Cartwright[5] has shown that in general the population want a general practitioner system, yet there is equally evidence that the relationship between parents and general practitioners is not as good as it should be. To some extent the differing attitudes may be related to maldistribution of doctors with excessive workloads leading to lower standards. But we sense too that many doctors may not fully appreciate the difficulties some parents feel about consulting them. They are afraid of making unnecessary calls, and feel that the doctor does not appreciate the fear, distress and panic which they experience when faced, especially at night, with unexpected pain or fever in their child which they cannot understand.

---

[1] Miller, F J W, Court, S D M, Knox, E G, and Brandon, S (1974). *The School Years in Newcastle on Tyne*. OUP, London.

[2] Logan, W, and Cushion, P (1958). *Morbidity Statistics from General Practice*. General Register Office, Studies on Medical and Population Subjects, No 14. HMSO, London.

[3] Joseph, M, and MacKeith, R G (1966). *A New Look at Child Health*. Pitman Medical, London.

[4] Stark, G D, Bassett, W J, Bain, D J G, and Stewart, F I (1975), Paediatrics in Livingstone New Town. *Brit. Med. Jour.* 4, 387.

[5] Cartwright, A (1967). *Patients and Their Doctors*. Routledge, Kegan and Paul, London

4.9 General practice has a continuing 24 hour responsibility for the therapeutic care of its patients. The organisation of services to provide 24 hour cover in a society where patterns of work and leisure have undergone a marked change has produced problems which the development of group practice is only partially solving. GPs worked in partnership long before the NHS commenced but the organisation of group practice is of more recent origin and has been encouraged by schemes to facilitate the financing of group practice premises and by the development of health centres. Between 1965 and 1974 the number of single-handed practitioners has decreased from 24% to 18%; and of those in group practice, the proportions in partnerships of 4 or more has almost doubled, to 44% (Statistical Appendix, Table F1). There has also been a significant increase in the number of health centres, which numbered 632 at the end of 1974, when 15% of GPs were working from them. Despite these developments deputising services have increased; as many as a third of GPs working in group practices now use them; and older GPs and those working in single-handed practices and in urban areas use them more than others. These services cause further problems for parents, who find themselves consulting a doctor who is a stranger to the child and to them and whose experience with children is an unknown quantity. Moreover in central urban areas, where the more disadvantaged families are likely to be living, and where consistent care and continuity of care are most important, deputising services are most in evidence.

4.10 The number of general practitioners practising in a given area is controlled by the Medical Practices Committee. There is an inducement scheme to encourage doctors to practice in under-doctored areas but even so maldistribution continues. Poverty and ill-health are fellow travellers, while health services tend to travel in the opposite direction. *The inverse care law still operates and there are fewer GPs, home nurses and health visitors in the areas where they are most needed.*[6]

The Development of Special Interest

4.11 Before 1948 basic qualification as a medical practitioner was sufficient for entry into general practice. In the early 1950s a voluntary training scheme was introduced offering preliminary appointment as a trainee to a general practitioner who was recognised as a "trainer" by the Local Medical Committee. More recently, voluntary 3-year vocational training programmes for doctors wishing to work as general practitioners have been introduced, and under legislation now before Parliament this will become in the next few years mandatory for all doctors becoming principals. At present about 90% of vocational training programmes provide up to six months specific training in the care of sick children. Welcome though this development is, it will take time before its effects are widely felt and studies show that many general practitioners currently in practice have had no specific training in paediatrics. In a representative sample in 1969, 54% had a basic medical qualification alone and 3% had the Diploma in Child Health.[7] In another enquiry[8], in 1968 among general practitioners

(6) West, R R, and Lowe, C R (1976.) *Regional Variations in the Need for and the Provisions* and *Use of Child Health Services in England and Wales. Brit. Med. Jour.* 2, 843–846.

(7) Irvine, D, and Jefferys, M (1971). BMA Planning Unit Survey of General Practice, 1969. *Brit. Med. Jour.* 4, 535–543.

(8) Wright, H J (1973). Primary Paediatric Practice in Industrial and Rural Britain. *J. Roy. Coll. Gen. Pract.* 23, 815.

in partnership or group practice in industrial areas, 36% had had no formal training in paediatrics beyond that given to medical students.

4.12 To a limited extent the development of the concept of "special interests" by individual practitioners has helped to counteract this deficiency. "Special interest" is not a new idea, but was commended in the Gillie Report in 1963[9] and again in the Report of the Sub-Committee on Group Practice[10] which argued the need for a generalist in the system of health care but also envisaged the opportunity for individual members of group practices to develop special fields of interest which would strengthen their own work and that of the group. The growing establishment of group practice has offered increased opportunities to develop such special interests, but it has been left to individual doctors and their partners to decide on the extent and the manner in which it is expressed within each group practice. Sometimes it has included sessional work as a clinical assistant in the appropriate specialist department of the District General Hospital, or in the child or school health service. It has been essentially a personal pursuit of knowledge in a particular field of medicine shared within the practice, but carrying no assumption that one day all children would enjoy this special pattern of care. It has not, for instance, so far required specific additional training in paediatrics or professional recognition of special expertise, as in the case of obstetrics.

4.13 Inevitably there is considerable variation in the quality of general practitioner services for children. This has no doubt been one of the factors, along with traditional patterns of use of hospital services in certain localities, maldistribution of practitioners and difficulty in providing 24 hour cover, which has resulted in parents, and not only those in areas of disadvantage, tending to use hospital accident and emergency departments—often at considerable inconvenience—as a source of help which it should be possible to provide more locally, more frequently and more effectively from the general practitioner.

The Changing Rôle of the General Practitioner
4.14 It is important not to underestimate the extent to which general practice has been changing. General practitioners for some time after the introduction of the National Health Service felt that their rôle was uncertain. This uncertainty was increased by the decline of general practice particularly in the United States of America and compounded by the emphasis placed upon hospital services within the National Health Service. Changing patterns of mortality and morbidity, however, together with advances in medical knowledge were already beginning to alter the emphasis of the practitioner's work which was increasingly concerned with chronic illness, handicap and the social and emotional problems associated with illness. The adminstrative organisation of the National Health Service also provided the general practitioner with a readily definable list of patients and thus opened the way for an involvement in preventive medicine. In the 1950s many doctors began to see a new and vital rôle for general practice within the National Health Service. The foundation of the Royal College of

[9] Central Health Services Council, Standing Medical Advisory Committee: Report of the Sub-Committee on the Field of Work of the Family Doctor (Chairman: Annis Gillie) (1963). HMSO, London.

[10] Central Health Services Council, Standing Medical Advisory Committee: Report of a Sub-Committee on the Organisation of Group Practice (Chairman: Robert Harvard Davis) (1971). HMSO, London.

General Practitioners was an important expression of this re-vitalising process and the College has since played a major part in the changes that have and are still taking place in primary care. *It is important to appreciate the rate at which general practice has evolved in the past 25 years, because health care systems do not usually change so rapidly, nor is major progress often achieved quickly without creating problems and highlighting deficiencies.*

4.15 The new rôle of the general practitioner, first defined in the Gillie Report, has recently been summarised as follows: ([10])

"1 The diagnosis and management in or near the home of undifferentiated illness in a defined population of individuals or families to whom he is directly accessible and for whom he accepts a continuing responsibility.

2. The prevention of disease and the maintenance of health both physical and mental including the detection of the earliest departure from normal in the individuals and families of this population."

4.16 It soon became clear that practitioners could not sustain these functions within the traditional organisation of the general medical services. They needed purpose-built or adaptable premises, and they needed to work closely with other doctors and with other professions such as nurses, social workers and therapists. It was these pressures which led not only to the development of group practices and the building of health centres but also to the attachment of health visitors and district nurses, and hence to the concept of the primary care team, a functional arrangement whereby general practitioner, nurse and health visitor work together from the same premises and see the same population i.e. the patients registered with the doctor. *The advent of the primary health care team has been of particular significance for the development of health services for children.* It was a step not only towards the coordination of the health services provided by Executive Councils and Local Authorities, but also towards the combination of preventive and theraputic health care. In 1971 just over half of all GPs were working in primary health care teams with HVs and HNs.

Preventive Health Services
Links with other Services
4.17 Although these changes have laid the foundations for the involvement of general practice in preventive work, the basic responsibility for developmental and preventive surveillance of young children has rested with an entirely different service, provided till 1974 by the local health authority. Some general practitioners do regularly undertake such surveillance of their child patients. It is estimated that between 10 and 20%([7,11]) of GPs organise their own child health clinics, although as often as not it is the health visitor attached to the practice who conducts the clinic in the practice premises. Such clinics normally serve only children registered with the practice. We were told however that there was some evidence when GPs do conduct their own child health clinics the consultation rate for illness in children under the age of 5 falls; also that attachment of health

---

([11]) Steiner, H (1975). Paediatrics in Hospital and Community in Newcastle upon Tyne, In: *Bridging in Health*. OUP, London.

visitors has apparently led to an increase in the number of general practitioners taking on this work. More than a quarter of the medical sessions in area health authority child health centres are undertaken by GPs employed on a sessional basis. In these circumstances however the general practitioner will see any child attending the clinic, and may thus be involved in the surveillance and the giving of advice to children for whom he has no responsibility as a general practitioner.

4.18 Some mothers may therefore be fortunate in having a general practitioner who is also involved in the developmental and preventive surveillance of her child, or who shares this with the practice health visitor. The majority however, still seek this service from a completely separate part of the health service, involving different personnel. Most mothers today have their babies in hospital. They will therefore already have received from the staff of the maternity and paediatric departments, advice on a wide range of aspects of baby-care. Sometimes they will also have had advice from their general practitioner and health visitor, if these are providing antenatal care as is usually the case. Evidence we received emphasised the importance attached by mothers to continuity of care and the avoidance of contradictory advice when they return home to the care of the general practitioner and the child health services. We were left with doubts as to whether communication and coordination between services was always as good as it should be at a time when mother and child are so vulnerable, and this is a point we return to in more detail in Chapter 8.

The Scope of the Pre-school Services
4.19 While seeking help with what she considers to be illness in her baby from the general practitioner, the mother looks to the preventive child health services as a source of information and advice on the feeding, health care, development and management of her infant or young child. Child health clinics provide regular sessions for routine examination and screening of the pre-school population. They offer health education on a personal basis for mothers and a programme of immunisation for children, currently covering diphtheria, tetanus, pertussis, and poliomyelitis. In some cases clinic premises are also used for the distribution of certain welfare foods. Parents have open access to these services, not only for advice about health care but also for help about any problem relating to health and management; additionally in many areas the services invite the parents to bring their child to a clinic for "birthday checks" on health and development. Since the widespread introduction of a routine screening test of hearing at the age of 6–9 months, these annual interviews have often included more extensive and systematic developmental screening.

4.20 These services have been provided to a large extent by health visitors, on home visits or in child health clinics, and to a lesser extent by clinical medical officers both of whom were employed prior to 1974 by local health authorities. In 1973 local health authorities employed 3,250 clinical medical officers on a full-time or part-time basis, for clinical work in the child health and school health services. Of these 38% worked only in the child health but not in the school health service. In addition they employed

72

1,648 GPs on a sessional or part-time basis, of whom 48% worked only in the child health services. The whole time equivalent number of HVs employed in 1974 was 9,137, of whom 2,236 were employed within the school health service. Essentially the child health services are advisory but they still constitute a personal service to individual parents and their children. Their quality depends on the clinical skills and training of the health visitors and doctors concerned. At present, neither clinical medical officers nor general practitioners who do sessional work in child health clinics are required to have postgraduate training or planned experience in infant and pre-school child health care. Some medical officers, probably less than 40%, hold the DCH, and some will have attended short courses in developmental paediatrics, but many are inadequately trained for the work they have to do and the quality of the service that parents receive is variable. Most of these doctors are at present also carrying out a variety of other tasks in the field of community health, such as family planning or cytology screening and are therefore working as generalists in preventive work rather than concentrating solely on work with children. This was recently argued as a justification for maintaining a separate community service.([12])

4.21 The health visitor is an SRN who holds a qualification in midwifery and has undergone 12 months full-time training for the Certificate in Health Visiting. This latter training includes theoretical and practical work in relation to child health care. The health visitor thus has a training which gives her specific skills in child health work, and she has become a key figure in the preventive services. Health visitors are however now seeing fewer children. In 1974 health visitors attended 2.8 million children under 5, 77% of that age group. In 1963 they saw 93%. This trend began in 1946 when the HV was designated a "family visitor" and consequently assigned increasingly to adults and the elderly. It has been accelerated by the attachment of health visitors to general practice, and more frequent requests from GPs for involvement with patients, three-quarters of whom are adults nowadays living to an older age. It is estimated that work with the under 5s now accounts for only some 59% of the HV's time. Behind the assertion that too few GPs appreciate the independent responsibilities of the health visitors, we believe lies evidence that her special skills are too often being used for help of a kind more properly sought from social workers, and used increasingly for patients other than children and families.† However it is also a reflection of some uncertainty about their rôle on the part of the health visiting profession itself.

4.22 The preventive services are in general population oriented. They have a strong tradition of going out and offering their services, rather than waiting to be consulted and have been organised on a territorial basis to facilitate this. Many authorities operate computer-based systems to remind

---

([12]) Report of a Special Working Party on Public Health Clinical Medical Officers (1974). British Medical Association, London.

† As we were completing our report we were interested to see that the need to emphasise the health visitor's work with young families was one of the issues raised at a conference on the rôle of the health visitor organised by the Department of Health.

parents to bring children for examination or vaccinations at specified times, and area health authorities still have a statutory duty to ensure that a mother is visited by a health visitor after the birth of a baby. *Traditionally the health visitor had a special responsibility for families with young children in a given geographical parish, but the attachment of health visitors to general practice has eroded their "territorial" responsibilities, and made more difficult the task of locating and offering help to mobile families and others who make ineffective use of the health services.* Moreover while attachment has strengthened the "family" dimension of her work by enabling her to work for children alongside their general practitioner, it has also created difficulties in relation to continuity of care since mothers who attend the local clinic can no longer be certain of seeing their practice health visitor.

The Use of Services

4.23 *Less than half the child population under 5 years attended local authority child health clinics* (Table 1). This national average conceals wide variations in different areas and in different age groups. Table 1 shows that on average three-quarters of children under the age of 2 years attend each year but three-quarters of 2 to 4 year olds do not; a plateau seems to have been reached in national attendances of children in all 3 age-groups. In terms of educating the mothers of young children and also of their children's health, this is a very unsatisfactory state of affairs. The stated reasons for attendance in one local authority area are shown in Appendix D, Table 1 but the reasons why some mothers never attend or cease after a few weeks must also be sought.

TABLE 1

Children attending local health authority child health centres by ages, (England and Wales) Percentage of Age-Group Attending

Year	Children under 1 year	Children aged 1 year	Children aged 2–4 years	Children under 5 years
1964	74.6	67.4	19.8	46.3
1966	78.3	70.9	27.9	46.8
1968	78.6	70.1	28.5	46.5
1970	82.5	71.2	28.4	46.9
1971	80.0	71.4	28.3	46.3
1972	79.4	72.4	27.5	46.5
1973	80.0	73.0	28.0	46.6

4.24 Recent studies confirm that among clinic non-attenders in the first 2 years of life there are a disproportionate number from families in social classes IV and V. It is among this section of the population whose needs may be least well met within their own families, that disadvantaged children are most often found. There is also a disproportionate number of children from social class I among non-attenders. Failure to attend a clinic is not necessarily evidence of lack of proper attention to the care of babies and young children. It is possible that non-attending children might be visited by a health visitor more frequently than usual in their own homes as a matter of policy but such evidence as there is indicates that they are not.[13][14][15][16] Alternatively, their parents may prefer to take them to their own family doctor. This was the case in 20% of non-attenders in one survey[16] but another 30% used neither their general practitioner nor clinic services. In a study of disadvantaged families[15] most mothers saw child health centres as hostile places where injections were given, and where children were more likely to pick up infections than be protected from them; 1 in 3 had no contact with a health visitor and among these were the mothers who made least use of their general practitioner.

4.25 Such attitudes may partly account for the incomplete take-up of programmes of prophylaxis against infectious diseases. Of the children in England and Wales who had their second birthday in 1973, 20% had not received immunisation against pertussis, diphtheria and tetanus, a similar proportion had not been vaccinated against poliomyelitis, and 50% had received no protection against measles (Statistical Appendix, Table E3). No doubt these figures conceal similar variations to those reported in the National Child Development Study of 7 year old children[14] which showed that progressively higher proportions of unprotected children are found as one moves from south to north of the country and from social class I to V.

4.26 Many parents may simply be confused about the rôle of the clinic, particularly in relation to general practice, or have little idea of the rôle of the health visitor and fail to see her as a specialist source of advice and support in the care of babies.[17] The range of advice and help that parents do seek from health visitors and doctors in child health clinics is evident from the Tables in Appendix D. The frequency with which particular items of service are sought or provided varies widely from place to place, reflecting for instance, local custom, the availability of alternative services from their general practitioner as well as the organisation of individual clinics by the health visitor or doctor concerned. The general pattern of use of clinic services is broadly the same today as it has been over the last 15 years, except perhaps that fewer parents nowadays attend clinics only to buy subsidised foods and more children are brought for developmental interviews.

4.27 Of particular significance is the extent to which mothers take their children to health clinics with what are essentially problems of ill health for which treatment will be required. In one study[18] one in 8 mothers consulted both their general practitioner and clinic doctor for the same problem. The rôle of the clinic doctor has however been regarded as advisory only and he has been expected to refrain from treating children seen in clinics. Medical

[13] Douglas, J W B, and Blomfield, J M (1958). *Children Under Five*. Allen and Unwin, London.

[14] Davie, R, Butler, N and Goldstein, H (1972). *From Birth to Seven*. A Report of the National Child Development Study. Longman, London.

[15] Wilson, H (1973). *Child Development Study* (Birmingham 1968–1971): A Study of Inadequate Families. Centre for Child Study, University of Birmingham.

[16] Radford, I and Pemberton, J (1975). *The use of Infant Welfare Clinics*. Evidence submitted to the Committee.

[17] Moss, P, Tizard, J and Crook, J (1973). Families and Their Needs. *New Society*, 22 March.

[18] Anderson, J A D (1968). Overlap of Child Health Services. *Medical Officer*, 22 March, London.

officers are not allowed to make out NHS prescriptions, (since they are not on a prescribing list) or to refer a child for specialist investigation and opinion (strictly speaking) unless the child's family doctor consents. This is confusing for parents, and the position is made more difficult by the fact that in some areas the general practitioner and the clinic doctor have overlapping functions, for example in the provision of vaccination and immunisation services. In one sense overlap may be desirable as it offers parents a choice. At the same time it is clear that *the broad distinction between services is not well understood and it is questionable how effective preventive and developmental surveillance can be when it cannot be followed through with treatment.*

The School Health Service

4.28 Going to school marks an important stage in a child's development. Development is a continuing process and the child's reactions to school, and his adjustment to perhaps his first contact with a form of "institutional living" will be influenced by his development in the pre-school years. It is however at just this stage when continuity of surveillance is particularly important, not only for the child and his parents, but also for teachers who will be working with the child for the first time and who will need advice and help in understanding the child's pre-school health and development, that a further separate area of the community health service becomes involved.

Organisation and Staffing

4.29 Prior to 1974 each LEA had a duty to provide its own school health service. The scope, organisation and structure of these services were fully described in the reports of the Working Party on Collaboration between the NHS and Local Government (1973 and 74).[19] Their function is no different now that it is the duty of the AHA to provide them. (The details are set out in Appendix E.) In short their purpose is to ensure as satisfactory a standard of health as possible for every pupil so that they can make the most of their education in school. These services have been provided by school medical officers and school nurses, now employed by Area Health Authorities and by health inspectors employed by local authorities. Between 1944 and 1974, except in central London, the same local authority administered both school health and local health (including child health) services. In practice, the principal school medical officer administering the school health service and the medical officer of health of the local health authority were except in two local authority areas, the same person. In most areas also the management of the school nursing service was the responsibility of the local authority's Director of Nursing Services. The responsibility for the day-to-day management of the school health service almost invariably devolved on a senior medical officer, who usually devoted all his time to this one service. In isolated instances one senior doctor had responsibility for the management of the local authority's unified child and school health service,

---

[19] Three Reports from the Working Party on Collaboration between the NHS and Local Government: 1972–74. Department of Health and Social Security 1973 and 1974, HMSO, London.

but for the most part progress towards integrating the two parts of the local authority service was slow, despite the fact that in practice there was a considerable measure of overlap amongst the staff involved, 80% of school doctors being involved in pre-school work, and 60% of doctors involved in pre-school health also working in the school health service. There has also been a marginal link in terms of manpower, with the general practitioner services, with 8–9% of school medical work being carried out by general practitioners employed on a sessional basis. This contribution has been concentrated in London and the South East of England where half the general practitioners doing school work were employed. This sharing of man-power has only exceptionally resulted in the provision of a combined thera-peutic and preventive service, with the GPs providing school medical services for their registered child patients as was largely the case in Somerset and in Oxfordshire.

4.30 Neither clinical medical officers nor general practitioners are required to have undergone any special training either in paediatrics or educational medicine before working in the school health service. A few LEAs have organised short induction courses for doctors without previous experience, and many clinical doctors have attended refresher courses for school doctors, but only those school doctors called upon to examine children who may need formal 'ascertainment' as educationally subnormal pupils have to have special qualification, obtained by attending a 3 or 4 week approved course. Since 1946 school nurses have in principle been required to be fully trained health visitors, and this training involves, in addition to child care theoretical and practical instruction in school nursing. By 1974 however almost half the nurse-time in schools (2,139 wte out of 4,375 wte) was provided by nurses who were not qualified health visitors, a reflection of the general shortage of health visitors. The strength of the service has been made up by the employment of SRNs or SENs, but neither of these receives specific training in school health work, and although a number of LEAs have provided in-service training for their own nursing staff, there is no recognised course of training for this work other than the certificate in health visiting.

Development as an Advisory Service
4.31 The 1944 Education Act obliged LEAs to ensure that free medical treatment was available to pupils, as well as medical examinations. Since the introduction of the NHS in 1948, LEAs have relied extensively on the NHS to provide treatment facilities, especially for acute, episodic illness and have subscribed to the principle that any medical treatment a school doctor may think a pupil needs should be provided by the general practitioner or hospital services. However, prior to reorganisation of the NHS in 1974, LEAs retained both their duty to see that treatment was available and their right to provide it if necessary and if they so wished, and many of them maintained (though on a diminishing scale) certain treatment facilities established before 1948, eg minor ailment and speech therapy clinics, and even set up others, eg for audiology, enuresis, asthma, obesity. In addition, LEAs have continued to provide such diverse items of treatment

77

as commercial hearing aids; electric bell apparatus for enuretic children; incontinent pads; extra milk for diabetic children and gluten-free bread for those with coeliac disease, and convalescent care. These facilities either originated or have been maintained in response to a need that the general practitioner and hospital services have either not sufficiently or conveniently been able to meet. They have been provided by school doctors and nurses in special clinics, or in schools. Some have been established in conjunction with regional hospital boards (prior to 1974), when the hospital consultant in the specialty concerned has attended.

4.32 The school health service has consequently become primarily a health advisory service, and an ascertainment service for handicapped pupils. Nurses have played the major rôle in the former, through annual hygiene inspections and involvement in health education; so far as the 'normal' child is concerned the school doctor has provided intermittent support to the nursing staff through routine and selective medical inspections, and has become increasingly concerned with work with handicapped children. *Parents and teachers have found themselves faced with a school health service which knew something of the child's health at school and had skills in educational medicine—but could rarely provide treatment and had no firsthand knowledge of the child's behaviour or development out of school; and a general practitioner service which could provide treatment but had no opportunity to study the child's behaviour in school and to discuss problems of health and adjustment with the teaching staff concerned, and had no experience of educational medicine.*

Current Problems
4.33 There has been growing concern about the school health service. Critics have suggested that in many areas its nature and organisation and its concentration on regular medical examinations have restricted its ability to meet the current needs of the children in school and their teachers and parents. In particular the services have attempted to serve the interests of the adolescent indirectly through advice to parents and teachers but rarely to meet his needs as he himself experiences them. There is concern too at the lack of appropriate training of most doctors and nurses who work in the service, and at the changing rôle of the health visitor. All these are reflected in a lack of satisfaction with the service, although this is not uniform because of the wide variations between LEAs in the philosophy, methods, staffing levels and quality of their services. We believe all those involved recognise the need for better communication, for more simple direct and honest talk between doctors, nurses, parents, teachers and pupils, and especially for more practical advice to teachers in relation to day to day problems in the classroom.

4.34 The professional staff are generally well aware of the difficulties and appreciate that they will be more effective if they work more closely together in the interests of individual pupils. However, there is uncertainty and some anxiety about the organisational implications of doing this and about the contribution and status of different professions. *There is still a striking lack of any national or local policy aimed at achieving rational, efficient cooperation between general practitioners and school doctors or resolution of the underlying dichotomy between promoting health and treating illness.* The staff have also suffered from the lack of a satisfactory career structure in their field of medicine, and the problems of professional status and organisation have been made the more acute by the reorganisation of the health service. They have also had to work largely in isolation from the specialist services which have been relatively slow to apply the increasing knowledge of developmental and educational medicine.

The Hospital and Specialist Services

Developments in Paediatrics

4.35 *The creation of a unified hospital service and the provision of general hospitals in every district has been the most successful aspect of the National Health Service.* Within this wider hospital setting paediatrics, the general and specialist medicine of childhood, grew and spread to all parts of the country. Progress was slow and we still have a smaller number of trained paediatricians in relation to our child population than any other comparable country. With their limited numbers and faced with an unmet need for better care of the new-born and the acutely ill, paediatricians, many of whom were for many years single-handed, initially confined their work mainly to hospital. In the last 15 years in response to the changing balance of illness in childhood professional attitudes have changed. Paediatricians are increasingly aware of the developmental and social aspects of their work, and have seen the necessity for closer links with primary care, for the better care of the handicapped and for a trained paediatric contribution to educational medicine and to the social services. This expansion in attitude and professional responsibility is slowly taking place, but limited numbers and the failure to include experienced doctors from the child health and school health service has meant that a specialist paediatric contribution beyond the hospital still lags far behind the need.

4.36 Between 1964 and 1974 the number of consultant paediatricians increased from 231 to 393 (Statistical Appendix, Table F6), and there has been considerable improvement in their distribution, although 48 of those working in district general hospitals still do so single-handed. In the University teaching hospitals the growing recognition of the special nature of children's illness has resulted in a further degree of specialisation with the development of paediatric specialists in perinatal paediatrics, neurology, cardiology, nephrology, gastroenterology, haematology, endocrinology and oncology. Seventy of the 393 paediatricians work in these fields. Similarly although children's surgery both general and specialist is undertaken by surgeons whose main activities are in adult surgery, some 25 with special expertise give their whole time to children as paediatric surgeons. There are some 20,000 children's nurses on the Register of Sick Children's Nurses but the number actively engaged in sick children's nursing is unknown. Our evidence suggests a serious shortage and an uneven distribution. Despite the recommendation made 18 years ago by the Platt Committee that the Sister in charge of any ward or department where children are nursed should have the necessary training in the care of sick children, 43% of those in such posts are without this qualification (Statistical Appendix, Table F15).

Facilities for Children
4.37 In terms of organisation and facilities, some progress has been made in the building of a small number of new purpose-built children's departments, and the improvement of many others, albeit too often on a "make-do-and-mend" basis. There has been less progress towards the ultimate goal of bringing all children in hospital together in paediatric departments under the clinical care of the responsible specialist and under the general surveillance of paediatricians. The concept of the district general hospital provides the right framework for this but *we are a long way from achieving the comprehensive children's departments in them which has been the policy of the Department of Health since the Platt Report of 1958.*

4.38 There are still moreover many aspects of hospital care where the special needs of children are not recognised. Between a quarter and a third of patients attending accident and emergency departments are children, yet special arrangements for their reception are rarely made. Of 50 such departments studied in Wales[20] only 2 had separate facilities for children. In almost all children could not be shielded from adverse sights and sounds. Yet these departments are inevitably busy, restless, distressing and at times frightening places, even for adults, still more so for children. There has been a steady increase in the provision of out-patient services and the Welsh survey also provided a picture of accommodation for children in these departments. In only 23% of hospitals were separate out-patient departments provided for children: most of these were paediatric general and specialist clinics and only 9% of the allied specialties provided special clinics for them. Moreover of the 80 clinics for children a mere 22 had separate accommodation.

4.39 Each year some 6% of children are admitted as in-patients (excluding those with psychiatric disorders). In a survey carried out by National Association for the Welfare of Children in Hospital in 1970 18% of children in hospital were in adult wards, although in 3 out of 5 of these wards the children were segregated. Of the 325 paediatric departments in hospitals in England in 1973, 77 had less than 10 beds and 129 had between 10 and 24—too small to provide an effective paediatric service (Statistical Appendix, Table E20). The Department of Health and Social Security's memorandum (HM(71)22) emphasised the need for all children's departments to have accommodation for parents, and arrangements for unrestricted visiting of children. It also urged that play space and equipment be available, and reminded hospital authorities of the need to make arrangements with local education authorities for children of school age to receive education if they were fit enough. The most recent information as to how far this advice has been implemented comes from a survey carried out by NAWCH, in 1973, extending to 654 hospitals in England and Scotland. Among the 710 wards (and 9 hospitals not replying in terms of wards) in the English sample

[20] Children in Hospital in Wales, 1972. Unpublished report produced for the Welsh Hospital Board.

only 2 out of 3 were able to provide overnight accommodation for the parents of at least one child in-patient. Only about half had unrestricted visiting (ie not less than 12 hours per day) and 8% allowed less than 6 hours daily.

4.40 A special census in 1969 admittedly now 7 years ago, examined the position of 1400 children under 15 who had been in non-psychiatric hospitals for longer than 4 months. Sixty-nine hospitals were involved, 30 general and 15 orthopaedic. Twenty-seven had no indoor play-space other than in the wards. Thirteen did not have an outdoor playground. In only 27 hospitals was unrestricted visiting allowed although all but 2 of the remainder allowed such visiting outside school hours. Rather less than half the hospitals had overnight accommodation for parents. Less than 40% had a paediatrician with general oversight of the care of the children, and half the hospitals had no RSCN allocated to the children's wards.

4.41 Despite the fact that the hospital service has played the major rôle in the development of paediatrics, and had a greater share of resources in money and staff compared with the community services, there are still many areas where the special needs of children are not recognised in the actual provision of hospital services. It is important here to recognise the contribution that social services can make in the sphere of social understanding of children's needs. The extent to which these social needs have not been met may, to some extent at least, reflect the shortage of social workers with a knowledge of child care working in the hospital services.

Links with the Community
4.42 Paediatrics is beginning to move beyond the old hospital-bound concept, but progress has not been as fast as the needs require. Day care services have developed slowly and have only rarely been backed up by paediatric home nursing schemes, despite the obvious advantages of avoiding separation from family and home or shortening the length of stay in hospital. Where a child needs nursing at home this is normally the responsibility of the home nurse, like the health visitor, formerly employed by the local health authority and now increasingly attached to general practice as a member of the primary care team. These nurses are SRNs, and although the current training syllabus for district nursing includes the special needs of children and their parents, the time that can be allotted to the subject is, inevitably, minimal. A mother may look to the health visitor attached to the practice for advice on the care of the sick child but the health visitor rarely undertakes the practical nursing care of children in their homes, despite the fact that she is by training a registered nurse. It is exceptional for the primary nursing staff to have ready access to the specialist nursing advice from the hospital, and equally RSCN training provides the paediatric nurse with only limited community nursing experience.

4.43 On the medical side steps have been taken to forge new links with community services particularly with the work with handicapped children carried out by the child and school health services, through the development

81

of comprehensive assessment centres. These centres, in district general and University hospitals, now number about 80. They have been used chiefly for the investigation and assessment of young children, and have provided a joint approach to their problems, bringing together paediatricians, senior child health doctors, educational and clinical psychologists, remedial teachers, social workers, therapists and the appropriate medical specialists.

Psychiatric Services

4.44 Since their inception, child psychiatric and child guidance services have provided facilities for the multidisciplinary investigation and treatment of children with behavioural and emotional disorders. The child psychiatric service has formed part of the hospital specialist services and been staffed by child psychiatrists, clinical psychologists, psychiatric social workers and therapists employed in the past by regional hospital boards and hospital management committees. The child guidance service has been organised by local education authorities, who have employed their own educational psychologists and social workers (though the latter are now usually seconded from local authority social services departments); consultant psychiatric sessions have usually been provided by regional hospital boards. Not unexpectedly in our divided system, the local authority child guidance services have been largely unrelated to the child psychiatric services based on the hospitals, though both have sought to achieve effective liaison between health, education and social work professional staff. The staff of the child guidance clinics have rarely been involved in the work of the child psychiatric service in hospital while those of the child psychiatric service have rarely contributed to the community child guidance service or worked in schools. Furthermore, the establishment of these special services to deal with "maladjusted children" has resulted in clinical medical officers, health visitors and school nurses having little involvement with this large and important group of children.

The Problems for Children and Parents

4.45 Parents, even if their child has few problems, find the existing pattern of services confusing, and teachers often find it difficult to obtain easy access to doctors who can explain to them the educational significance of their pupils' developmental and health problems. Both are faced with a conglomeration of professionals, the majority working in separate unco-ordinated services with limited rôles and limited communication with each other, and few of whom are specially trained to work with children. Not all are equally accessible, and parents often do not know to whom to turn for help. They see their child as a whole person and find it difficult to see "health" as distinct from "development", or behaviour at school as something distinct from behaviour outside it, or to appreciate the logic of a service which has doctors who advise but do not treat or prescribe.

4.46 It is children with most need of help upon whom the deficiencies and illogicalities bear most hard. Children with chronic disease and handicap present problems in health care and make demands on family cohesion which are outside the comprehension and experience of the average family. Those with gross disorders are usually identified early by the specialist services, and the measures for comprehensive assessment and planned care undertaken increasingly in the comprehensive assessment centre, but the latter rarely see children of school age. However the majority of handicaps are not gross, and therefore not usually identified until they cause problems in learning or behaviour at school. Children with problems of learning and behaviour are too numerous to refer to consultant paediatricians yet the examinations carried out by school doctors for formal "ascertainment" as a handicapped pupil are rarely adequate as an investigation of their total health needs. As new problems in management arise the family naturally turn to their general practitioner; but as we have seen his training in paediatrics and particularly in this aspect of it may be limited and will have been geared to the provision of curative care and not to developmental paediatrics and the management of chronic handicap. Many general practitioners have never developed an interest in these problems, and tend to refer the child to the hospital consultant services. Since the latter are tempted to take over the continuing care of the child's principal disorder, the practitioner rarely sees the child except in the event of inter-current illness. Yet few hospital specialists have the time to provide the care these children and their parents need. Moreover until relatively recently paediatricians have been predominantly concerned with acute illness and the majority are not trained in the overall health and educational care of handicapped children, and doctors in the present school service who have acquired considerable skills in general management, parental guidance and educational advice and can see the children in school, are isolated from both primary and specialist paediatric services and from research. So parents fail to obtain the ready help and support for which they constantly and sometimes desperately feel the need.

4.47 Difficulty in providing adequate support in the community, including a serious shortage of day care and residential care facilities (the responsibility of social service departments), means that there are still too many mentally and physically handicapped children not needing medical and nursing care in hospital who nevertheless remain for years as long-stay patients for social reasons. Sadly it seems to us from the visits we have made and the well-documented evidence we have received that the variable progress in meeting the special needs of children in hospital has been least satisfactory in this area. We have seen for ourselves how hollow the lives of these children can be. Early to bed, and early to rise, with few toys and little education and nothing to do at weekends, their quality of life and standard of care are all too often subordinate to régimes and staffing dictated by the organisation of a large institution. We have also seen the caring devotion of staff struggling with professional isolation as well as lack of facilities. The primary responsibility lies not with them but with an insensitive society which chooses to ignore the problem.

Conclusion

4.48 With all their shortcomings the present services do provide the foundations on which to build a new service. We have in general practice a strong tradition of family-based care, whose practitioners are increasingly trained to see their patients in the context of their home and social environment. We have inherited from the former local health and education authorities a tradition of preventive medicine, committed to ensuring that services reach those in need, even when they do not seek them, and clinical staff who are skilled in developmental and educational medicine. Within the hospital service we have the specialist disciplines of paediatrics and paediatric nursing with their recognition of the need for special skills and training for those working with children. Alongside them are child psychiatrists, paediatic surgeons, and adult specialists involved in the care of children. All are necessary for an effective service for all children. Yet expertise, and understanding of the problems of children and their families acquired in each part of the service have been confined to that branch, so that each has but a partial understanding of the whole. And so many sick and disabled children do not receive the full benefit of all that has been learnt about the way to treat their illness, prevent their disability and promote their health. Often those at greatest risk have little contact with services at all. It is against this background that we have endeavoured to set, in CHAPTER 5, new objectives for the future.

CHAPTER 5

OBJECTIVES FOR TOMORROW

5.1 In the preceding chapters we have looked at children and families in our society, the changing pattern of childhood illness and the services which are available to deal with it today. In this chapter we identify certain principles derived from these considerations and set out the objectives which should determine the further development of health services for children.

5.2 *Children are full citizens with an equal right to health and to health services, whatever their age and wherever they live.* Developing and dependent, their changing needs call for services which are both specific and adaptable. Children live and grow in families and their health is strongly influenced by family circumstances and parental competence and responsibility.

5.3 The health of children has wonderfully improved; but a great deal of illness remains and this is increasingly seen in chronic forms, as physical and mental handicap and as psychiatric and social disorder. Professional training must reflect the change. Understanding of the causes and the treatment of illness and of the conditions necessary for health is increasing rapidly and the gap between knowledge and practice has widened. The professions involved in the health care of children have not fully grasped how far they have fallen behind and the educational effort which will be necessary to catch up. There are barriers within the professions and between professions, and between professionals and parents, which must be broken down so that a new quality of understanding, respect and cooperation is achieved.

A Child and Family-Centred Service

5.4 The special needs of children which arise from the fact that they are growing developing persons should be reflected in the facilities that are provided for them and, perhaps more important, in the training of those who care for them. *We want to see a service which is child-centred and we believe that this must be a service in which the professional staff are adequately trained and experienced in the special needs of children.*

5.5 Children grow up in families and their parents are the primary guardians of their children's health. This rôle is assuming greater significance for the health services as society increasingly acknowledges the importance of family and environmental circumstances as a determinant of health. The family environment may adversely affect children's health through poverty, ill-health and other forms of disadvantage, or because of parental ignorance or failure to understand and make use of the services available or to appreciate what steps are necessary to protect their child's health and development. At the same time parents are increasingly involved in the management of childhood illness as they shoulder the burden of long term care at home of children with chronic or recurrent illness. *The importance of the family must be reflected in the organisation and delivery of health services for children.*

85

5.6 This has implications first for the attitude of professionals. They should see their task not as usurping the responsibility of the family but as encouraging it, so that families are better able to exercise their responsibility for their children. They should see themselves as partners with parents: prepared and willing to give them explanation and advice about their children's health. And because parents have differing aspirations and backgrounds, they should help parents to make plans in ways which take account of family identity and individuality. Parents' understanding of children's development and illness varies widely and this is due in part to the poverty of professional communication. There can be no doubt that all too often parents feel they are passive bystanders rather than active partners in the care of their children. *The need is for a service that is geared to ensuring that parents are well informed and increasingly involved in their children's development and health, and which from the start will enable them to feel confident in their ability to care for their children.*

5.7 This has implications for all those who come in contact with parents whether in the primary or specialist services and for services other than the child health services. Antenatal care is concerned with the health of the future infant and the early education of the prospective parents in the care of young children is as much part of good obstetric practice as the monitoring of maternal and fetal health during pregnancy and birth. Once pregnancy and birth are safely over mothers need access to professional guidance about the growth and development of their babies; advice about bringing up a family and how to recognise signs that something may be amiss. The need for such help often arises in an acute form on the mother's return home, and there must be the closest possible liaison between doctors and nurses in hospital and in the community, and between the maternity and child health services. Thereafter it should be part of the continuing responsibility of all those professional staff concerned with the health care of the young child to use any and every suitable contact with the parents as an opportunity for appropriate teaching and exchange of information on the child's health and development.

5.8 Information and communication is but one aspect of a family-oriented service: parents can only be asked to accept their responsibilities if they can be confident that they will have adequately skilled professional help available to them, when they need it. *This will require a considerably greater level of paediatric competence among those doctors and nurses, who are going to be the parents' first point of contact when they seek help for their child, than exists at present.*

5.9 *Services should not only be readily available to parents, but they should be easy to use.* This is to some extent a matter of sensible organisation which is understood and can be relied on. It is a question of, for example, organising child health clinics at times which are convenient for mothers; providing them in premises that are convenient and easy to reach and which offer facilities for relaxed discussion.

An Integrated Service

5.10 It is also a matter of providing a service which sees the child as his parents see him, as a whole person, whose life is a continuum rather than a series of segments. Parents should not have to draw distinctions between 'pre-school' and 'school'. *There should be one service which follows the child's development from the early pre-school years, through school and adolescence.* School may often present particular problems: if the child suffers ill-health a parent wants to be confident that his teachers will understand and be advised by doctors and nurses of the implications for his education and his care whilst in school. Parents should of course have ready access to the appropriate teacher, but they need doctors and nurses who can guide them with educational difficulties and unusual behaviour, and make sure that the child is not struggling with a developmental disorder or with physical illness, rather than with an educational difficulty. There is therefore a need for professional staff who not only have an understanding of educational medicine but can interpret the child's behaviour at school in the light of his behaviour out of it. A strong health service in school is an essential part of a good child health service. Similarly adolescence often produces renewed parental concern about personal behaviour. At a time when conventional adult attitudes and the authority of those who hold them many well be rejected, conventional health care may be rejected too. Yet professional help is often needed, and it has to be offered in ways which show understanding of the adolescent's particular problems of development and adjustment to the adult world.

5.11 *The need for an integrated approach to health care is particularly great in the case of the handicapped child.* Parents understandably want a single door leading to assessment, explanation and treatment. They need a coordinated service of care, therapy and education, with regular reviews of the child's progress leading to advice and support. They need an extension of services beyond the normal school leaving age until their child is effectively cared for by health services for adults, and by the Employment Medical Advisory Service. They also need ready access to the professional staff involved in treatment, especially to someone who has accepted personal responsibility for their child.

5.12 Equally parents should not have to attempt in making their first approach to the health services to draw a distinction between "treatment" and "prevention". *The child health service should be able to provide families with a single identifiable source to which they can turn for skilled advice and where necessary treatment,* whenever they feel that they need to.

5.13 Some children will need specialised assessment and treatment. *So far as possible primary and specialist care should also be seen as a coordinated service.* Parents should not feel that there is a break in continuity of care when they are referred to the hospital-based services. Paediatric and specialist services are still for the most part hospital-based and concerned mainly with the treatment of acute illness. *In future we see these services having closer contacts with families, schools and communities in which children*

87

grow up. They must continue to extend specialist interest to the problems of chronic illness, handicap, and problems of disturbed behaviour.

5.14 Equally if the specialist services are to play a full part in the child health services, *further efforts must be made to strengthen the practice of paediatrics within the hospital services.* Despite the fact that paediatrics, the recognition of the special needs of children, has largely developed in a hospital setting, there is still much that needs to be done to give practical effect to the principles on which it is based. Whenever admission to hospital is required it should be to a children's department which should be able to accommodate not only children with paediatric problems but those of the allied specialties too. Whatever hospital department a child attends the surroundings and facilities should be appropriate for children. There should be staff trained to meet both the personal as well as the technical needs of the child, and the need for play for younger, and teaching for older children, and for explanation and for comfort from a resident parent or visiting family, should be recognised. Above all these principles need to be applied to the care of the long-stay patient, and in particular to the handicapped.

5.15 We have argued that parents should feel that whether their child's problem is simple or complex, whether their need is for treatment or advice, guidance and support, and at whatever stage in his development it occurs, they are dealing with an integrated service. But the case for a more closely coordinated child health service can also be strongly supported on professional grounds as well. There is no place for hospital services which are separate from community services or community care which cannot move easily into a hospital setting. There is no place for developmental medicine which does not see the child also in educational terms. There is also no place for preventive or advisory services which are wholly divorced from treatment services. All trained doctors who are involved in the clinical care of children must be empowered to treat as well as to ascertain, diagnose or advise. Our argument rests on the nature of current health problems. Since so many of these have their origins in family or environmental circumstances, since so many have long term implications for a child's development, his ability to learn and benefit from education, we believe that their successful treatment and management cannot be carried out without understanding of the developmental aspects of child health and of the two major formative influences on a child's development, his family and his school. *An integrated service must include at every level both developmental and educational medicine as well as the treatment of acute illness.*

The Need to Reach All Children

5.16 We have also been concerned that services should reach every child. The majority of parents will make good use of the child health services; a minority of limited and unsettled parents, perhaps suspicious of authority or unable to make the system work, often living in the disadvantaged areas of large cities will not. We have been concerned at the evidence of the extent to which some parents fail to make contact with services and equally of the extent to which, in some areas, the services available to them are less than

88

adequate. At local level we consider that a good child health service, must as the local health authority services have tried to do in the past, accept a responsibility for taking services to these families—albeit a minority of their clients—who need help, but who have difficulty in using existing services. *This in turn means that there must be effective means of defining the child population and greater emphasis on services being territorially planned and organised.*

5.17 However, a major obstacle to a satisfactory health service which meets the needs of all children is the regional, area and district variation in facilities. There should be better distribution of manpower, and equally a more rational sharing of work among the professions. The achievement of the objectives outlined in this chapter will involve increases in professional staffing and investment in facilities and training. But we shall certainly deceive ourselves if we think we can equalise health opportunity in child-hood by simply expanding the National Health Service. The priorities begin at the centre with (i) the decision about how much money shall be allocated to the NHS and how much to housing, education, social services and other services affecting child health, (ii) how much of the resources allocated to the NHS should go to child health, (iii) within child health, how resources should be divided between treatment, prevention, care and research.

5.18 This brings us back to the social factors which have influenced our thinking throughout. Children's growth and their experience of illness and health are profoundly influenced by the social circumstances in which they live. *Economic prosperity, a sufficient family income, adequate food, satis-factory housing, a widening education and a safe environment are still the foundation of good health in childhood and of services designed to maintain it.*

5.19 *The final problem then is how to employ scarce resources to the best possible effect.* Left to themselves resources simply do not flow where health care needs are greatest. The first necessity is the provision of a sound frame-work for estimating local needs, in the light of available resources deciding priorities and planning collectively to meet them. We believe the advisory and administrative machinery created by the re-organisation of the NHS and described in Chapter 21 will prove satisfactory for this purpose.

5.20 Tomorrow's services are for tomorrow's children. Children do not easily formulate their views and have no forum where they can express 'them. Politically they are seen but not heard, and have no voice in the decisions which effect their health. We hope this will improve in future as the conditions for health and the nature of health services are increasingly part of social education. But always parents must speak for them. They are doing so through local community health councils, and in a variety of parent groups and societies. *A way must be found for children's rights to be more clearly defined and for their needs to be made regularly known to the relevant Departments of State and through them to Parliament.*

Prevention

5.21 Lastly, we think that in future much greater emphasis must be placed on prevention. Following the success of environmental control, improved mother and infant care, and immunisation against infectious diseases we are now in what has been described as the fourth preventive stage when individuals must modify their behaviour to improve their health.[1] This concept is valid and helpful, but requires interpretation in relation to children. The arrival of the fourth stage of prevention does not mean we can ignore the other three. THERE are still major hazards for children in the contemporary environment.[2] We face continuing problems with infant feeding and child nutrition and the provision of adequate advice on child-rearing to the mothers of all young children. Immunisation must be maintained against diseases increasingly unfamiliar to parents and doctors and specific preventive measures are not available for respiratory infections, the major infective cause of illness and death in childhood. If we are to prevent the dangerous heart and lung diseases of adult life through sensible eating, continuing exercise, the rejection of smoking, then the necessary habits must be accepted by children. Our main method will be education: the education of all concerned, but with a special responsibility for doctors and nurses working in the home, the school and the child health clinic.

5.22 The task is a challenging one but the personal and economic benefits are immense. And the way lies through identifying the hazards to health at every age and finding ways of identifying the groups who are at special risk. *The greatest single need in medicine in the next 25 years is to give prevention the degree of scientific and educational attention that has been given in the last 25 years to treatment.* In this context we particularly welcome the Department of Health's recent publication, "Prevention and health: everybody's business".

5.23 The achievement of some of our other objectives should in themselves help to achieve a new emphasis on prevention—in particular the development of better understanding between parents and professionals, the increasing acceptance of responsibility for comprehensive cover in primary care services and hence the identification of those at risk, and the closer involvement of specialist paediatric services with what we have in Chapter 2 referred to as "social paediatrics".

Conclusion

5.24 We can summarise our objectives quite simply: we want to see a child and family centred service; in which skilled help is readily available and accessible; which is integrated in as much as it sees the child as a whole, and as a continuously developing person. We want to see a service which ensures that this paediatric skill and knowledge are applied in the care of every child

---

[1] Building upon our Assets. Interview with Sir George Godber, 1976. *Brit. Med. Jour.* 1, 638–640.

[2] Barltrop, D, ed (1975). Paediatrics and the Environment. *Fellowship of Postgraduate Medicine,* London.

whatever his age or disability, and wherever he lives, and we want a service which is increasingly oriented to prevention.

5.25 Our remit is limited to the health services: but it follows from much of what we have already said about the needs of children that just as doctors and nurses and therapists must work as a team within the health services, so the health service must work in partnership with education and social services. Many of the children with the most complex problems, and the most severe handicaps will require help from all three services. The planning and development of an integrated health service must therefore be done in such a way as to facilitate at every level the closest possible working relations with these other services.

5.26 Despite the difficulties of moving towards new patterns of service we believe it is possible to achieve our objectives. In Chapter 7 we consider the ways in which the organisational framework might be changed to this end.

CHAPTER 6

WHAT OTHER COUNTRIES ARE DOING

6.1 In previous chapters we have outlined changes that have taken place in Britain, especially since the second world war, and have pointed to the effects they have had on the growth and health of children. Similar changes have occurred in all other industrial countries, and the evolution of their health and welfare services has, in most respects, followed similar lines. There are however differences between countries which arise not only out of different rates of development, and differences in the history of how their health services have developed, but also from different cultural values and professional attitudes. Any comment on services in other countries must take these into account. It is essential also to realise that similar terms may be used with different meanings so that national statistics for example may not be comparable unless adjustments are made.

6.2 All industrial countries have achieved high standards of child health: standards scarcely even envisaged before the second world war. The rise in standards has come about primarily because of an increase in prosperity, accompanied by better education, and through the introduction of well developed systems of social security, available to the whole population. However, better health services have also contributed increasingly to this improvement and some countries have been conspicuously successful in reducing child mortality and morbidity.

Mortality and Morbidity

6.3 As implied in Chapter 2, and shown in the Statistical Appendix, Table C4, mortality at birth and in the first year of life has declined in most, if not all, European countries since 1965, but in some countries the decline has been faster than in others. The reason is not that countries showing the smallest rate of decline are necessarily those in which mortality rates are already so low that further improvement is scarcely possible. On the contrary as Pharoah[1] has pointed out, Sweden continues to lead the international league yet her infant mortality still shows a continuing decline. In England and Wales however, the decline has been less rapid than in most other comparable countries at least until 1974/75 when there has been some improvement, and our rank position has worsened in relation to the post-neonatal mortality rates and the infant mortality rate as a whole. The trend in the neonatal mortality rate in England and Wales is similar to that of infant mortality as a whole except that neonatal death rates have continued to decrease slowly. The post-neonatal mortality rate has however 'failed to show any significant improvement over the past 15 years in contrast to that in many other countries'. Table C2 shows that within the post-neonatal period it is the deaths in the period 4 weeks to 6 months which have been largely responsible for the relative lack of improvement in our infant mortality rate.

---

[1] Pharoah, P O D (1976). International comparisons of perinatal and infant mortality rates. *Proc. Roy. Soc. Med.*, 69, 335.

6.4 There is a lack of reliably comparable data on morbidity of children in European countries and statistics at the level of primary care are available only from sporadic morbidity surveys of the type of the "General Household Survey" and the "National Study in Morbidity Statistics from General Practice" in our country. Attempts are being made to improve comparability of hospital data by WHO European Regional Office (Copenhagen) and to gather national data on congenital malformations and biochemical defects among live-born children in countries of the Council of Europe Partial Agreement. Also the EEC of which Britain is a member are contemplating a project to develop comparable methods of recording in small areas of each EEC country in order to record and to follow-up studies of malformations, various biochemical abnormalities and twins. Finally WHO Geneva are conducting an International Perinatal Mortality Study with Sweden, Hungary and England and Wales as the European Countries.

6.5 There are no comparable data about the growth of children and what exists about birthweights shows that England and Wales appear to have more smaller babies and more larger babies than Scandinavian countries for which data are available.

6.6 Despite the lack of unambiguous data which would permit critical evaluation of our own services and better international comparisons, it is clear that we can learn from what other countries are doing; and by studying the varieties of practice in Europe and elsewhere we can gather clues as to how to improve our own services.

The Organisation of Services

6.7 All well-developed health services make a distinction between primary health care services and specialist and hospital services. In Britain the primary health care physician is the general practitioner who treats patients of all ages registered with him for services. Some general practitioners undertake developmental surveillance of children and run their own "well-baby" or child health clinics, but for the most part these "preventive" services have in the past been organised by local authority health departments. They are today, since NHS reorganisation, organised by area health authorities.

6.8 The area health authority also organises and maintains the school health services. Like the child health clinics these remain a largely separate branch of the child health service having only tenuous links either with primary medical care (general practice) or the supporting, mainly hospital-based, specialist services. How best to integrate primary and supporting services poses problems for the organisation of health services everywhere.

6.9 On the continent of Europe practice varies from country to country. In general the main difference from this country in the medical services is the existence, in varying numbers, of paediatric practitioners providing paediatric primary care alongside general practitioners and community doctors. The general trend would seem to be a loss of ground by general practitioners to paediatric practitioners. Sweden, Finland and West Germany are moving towards a separate comprehensive paediatric service. In France group general practice is increasing, but there are more than 1,300 paediatricians who also provide sickness care and play a major part in the preventive services. The pattern in Holland is more varied but it resembles this country in the persistence of general practice and in being one in which paediatricians are consultants and teachers working essentially in hospital. In the Soviet Union there is a separate child health service, organised on a district basis, domiciliary practice being organised in microdistricts each serving a population of about 900 children. The microdistrict units are staffed by a paediatrician, a medical sister or *feldscher* and a nurse. This primary health care team refers patients where necessary to the polyclinic at district level; children with a particular disease or group of diseases are treated at dispensaries (outpatient units) or hospitals. Supporting care is highly specialised and is concentrated in large units.

School Health Services

6.10 All countries stress the importance of the school health service, but the maintenance of traditional patterns and the lack of experiment suggest uncertainty about its contemporary rôle. We are uncertain as to how far the school health services in different countries extend into "educational medicine"—the growing area of knowledge concerned not only with individual children but with schools as institutions, rooted in local communities, and linked with locally based primary care services, with psychology and social work services, and above all with parents and neighbourhoods. Holland maintains a separate whole time "local authority" school health service. Denmark includes school health in its comprehensive general practitioner primary care. In Sweden it is provided in the rural areas by the "district medical officer" and in cities by paediatricians or general practitioners. In 1972 Finland expanded her school health service to cover all schools but left it as a separate provision by local authorities. The Soviet Union health services for children in schools, kindergartens and nurseries are separate from, and additional to those available at polyclinics and employ their own paediatric staff.

Hospital Services

6.11 The trend, on the continent as in this country, is towards larger obstetric and paediatric units. Only in well-staffed, well-equipped, concentrated units can a satisfactory 24-hour obstetric and paediatric service be maintained. The necessity for this has resulted in a closing of many smaller, isolated maternity and paediatric units all over Europe.

6.12 Almost all European countries with the exception of Holland favour birth in hospital. In Finland, for example, a country larger than the British Isles but with a population of only 4.3 millions, 99.8% of births took place in hospital in 1971 compared with 89.0% in England and Wales: this despite the fact that most of the country is snowbound for five or six months or more, and that the distance from home to hospital may be over 100 miles or even 200 miles in northern Lapland—where in winter it is dark 24 hours a day, temperatures are low, the snow deep and snowstorms frequent. Like other, more heavily populated countries Finland too is closing its small maternity units in order to concentrate all deliveries in large central units capable of dealing with any medical emergency.[3]

6.13 An outstanding exception to the practice of aiming for all children to be born in hospital is Holland. A country with one of the lowest perinatal death rates in the world, Holland has shown that home confinements can be safe, given a highly trained domiciliary midwifery service and quick and efficient transport to a specialist hospital unit should an emergency occur. Even in Holland however the proportion of hospital births is increasing, though at almost one half it still remains low compared with that in other European countries. In 1963, 22% of births took place in hospital; in 1972 47%.[4]

6.14 It is clear from a study of the diverse patterns of organisation of the health services in European countries that no single pattern can be said to offer outstanding advantages over others. *A central impression, however, is that the countries which have made the greatest advances in reducing mortality in children and providing services which reach the whole population are those in which the health of children stands higher in the scale of social priorities than in our own.* Thus the French government admitted that they found the pressure for improved services for mothers and children from family organisations, voluntary societies and paediatricians, irresistible.[5] Similar comments are to be found in official reports from other countries: in this respect the rest of the world is, not surprisingly, no different from us, though some countries have got closer to their objectives than we have.

6.15. The differing patterns of delivery of health care are of great interest in themselves, and an awareness of what other countries are doing informed our discussions about our own problems. It is however neither necessary nor appropriate to attempt an overview here. Instead we comment briefly on a few major topics of special relevance to our own task.

Primary Care

6.16 As we have mentioned, there are marked differences between countries in the extent of specialisation in primary *medical* care. In the Soviet Union for example all paediatrics is a separate specialty; in Sweden, Finland and West Germany paediatric practitioners are becoming more popular; France in a sense has two competing systems; the Dutch system resembles our own. We thought that Denmark's approach merited separate description.[6] We understand that since 1946 general practitioners have been responsible for both health and sickness care; their preventive responsibilities include a "contract" to provide ten developmental examinations between birth and six

---

[3] Wynn, A, and Wynn, M (1974). A study of the services for pregnant women and young children in Finland with some comparisons with Britain. Council for Children's Welfare, London.

[4] Central Bureau of Statistics. Ministry of Public Health and Environmental Hygiene, The Netherlands.

[5] Wynn, A. *Personal Communication.*

[6] Danish Information Handbooks: *Special Education in Denmark* (1970).

years. They make the main contribution to the school health service and must accept special instruction before appointment. Specialist advice is readily available especially for children needing special education. We cannot comment on the quality of preventive and educational care the general practitioners provide, nor have we knowledge of the content of their preparatory training. However Denmark's health indices are among the best in the world, and the persistence of the system for thirty years suggests that, though doubtless it could be improved, it has worked and is acceptable.

6.17 Whether, or to what extent, England and Wales would gain from the introduction of a primary medical care service for children in which the physicians were full-time or nearly full-time paediatric practitioners was a matter we debated at length. Our conclusions and the grounds on which they are based are set out in the Chapter that follows. Similar issues were raised regarding the future of the Child Health and School Health Services. Can these function effectively except as part of primary care? If not, how are these essential preventive, assessment and advisory services best to be linked with a primary care service which is at present largely taken up with consultations about, and treatment of, illness?

6.18 We discuss these issues in Chapters 17 and 19 but some comment is in order here. We are convinced, both by what we have learned about services in Europe and from our knowledge of needs in this country, that means must be found to ensure that health surveillance and prompt treatment are available to all children. For children of school age casefinding through the schools presents no problems in principle, though the complexity of educational failure often calls for a multi-professional specialist team drawn from education, psychology, paediatrics and social work which no country, as far as we could discover, is as yet satisfied that it is able to provide for all its children. For infants and young "preschool" children there is no social institution, comparable with the school, which they are obliged to attend and in which their health needs can be appraised by adults other than their own parents. But most other European countries place much greater emphasis than we do on the regular supervision of all children throughout childhood, especially in the preschool years. The number and frequency of "examinations" vary; France[7] has 9 in the first year, 3 in the second and then twice a year until the age of six; Finland monthly for the first year, and then annually until 7; Sweden[8] regularly, and with almost total coverage, in the first two years, and a comprehensive examination at 4, with the parents present and involving doctor, psychologist, nurse and dentist. Doctors take part in health surveillance in all these countries but most of the work is done by community nursing services. We are uncertain what proportion of the health budget for children is used in this way, and to what extent critical evaluation is taking place. There is certainly a strong belief in its value; in France to the point where three substantial lump sums are given on proof of attendance for specified examinations when the child is 8 days, 9 months and 2 years

---

[7] Wynn, A, and Wynn, M (1974). *The Right of Every Child to Health Care.* Council for Children's Welfare, London.

[8] Sjölin, Stig, and Vahlquist, Bo (1974). *Acta Paediat.,* 63, 485.

old. In the Soviet Union "the national resources devoted to the medical care of children are vast by any standards and the domiciliary and preventive services must be the most comprehensive in the world".(⁹)

Health Visitors and Home Visiting

6.19 How can very high rates of attendance at routine medical examinations be achieved? The answer is in large part the availability and accessibility of a service of high quality. This is maintained to a greater extent than in this country, by the use, especially during the period of early childhood, of adequate numbers of well-trained children's nurses based on local clinics or health centres, providing nursing care and health education, and with home visiting a priority. In France an earlier decision to put family surveillance in the hands of social workers has been reversed in favour of paediatric nurses; and Finland considers that the most important factor in the remarkable improvement in the health of children that has taken place there in the last decade has been the increase in the number and quality of community nurses. Where numbers are adequate, as in Finland, we understand that the children's community nurses (our health visitors) are appointed on a standard population basis and therefore probably serve a well-defined catchment area. They undertake frequent home visiting, especially where the parent fails to bring a child to the clinic. Home visiting by children's community nurses at other times is also encouraged; it is considered to have great educational value quite apart from its use for routine medical assessment. In France, as in Britain, there is less home visiting because of the shortage of staff. To ensure universal surveillance of the health of young children, the French introduced in March 1975 the financial incentives to which we have already referred and it is as yet too early to assess their effectiveness. They have also passed a permissive legal power to withhold payment of family allowances, the single wage allowance and the "mother at home" allowance for failure to bring the child to 3 of the 14 medical examinations in the first 2 years. It should be noted, however, that the permissive power has never been used. In most other countries there are no sanctions attached to failure to attend antenatal care or to bring children for examination. Rather, where high attendance rates are achieved success is attributable to the high quality of service provided, the use of children's community nurses to persuade defaulters to come, and the high level of parental education in child care which prompts them to make full use of services they believe will help their children. How in this country we can reach comparable levels of attendance is a matter we discuss in Chapter 9.

6.20 Despite the importance given to trained children's nurses in every other aspect of child health, the rôle of the specially trained school nurse appears to have received little attention in most countries including our own.

Handicapped Children

6.21 The organisation of services for handicapped children and their families differs from country to country, but in the development of services

(⁹) Bamford, F N, and Mitchell, R G (1976). Child Health and Paediatrics in the USSR. *Dev. Med. and Child Neur.,* 18, 3.

on the continent, as in Britain, increasing attention is being paid to problems of early diagnosis and treatment (including helping parents to treat and manage their children). France, a country which has for two hundred years been a leader in work on behalf of the handicapped, is making most strenuous efforts to prevent handicaps from occurring, and to identify and treat those that do, from the earliest age. Cost benefit analysis has convinced the French Government that expenditure on the prevention of handicap not only reduces suffering but leads to substantial financial saving. France is therefore directing an increasing proportion of its health expenditure into "preventive obstetrics and paediatrics". The emphasis in management is on the trained specialist both in paediatrics and nursing.[5] Excellent facilities for handicapped children have also developed in Holland and Sweden and in the USSR. Our own proposals are set out in Chapter 14 of this Report.

Records
6.22 We noted general support for standardised record cards maintained from birth to adolescence or early adult life. In some countries use of computers allows events recorded in different parts of the health care system to be more easily linked than is possible in Britain. Of equal interest is the personal record card maintained at district level as in the USSR and Finland, or kept by the mother as in France. The French *carnet de santé*, given to the mother when the child's birth is registered with the local authority, is intended to provide an ongoing record of the child's circumstances and health, including the results of medical examinations from infancy through early childhood and the school years. It becomes the property of the child when he reaches the age of 21.

Evaluation of Services

6.23 In all countries there is a growing awareness that records should be in part designed and used for appraisal of the quality of the services recorded. We are not sure how far the concept of clinical and administrative review (medical audit) which is slowly spreading in general practice in this country is developing elsewhere in Europe—and valuable though it is, internal assessment alone is unlikely to satisfy completely either public concern or professional standards. In Holland both the State Sickness Fund and the Private Insurance Schemes employ doctors to see that standards are satisfactory: we are unable to judge the acceptability and effectiveness of this. We did however sense that there is, throughout Europe, widespread discussion about the "accountability" of professional workers to their clients and about how best to maintain and monitor the quality of the services provided.

Conclusion

6.24 The child health services in different countries all present individual strengths and weaknesses. Our own NHS is no exception. We are not blind to its deficiencies, but we believe that it offers an adequate framework for the delivery of services for families and children even though at times it lacks the data required to analyse needs. Within the structure of the reorganised NHS we should be able to avoid professional division and the duplication of services and achieve a unity of preventive and curative medicine which includes partnership with parents and with the sister professions of education and social work.

6.25 We have taken into account what some other countries are doing; we hope they will find that our remedies are relevant to some of their needs.

CHAPTER 7

AN INTEGRATED CHILD HEALTH SERVICE

7.1 In Chapters 1 and 2 we described the changing picture of children's health and the nature of the families and communities in which they live. In Chapters 3 and 4 we saw how the present services had arisen and we considered their strengths and weaknesses. In the light of that analysis we attempted, in Chapter 5 to set out the broad principles on which services should be based if they are to meet the needs of children and their families adequately in future. Translating these principles into action will depend—as always—on the knowledge, skills and attitudes of those who actually provide the services, their willingness to adopt new approaches and to see their relationship with children and their parents in a new perspective. At the same time it is the responsibility of those concerned with the overall planning and development of services to ensure that the basic structural organisation within which doctors, nurses and other therapists have to work is one which fosters rather than frustrates the best kind of professional practice. In seeking therefore to achieve the objectives we have set, namely the provision of an integrated child and family-centred health service for all children, we have asked ourselves firstly whether there is a need to change the existing pattern of service.

Retaining the Present Pattern

7.2 Reorganisation is generally a painful process: it is unsettling for the staff concerned and inevitably involves a considerable amount of administrative work and expense. The health services and particularly those parts of them that were, prior to 1974, provided by local authorities have already suffered the stress of the simultaneous reorganisation of the health service and local government. We would therefore not wish to propose further reorganisation unless we were convinced that it was impossible to achieve our objectives without it and equally if we did not think that to expect the medical staff of the former local authorities to maintain and improve their services while remaining in professional isolation and administrative uncertainty would not prove equally stressful in the long term.

7.3 The present pattern consists of three interrelating but still functionally separate components. Clearly there are a number of steps that could be taken, short of reorganisation, to improve their individual effectiveness and the degree of coordination between them. It would be possible to introduce mandatory training for community clinical doctors and school nurses, to require that vocational training for general practitioners, and training for health visitors and district nurses should include a larger component of paediatrics, and to restore the territorial responsibilities of health visitors. Individual general practitioners could develop a special interest in paediatrics (as indeed a number have), and spend a large proportion of their time in dealing with children. Given goodwill and mutual respect, both of which are essential whatever the pattern, liaison between general practitioners and clinical medical officers might be such that management of child patients

100

could be shared according to the circumstances. Similarly changes in the hospital service could lead to easier communication and integration with the services outside hospital. For example, consultant paediatricians could more frequently undertake out-patient sessions in selected health centres. Links between the preventive and specialist services could easily be strengthened through a more extensive participation (already developing) of community clinical doctors in hospital assessment centres for handicapped children. If in addition, there were a satisfactory career service structure in preventive paediatrics, associated with special training, this might lead to the recruitment of increasing numbers of able and interested staff to this part of the service.

7.4 All of these could be valuable in themselves and would lead to improvements in the standard of service. We examine this situation more fully in Chapter 19. We doubt however whether, without considerable changes in the attitudes of professional staff, it would be possible to achieve within such a service the degree of functional integration which the changing needs of children and parents indicate are essential. Knowing is not doing. While doctors working in one part of the threefold service may be trained to understand and respect the contribution of the others, we do not believe that continuing fragmentation can be a satisfactory substitute in terms of either patient or professional satisfaction, for a service in which doctors and nurses practise paediatrics in its therapeutic, developmental and educational aspects as a single activity. Moreover, in practice, there would be a real danger that measures to strengthen each part of the service, while retaining the present fragmented structure could lead to the divisions becoming sharper rather than blunted, the very reverse of what we desire. We certainly understand those who in present circumstances advocate a continued policy of "liaison and cooperation"; however the evidence from the report "Working Together"(¹) has suggested that while genuine attempts have been made to achieve coordination between the three existing branches of the service, the efforts required were out of all proportion to the results achieved and far from uniform in their results. Reluctant as we are therefore to propose further reorganisation, especially one affecting those who more than any others have suffered from past administrative upheavals, we are in no doubt that to give effect to the principles we believe to be fundamental will require a more radical approach. We describe this separately in relation to medical and nursing services for the sake of clarity. We strongly support in practice the concept of medical and nursing staff working as a health care team.

The Reorganisation of Primary Medical Care

7.5 We start from the premise that first-contact care and hospital care are the two essential organisational components of an integrated child health service. Furthermore we inherit a situation in which the hospital component is organised directly by AHAs and includes the provision of services by doctors who are specifically trained and work exclusively with children.

(¹) *Working Together:* A study of coordination and cooperation between general practitioner, public health and hospital services (1968). King Edward's Hospital Fund, London.

We would not want to see any change in this basic pattern of hospital care though we do see a need for modifications in detailed arrangements that would increase the range and degree of consultant paediatric participation in services in the community (see paragraph 7.33).

7.6 It is in the organisation of first-contact services that significant changes are necessary, in order to achieve a higher calibre of comprehensive primary child health care—a term we use to describe an overall responsibility for the therapeutic and preventive (including developmental and educational) health care of individual children by the same medical personnel.

7.7 There are two issues here, that overlap:

First, whether the existing preventive child health services, organised directly by the AHAs and staffed by clinical medical officers, should assume responsibility for providing therapeutic services to children or whether the existing primary health care services, provided by general practitioners under contract, should incorporate all preventive services for children, including those in school;

Second, whether the comprehensive primary child health services, however they may be organised, should be provided by doctors specifically trained and exclusively working with children as in the supporting hospital services.

A Single Paediatric Service
7.8 In practical terms, the first issue resolved itself into the question of how practicable and desirable it might be for AHAs to organise both primary and supporting health care for children as a single paediatric service. Essentially this would be a service staffed throughout by doctors specifically trained for primary or supporting paediatric practice and devoting their time exclusively to this. It could provide first-contact and consultant care in clinics, health centres and schools, and certain specialised services in district general hospitals and university hospitals or regional children's centres.

7.9 This approach has some merits. As we have seen in the preceding chapter, such a system is already operating in other countries notably the USSR and Sweden appears to be moving deliberately towards it. A single paediatric service would make it easier to plan for comprehensive primary care to be arranged according to the neighbourhood in which children live and the schools they attend; and it would facilitate links with the local social and educational services. It would also make it easier to provide links between the hospital and community based services.

7.10 We have rejected this pattern of services for the following reasons. There would still be considerable duplication of personnel and facilities already provided by general practice; this would be wasteful and expensive. Major problems would in any case be likely to arise in the early stages of setting up such a service and running down the existing ones, particularly because of the number of doctors at present manning the preventive services and the proportion engaged in part-time work. There is some suggestion from East European countries that a higher doctor/patient ratio would be required in a single paediatric service than in general practice. Nor is there any evidence that such a service would be any more efficient, acceptable or available than existing services could be made by modification. It is also open to objection on the grounds of its total age-specialisation.

Age Specialisation in Primary Care
7.11 This is the second issue. We considered whether our objectives could be achieved by an age division of care at both the primary and supporting levels of care, so that the paediatric practitioner and the paediatric consultant alike gave their whole attention to children in the home, the consulting room and the hospital. Theoretical arguments have been advanced before in support of this approach to primary care; namely that competence in the prevention, recognition and treatment of disease cannot be maintained on too wide a front and that it is to the benefit of both patient and doctor that practitioners should specialise in the medical care of a limited age range. Applied to children this has obvious attraction in terms of the enhanced knowledge and skill which can be brought to bear in a setting of personal continuing care in or near the child's own home, and the reduction in numbers of primary care doctors working with children would help to achieve effective and continuing contact with other professionals and agencies responsible for children in the community and with hospital-based specialists.

7.12 We are, however, not convinced that the knowledge and time that are required if children are to receive the quality of primary medical care that we perceive to be necessary, can best be provided by doctors who devote the whole of their time to paediatrics. In proposing a re-organisation of the child health service our objective is to attempt to strike the right balance between the need on the one hand for a higher degree of knowledge and expertise in child health to be available at the level of primary care and on the other to ensure that those who have that expertise remain equipped to apply it broadly in a family setting, since it is one of our basic principles that paediatrics requires of its practitioners an understanding of the family as it affects the child's health and development. We do not consider it necessary for a practitioner always to be responsible for the primary health care of all of the parents of his child patients, but we do believe that he should have been adequately trained in the general medical care of adults. We believe too that a children's doctor can usefully maintain his skills as a family practitioner by continuing to treat some adult patients—who would generally be the parents of some of his child patients—and thus continue to bring an up-to-date knowledge of adult medicine and of parental attitudes and of the strains and stresses which parenthood brings, to his child health care.

7.13 *In our view therefore total paediatric specialisation in primary care for children fails to reconcile two essential and complementary needs: for greater paediatric skills and experience and for the care of sufficient parents*

103

to remain involved in the family context of child care. It is we note a system of care which has already been rejected by all the previous committees which have examined the issues in the U.K.([2,3,4,5]) and despite considerable critical attention([6]) has provoked little enthusiasm. We know of only two attempts to apply it and so far as we are aware the experiments have foundered. This would certainly suggest that there would be serious difficulties in attempting to introduce total paediatric specialisation within the existing primary care services. We have not overlooked in our discussion the fact that in the United States where this system has operated for many years there has been in recent years an increasing demand by patients for primary care from a general practitioner who will accept responsibility for all members of the family.

Comprehensive Primary Care based on General Practice

7.14 We are convinced that the correct approach to an improvement in the child health services in the UK would be one based upon the existing pattern of services but suitably modified to achieve the objectives which we have defined in Chapter 5. The changes which we see as necessary lie principally in three areas: —

The rôles of some staff in the service

The training required to fulfil these new rôles

The administration required to support the staff.

It would be foolish to deny that there are strong arguments in practice as well as in principle for basing the primary level of child health care in general practice, and that these have inevitably weighed heavily with us. There is little to be said in life for proposals which take insufficient account of both the constraints and the opportunities of the existing situation. An increasing number of general practitioners in the UK have in recent years recognised the opportunities for providing total health care for children, although many still lack the training, organisation and time to do so. Now would be the time to extend such arrangements and give them an organisational structure. Furthermore, the changes that we think are necessary could be more effectively achieved by building upon the developments that have been taking place in the field of primary care in recent years: a trend towards group practice, the emergence of the primary health care team, and the concept of general practitioners having a special interest in a particular facet of health care.

([2]) Consultative Council on Medical and Allied Services: Interim Report on the Future Provision of Medical and Allied Services (Chairman: Lord Dawson of Penn), (1920). HMSO, London.

([3]) Central Health Services Council, Standing Medical Advisory Committee: Report of the Sub-Committee on the Fieldwork of the Family Doctor (Chairman: Annis Gillie), (1963). HMSO, London.

([4]) Central Health Services Council, Standing Medical Advisory Committee: Report of the Sub-Committee on the Organisation of Group Practice (Chairman: Robert Harvard Davis), (1971). HMSO, London.

([5]) Report from General Practice, No 16: Present State and Future Needs of General Practice. *J. Roy. Coll. Gen. Pract.*, 25, 81–91.

([6]) McKeown, T (1965). Medicine in Modern Society. Allen and Unwin, London.

7.15 The care of children is numerically such an important part of the work of most general practitioners that *training in paediatrics should be a mandatory part of the vocational training of all general practitioners*. This training should encompass not only the management of acute illness but also the preventive aspects of child care and in particular the assessment of the normal development of children and the effect of emotional disturbance on the health of children. This policy is supported by the Royal College of General Practitioners and the British Paediatric Association and implementation can be started immediately. However, comprehensive primary care for children of the standard and range that we envisage, through pre-school years into adolescence will involve both special training and continuing experience through work not only within the group practice but also in a variety of settings outside the practice, for example in the schools, in relation to the social services and in hospitals. We have therefore, sought to make proposals which will both help to promote a higher quality of comprehensive child health care within a group practice and also provide for the necessary paediatric services outside the practice.

The General Practitioner Paediatrician

7.16 We therefore propose that the primary health care team would continue to be the service unit providing 24 hour first contact and continuing therapeutic and preventive health care for children, whether this be sought or advised, and calling where necessary upon the supporting service of consultant paediatricians and allied specialists in and from hospital and of other professionals, especially social workers. *We recommend that the concept of a general practitioner with a special interest become more formalised both in terms of responsibility and training.* We define our interpretation of this special interest in detail later in this chapter and believe that it would assist understanding of his rôle to call such a practitioner a *general practitioner paediatrician, a GPP*. Furthermore, *we propose that he should have working with him a Child Health Visitor, a CHV*, whose rôle we consider in greater detail below. Here it is necessary only to emphasise that she will have responsibility for health visiting and nursing services to all the child patients within a practice for whom the GPP has responsibility and also for providing health visiting services to their parents. She will thus be able to provide the GPP with the continuing and close understanding of the family circumstances of all his child patients, including those whose parents are not registered with him, which he needs to provide a family based service for children. We envisage that each group practice would have at least one GPP and child health visitor and we estimate in Chapter 17 that this might amount to 40% of the total number of general practitioners.

7.17 We have argued that our general practitioner paediatrician is a development of the concept of special interest within group practice. Hitherto it has been left to individual doctors and their partners to decide the extent of the special interest and the way in which it is expressed. Flexibility which fosters a raising and not a lowering of standards, and which encourages adaptation to local circumstances, is obviously valuable. We

105

believe, however, that if the GPP is to have the effect which we intend, both in enhancing the overall standard of primary health care for all children and in providing, at primary care level, the basis of an integrated child health service, then the nature of his special interest in paediatrics must be clearly defined and understood. The solution we are proposing is not a new one. The idea that general practitioners should provide comprehensive care for children has been repeatedly advocated for a quarter of a century. Why has it not been implemented? We believe the explanation lies in a failure to define the professional responsibilities involved, to provide the necessary training and to offer proper remuneration for the additional services required. We have been concerned that our proposals should not suffer the same fate.

7.18 A doctor practising as a GPP would in the first instance be a GP and in that capacity he would provide all necessary medical services to the children and adult patients of the practice for whom he has responsibility.

7.19 To be eligible to practise as a GPP a doctor must have successfully completed an appropriate training; this should lead to a formal recognition which we shall refer to as accreditation and which we consider in further detail in Chapter 20. Few doctors in general practice at present have had training in paediatrics and educational medicine at the required level and it involves greater experience in child care than is usually included in current vocational training programmes for general practitioners.

7.20 In his capacity as GPP he would normally have the following responsibilities:—

i. for ensuring the provision of developmental surveillance and preventive services to the children registered with the practice. Normally he would provide such services himself but there may be certain instances where this is not practicable. (The detailed arrangements are considered in Chapter 17).

ii. for a minimum commitment to the Area Health Authority to enable that authority to meet the requirements of the LEA and LASSD for medical services in respect of children. Although circumstances will vary between practices our estimate of needs of LEAs and LASSDs (see Chapter 17) suggest that this sessional commitment would in most cases be largely employed on work within the school health service. We would therefore expect that, as a general rule, a GPP would be involved both in developmental and educational medicine.

iii. for taking the lead in ensuring continuing education and maintenance of standards in child health care within the practice as a whole. His colleagues should then be able to look to him for advice on problems they encounter in the therapeutic care of their children and we would envisage close and continuing consultation between him and his partners on the health needs of children within the practice.

iv. for acting as a link between the primary care services for children and the child health services in hospitals. In addition to the usual professional contacts the GPP would thus have to be in effective communication with the consultant community paediatrician (see paragraph 7.33 below), the specialist in community medicine (child health) and those involved in the handicap team (see paragraph 7.35 below).

7.21 The precise nature of the GPP's work with the education and social services is described respectively in Chapter 10, Health for Education, and Chapter 17, the Organisation and Staffing of the Primary Care Services. Broadly, it is envisaged that in future the GPP would act as school doctor for one or two primary schools or one secondary school in the district in which his practice is situated. In performing this work the GPP will be dealing not only with his own patients but also with the patients of other general practitioners in the area; his rôle would be analogous to the rôle of the part-time industrial medical officer which is already performed by many general practitioners. For the social services departments he would primarily be concerned with the provision of advice to individual local area offices or with advice on problems affecting social services institutions for children. Professional services to individual children "in care" of social service departments would be provided, where such children were registered with him, under 7.18 and 7.20 (i) above.

7.22 We have considered whether, as a further concrete expression of "special interest", and as a means of ensuring the experience necessary to maintain standards, we should specify the amount of time a GPP should devote to child health, or, alternatively a minimum number of children who should be registered with him, thereby entailing a partial redistribution of patients in a practice so that the GPP had more of the children and his partners more of the adults. Although it is of the greatest importance that the GPP's continuing experience should be sufficient to sustain special knowledge and skills in child health, we do not believe that it is desirable or practical to make rigid requirements concerning workload. Nevertheless the evidence from practices where one or, in large practices, more partners take a special interest in child health, is that they spend a substantial part of their time with children. Moreover some of these practices have found it inevitable or desirable that their "prototype GPP" should provide both curative and preventive care for a larger share of the children (whether or not they are formally registered with him). We would expect that carrying out the responsibilities which we have set out in paragraph 7.20 (i)-(iv) would involve a GPP in spending the major part—probably of the order of 70%—of his time working with children.

7.23 We are well aware that the new pattern of service we are proposing will require a change of approach and a widening of responsibilities for general practice. We are confident, however, that these are changes which many will welcome as an opportunity to provide a better, and professionally more satisfying service for children, and that if our proposals are implemented they will ensure an overall improvement in the standard of primary child health care in the home, the practice and the schools and for local authority social services departments. We have been particularly encouraged

107

in this view by the speed with which group practice is growing, health centres have been built and vocational training including a paediatric component is developing. We have been equally impressed by the evidence we have of the willingness of members of general practice[5,11,12] to make self-criticism the for reform.

7.24 In Chapter 17 we discuss in greater detail the administrative arrangements which we consider would be necessary to give effect to our proposals, including the way in which the special responsibilities of the GPP would be translated into a contractual commitment.

7.25 We have already referred to the importance of the child health visitor working in partnership with the GPP; all those providing primary health care for children should see themselves as part of a wider comprehensive pattern of services for children, working in close cooperation with social workers, psychologists, teachers and therapists. The training of the GPP and the child health visitor should assist them both to appreciate the contribution which each can make to the other, and to undertand the complementary contribution which other professional groups make to the care and wellbeing of children. Such teamwork will be of particular importance in relation to handicapped children, and to children whose health is affected by social disadvantage.

Primary Nursing Care

7.26 The arguments for comprehensive primary health care, covering both preventive and therapeutic needs, apply no less to nursing than to medicine. The distinction between prevention and treatment in the present organisation of nursing services influences the different training required by health visitors and home nurses and their conditions of work. The main justification for this distinction has been that these different forms of nursing care cannot be combined without an unacceptable sacrifice of preventive work. However in clinical practice the distinction has never been rigidly applied. In other words, no self-respecting health visitor has ever withheld advice and practical demonstration to a mother in the nursing of her sick child, any more than a home nurse has refrained from giving advice and assistance in the prevention of further illness in her patient. It is wasteful, and confusing to the parents, to have different types of nurses visiting the family for purposes only ostensibly different. It also under-estimates the value to the family of having one familiar figure to whom they can turn for advice or help in health promotion and in the event of illness.

The Child Health Visitor

7.27 As with the primary medical care of children so we were again forced to consider the extent to which specialised knowledge, skill and concentration of experience—particularly if it were to extend to both preventive and curative nursing care of children, could be reconciled with the

---

[11] Irvine, D (1975). 1984—The Quiet Revolution. *J. Roy. Coll. Gen. Prac.*, 25, 399–407.

[12] Scott, N C H, and Davis, R H (1975). Clinical and Administrative Review in General Practice. *J. Roy. Coll. Gen. Pract.*, 25, 888–896.

responsibilities for patients of all ages which both HVs and HNs have at present. In primary medical care the solution to this dilemma emerged through the concept of 'special interest'. Within primary nursing care there is more scope for a measure of specialisation according to age and family structure. *We propose therefore that within community nursing there should be a distinct group of nurses with combined preventive and curative nursing responsibility for children and preventive responsibility in respect of their parents.* This way, the HV would retain her cardinal responsibility for child health care in the context of the family and ensure that a child's family circumstances are fully known to the GPP. The fulfilment of these functions does not depend upon the HV providing preventive health care to either elderly persons or adults who are not bringing up children. We have suggested that these nurses might reasonably be called *child health visitors,* because although this does not express explicitly the addition of curative responsibilities, it does emphasise the continuity with the present health visitor's tradition of special responsibility for children and parents, and her acceptability and accessibility to families.*

The School Nurse and Child Health Nurse

7.28 The scale of work entailed in comprehensive primary nursing care is such that it would be more than one CHV could do to provide this for as many children as one GPP could reasonably provide comprehensive primary medical care. Moreover, not all the tasks which such a service would include would require the specialist skills and training of the CHV. *For this reason we propose that the nursing duties in schools should be carried out by a specially trained school nurse* who would naturally turn for guidance to the CHV working with the GPP who was the doctor for the school.

7.29 *With her work in surgeries and health centres and in home nursing the CHV would be assisted by a child health nurse.* Her rôle and training are described in Chapters 17 and 20 respectively.

Territorial Responsibilities

7.30 We envisage that each GPP would have working with him a CHV. This system of "attachment" will not, however, in the short term make a significant contribution to ensuring that health care reaches all children. This could be overcome if primary care teams restricted their patients to those living within a geographically designated catchment zone. There is an obstacle here in general practice that for the moment we accept, though not without hope that as comprehensive primary care is increasingly provided in health centres and in relation to schools as well as homes catchment zones will tend to be determined by the parents. In the meantime, we are confident that a partial restoration to the CHV of the HV's traditional territorial responsibilities, together with improved administrative procedures for monitoring changes of address, can go a long way towards ensuring that all children are included in primary health care schemes. *We propose that the nursing officer who coordinates the activities of a number of CHVs*

* We recognise that this has considerable implications for the organisation and staffing of nursing services to patients who fall outside our remit, and we refer to this point again in Chapter 17.

should ensure that as best befits local circumstances the attachment for each CHV to a general practice obliges her to have a clear responsibility for a geographically defined patch, within which she will see that all children are known and registered either with her "own" practice or with a neighbouring one.

Supporting Medical Care

7.31 Our use of the term *Supporting Care* needs explanation. Reorganisation of the health service has brought a new terminology and new terms are arising in medicine and nursing partly by common usage and partly from Committee proposals. Primary health care was introduced by general practice to describe the widening services provided by group and health centre practice and health visitor and other professional attachments. There is no comparable term which covers the consultant, specialist and hospital service. Secondary, or even secondary and tertiary, care would seem the natural answer. Our concern for a single integrated service, rather than a hierarchy of care, suggested *Supporting Care* as the best expression of the relationship between its two elements that our proposals imply. We have used it to cover not only the contribution of consultants and specialists, paediatric nurses and therapists, but also that of other professions involved with child health. It is complementary to Primary Care; we have found it useful but make no claim for its wider adoption unless others agree.

7.32 As we saw in Chapters 3 and 4 it is within the hospital-based supporting services that the concept of paediatrics and the skills and expertise with which to practise it have been developed. The need to apply that knowledge more widely and to use it more effectively has been an important factor in our recommending changes in the pattern of primary care. Our proposals for the future of supporting care are concerned therefore not so much with change, but rather with strengthening paediatrics and the allied specialties dealing with children and extending their involvement into the community, in particular in respect of the developmental and educational aspects of child health and the care of handicapped children. In the light of our decision to develop a service based on primary and supporting care we have looked at ways of ensuring the closest possible integration between them.

The Consultant Community Paediatrician

7.33 Supporting care for children should continue to be a district service based on children's departments in district general hospitals, and consultant paediatricians and other specialists in hospital should provide continuing support to the primary care teams in their district. Where the association involves a necessary service or teaching the GPP could have a formal attachment to the children's department of the district general hospital. More important in our view is the extension of outpatient consultation to health centres and group practice. This practice is growing and its value in reducing referrals and in mutual education has been well demonstrated.[14] We do not however think it will be possible to achieve the degree of integration of

[14] Cain, A R R *et al* (1976). Consultant Paediatric Clinics in Group practice. *Brit. Med. Jour.*, 1, 33.

primary and supporting care for children which we consider essential without *the development of a new type of consultant paediatrician. He will in many ways be the specialist counterpart of the GPP with special skills in developmental social and educational paediatrics, and hold a special responsibility for supporting the GPPs in these aspects of their work.*

7.34 His work in educational medicine and with handicapped children would occupy much of his time and frequently take him into the community. Consequently, he would largely be functioning as a consultant community paediatrician. We want to make it quite clear, however, that we see him also engaging in selective aspects of traditional, consultant paediatric work, in the wards and outpatient departments of hospitals—just as we anticipate that other consultant paediatricians will in future spend more of their time in the community, seeing a variety of children with GPs and GPPs. We consider that there should be one such consultant community paediatrician in each health district. The largest districts may require more than one whole-time, the smaller perhaps somewhat less.

The District Handicap Team

7.35 *We also propose that in each health district there should be a special handicap team based on the district general hospital.* This team would work from a child development centre and would provide a special diagnostic assessment and treatment service for handicapped children, and advice and support for their parents, as well as having "operational" functions including the provision of training seminars etc. for other professional staff working in the district. The handicap team would thus represent a drawing together of the services provided at present for pupils in school by a small number of senior clinical doctors and nurses, and the specialist services provided by district and university teaching hospital paediatric services. It would create a single district supporting service functioning both inside and outside hospital. In the university teaching hospitals, the "district" handicap team would be additionally equipped to serve as a regional centre for severe and multiple handicaps. The consultant community paediatrician would be a key member of the district handicap team, and work with it would occupy a major part of his time. In this he would be joined by a Nursing Officer/CHV with a special interest in handicapped children, a social worker, a psychologist and a teacher. The Nursing Officer/CHV would be additionally trained and experienced in the nursing care of handicapped children in general. She would provide the team with CHV expertise and liaise with the CHVs who share with GPPs the comprehensive primary care of handicapped children. We would hope that the social worker would similarly have special training in handicapping conditions, their prognosis and treatment and in particular would be conversant with the implications for family management and functioning and community involvement and support.

7.36 The creation of a single district supporting service, that would assume existing commitments of area health authorities to a variety of services, in the community, including educational and social work services, would effectively increase the influence and accessibility of consultant

111

paediatricians and paediatric nurses outside the hospital. *Similarly we believe that there should be a single supporting child psychiatric service, that
would embrace the functions of the present child guidance services and the
hospital based child psychiatric services, and which would operate in a
variety of settings both in hospital and the community.*

7.37 These developments and a primary care service staffed by doctors
and nurses better trained than at present in the health care of children,
would lead to greater selectivity in the use of out-patients, accident and
emergency, and in-patient hospital departments. In communities where
accident and emergency departments were regarded as a necessary alternative
source of primary care, they would be properly staffed and organised for
the purpose in concert with the primary care service, though we would hope
this would be a declining rôle as the new comprehensive service from GPP
and CHVs developed.

7.38 University Children's Hospitals and departments would continue to
make their special contribution to an integrated child health service by
providing an exemplary clinical service, intensive peri-natal care, system-
specialist care, services from allied specialists, and above all facilities for
teaching and research.

Supporting Nursing Care

7.39 The need for specialist sick children's nursing in hospital will remain
and we believe that the standard ensured by the RSCN certificate should be
safeguarded. However, if the specialist nursing service is to play its full part
in an integrated child health service we consider that its influence will need
to be strengthened in two ways. In the first place the guidance given by the
Department of Health and Social Security in 1971, that the nurse in charge
of each non-psychiatric ward of the children's department and of the out-
patient services for children should be a paediatric nurse, must be fully
implemented. Secondly, we consider that the specialist paediatric nurse
should have a training which includes both hospital and community experience. We recommend this for two reasons; firstly because within an integrated service, the specialist paediatric nurse, though hospital based would
provide a consultancy service for the child health visitor and her staff in the
nursing care of sick children in the community and thus provide a further
important link between the primary and supporting care service. Secondly—
and this is a further reflection of our underlying belief of the importance
of social, environmental and family factors in relation to child health—we
consider that it is as important for nurses working mainly in hospital as for
those working in the community to have an understanding of this family
context. They must, for example, appreciate the special significance for a
child of being separated from his home environment on admission to
hospital.

The Transition to the New Pattern of Service

7.40 We have, in the preceding paragraphs, described our objective of a

112

reorganised, integrated child health service. We recognise that some changes will take longer to introduce than others. Even if our proposals are accepted at national level, there will be local variation in the rate at which, for example, responsibility for developmental and educational medicine are taken over from the existing services by GPPs and CHVs. We recognise therefore that there will be a transitional period before the essential concept of the GPP as we have described it in this chapter, is realised throughout the country. In a prolonged transition "interim measures" all too often become institutionalised and the ultimate objective lost. For this reason we have devoted this chapter to what we hope is a clear and unequivocal statement of how we think the child health service of the future should be organised. In Chapters 17 and 18 we describe the manpower and organisational implications of our recommendations and in Chapter 20 the training and retraining programmes that will be required. Chapter 19, however, we have devoted specifically to consideration of some of the important practical issues which will need to be considered if, in the transitional period, there is to be on the one hand satisfactory progress towards our objectives and at the same time maintenance of adequate standards of service, particularly in developmental and preventive paediatrics, parent guidance and in educational medicine. We have been particularly concerned to explore ways in which the skills and experience of the clinical and senior clinical medical officers can be brought within a developing integrated service, and Chapter 19 contains detailed recommendations for this.

7.41 In Part II of our report we examine in detail the way in which the needs of particular groups of children would be met within the integrated service which we have proposed, and we identify more precisely the specific tasks which individual members of that service would be required to perform, and the ways in which they will work with parents to provide a better service for children.

PART II

PARTICULAR NEEDS AND REMEDIES

CHAPTER 8
THE UNBORN AND NEWBORN BABY

Child Health and the Maternity Services

8.1 The prenatal period has well-recognised significance for future health, growth and development. The fetus is entirely dependent upon the mother, and her health and perhaps happiness are vital determinants of the well-being of the child. The event of birth should be an achievement and fulfilment for both but is still too often associated with tragedy and disappointment.

8.2 It is natural that we should begin with the unborn and newborn child. We recognise that the medical care of the mother and her fetus and the arrangements for both are largely the responsibility of the maternity services, and the part played by the child health services is less substantial but nonetheless of great importance. The maternity services were examined 6 years ago and the Government has accepted the recommendations of that enquiry.[1] We were not asked nor are we competent to review the maternity services in any comprehensive manner, but at the same time no review of the child health services could be considered comprehensive if it omitted the period of the child's life during which growth is most rapid, the risk of death is greatest and the foundations of subsequent development are laid. At this time the wellbeing of the child is almost inseparable from that of the mother and any attempt to distinguish boundaries between them would be as illogical in this report as it is undesirable in clinical practice. We did not have an obstetrician among our membership, and our account is therefore deliberately weighted towards those aspects of the maternity services which bear most heavily on the contributions which can be made by children's doctors and nurses, and which are of particular importance to the wellbeing of the child. Nevertheless this has not prevented our receiving and considering submissions concerned with mothers as well as babies and we have referred to these where it seemed helpful to do so.

8.3 Many advances in knowledge and skills in the fields of obstetrics and neonatal medicine have been made during the last 25 years and their successful application through the growing partnership between obstetricians, paediatricians, midwives and nurses together with other professional workers has been the most important factor in promoting the health of the unborn and newborn baby. It is from a wish to develop this partnership in both hospital and community that the comments and proposals in this chapter are made.

---

[1] Central Health Services Council, Standing Maternity and Midwifery Committee, Report of the Sub-Committee on Domiciliary Midwifery and Maternity Bed Needs (1970). HMSO, London.

The Child-Bearing Population

8.4 There are in England and Wales over 9 million women between the ages of 15 and 44 years. They are probably more physically fit, and as a group they can expect to live longer and more healthy lives, than their mothers and grandmothers. They are better informed and have justifiably higher expectations of the health care given to them and their babies during pregnancy, childbirth and the post-partum period. In early adult life and in middle-age they will be less occupied with child-bearing and child-rearing. Of particular significance for health services has been the decrease in the birth rate amongst women over 40 and those who already have several children, since older women and women of high parity have relatively greater need for antenatal beds and specialised maternity services. The former are also at greater risk of giving birth to babies with Down's disease. In 1974, only 1.2% of births were to women aged 40 years or more compared with 2.5% a decade earlier. So far as parity is concerned, in 1963 35.7% of all legitimate births were first children compared with 41.3% in 1973, while 8.6% were fourth or higher births compared with 3.7% in 1973.

8.5 Many of the changes which have transformed the lives of women and greatly reduced the mortality and morbidity related to childbirth have been gradual and cumulative. Some recent changes, the effects of which cannot yet be fully evaluated, have given us cause for particular consideration. In 1966 25.2% of live births took place at home. In 1973 the percentage had fallen to 6.1. (Statistical Appendix, Table A 10.) The hospital is now the place in which most of Britain's babies are born, with a concomitant reduction in the participation of the general practitioner and domiciliary midwifery services in care in labour. The development of simple and reliable contraceptive methods which have gained wide acceptance and official promotion has provided the means for family planning as well as enabling women to be fully sexually active without the fear of pregnancy. Following the Abortion Act of 1967 it has been easier to obtain a legal abortion and this has also furthered the sexual and social emancipation of women. The reticence and ignorance about reproductive matters which marked the attitude of sections of society, often the most influential, in the past has quite recently given way to the positive advocacy of "sex education" as part of health education. We have a particular concern over family planning, termination of pregnancy and sexual attitudes because of our knowledge of the vulnerability of illegitimate and unwanted children to a variety of medical, educational and social troubles, and of the special demands imposed on services by them. We are anxious that the family planning services and provisions for termination of pregnancy should be fully effective in reaching those most likely to benefit. We comment further on family planning services in a postscript to this chapter.

Preparation for Parenthood

8.6 In one sense preparation for parenthood begins in childhood. A high standard of physical health care during childhood and adolescence can do much to ensure that the possibility of genetic problems has been identified, the prospective mother has reached optimal growth and nutritional status, and is not susceptible to diseases such as rubella and tuberculosis which might damage the fetus. A high standard of treatment of medical and surgical conditions in the

115

mother is essential if impairment of fertility or reproductive failure and pregnancy wastage is to be avoided from such maternal conditions as diabetes mellitus, rheumatic heart disease, genito-urinary infection, rickets and the results of trauma to the pelvis or reproductive organs.

8.7 Perhaps of more importance to a greater number of persons, however, is preparation for the psychological, social and economic changes that can result from parenthood and this requires a contribution from parents, doctors, nurses, teachers and social workers at appropriate times during childhood and adolescence. We discuss this further in the context of health services for schools in Chapter 10. While we would emphasise the need for young people—particularly those whose experience of family life has been unhappy—to be prepared for parenthood, we recognise the difficulties in recommending more "education for parenthood" in any formal sense. There are problems in determining how information and advice should be presented to ensure that it is helpful and educative without necessarily being prescriptive, and in deciding how far it is justifiable to promulgate a particular set of values and attitudes about what constitutes good parenting. We are encouraged to learn that both the Health Education Council and the Department of Health and Social Security have taken some initiatives in this field. The former are sponsoring an Open University Course on "The First Years of Life" and have carried out an investigation of the ways in which adolescents learn their health behaviour, which is aimed at producing material which will stimulate discussion in education in personal relationships. The Department of Health and Social Security has commissioned a literature survey on "The Needs of Parents" which we understand should be completed later this year. We hope these initiatives will be followed up, in spite of the difficulties.

8.8 Preparation for parenthood becomes a reality for the mother, however, only when the fetus is conceived. The great majority of women have normal pregnancies and give birth to healthy babies. For them the rôle of the maternity services is to provide supervision and support in what is essentially a natural physiological event. There are however a small minority who will require for themselves or their babies highly skilled and specialised care if they are to survive or achieve an acceptable quality of life. A good maternity service must be able to respond to both types of need.

8.9 If it is their first baby the expectant mother and father will have no personal experience of childbirth and may have had little or no previous contact as an adult with the medical services. The quality of prenatal care which the mother receives has significance not only for the immediate outcome of the pregnancy but also for the parents' future relationship with the child and the professional services. This means that there is firstly an obligation on those concerned to ensure, so far as possible, that antenatal services reach those who need them and that once a woman has had her pregnancy confirmed the maternity services should endeavour to maintain contact with her. In particular prenatal care should enable the detection of those mothers and fathers whose social conditions or physical or emotional state may adversely affect their ability to offer proper care to their children. Social work help should be readily available to the general practitioner and to the health visitor so that other specialist social services can be made available where necessary.

116

8.10 Parents should be encouraged to develop a sense of responsibility for the health and wellbeing of their new baby, and this will entail giving them advice for example about the hazards of smoking during pregnancy, and the importance of diet and exercise. They will also need to learn about alternative methods of infant feeding, how to care for the new baby, and to be prepared for changes in their own psychological and emotional state of health. Their views will often be affected by what they learn from friends and neighbours, and by what they read in magazines and books, and it is important that doctors and nurses should appreciate the range of—often conflicting—advice that the prospective mother and father may receive and help them to feel confident about their future rôle as parents. A sense of responsibility and partnership is also more likely to be developed if parents are enabled and encouraged to discuss with their advisers the arrangements for the baby's birth and to express freely their preferences regarding such matters as the presence of the husband during labour and at birth, and choice of methods of pain relief and feeding practices. When clinical considerations limit the freedom of the mother's choice the reasons for this should be explained.

8.11 We were told that "parentcraft" classes during the prenatal period had great value in preparing expectant mothers for childbirth and introducing them to the hospital in which they were booked for delivery. They were also used to give information about nutrition and the care of the baby, and some obstetricians and midwives were enthusiastic about their beneficial effect on the expectant mother and her spouse. A somewhat contrary view was also expressed which stated that formal hospital-based classes could not replace, and might even conflict with, the continuity of care, advice, and support given by the primary health care team and in particular the health visitor.

8.12 It could be argued that both are necessary and desirable; however there are problems regarding resources and communication which militate against the ideal solution. Unfortunately we could find little objective evidence regarding the value of "parentcraft" classes or even evidence that their content had been systematically constructed. *In view of the importance of the subject we would like to see further study of this aspect of prenatal care aimed at providing those involved with clearer guidance both on what advice parents need during the antenatal period and how best to give it to them.* We are, however, clear that this kind of health education should not be confined to formal classes, however well organised, but that it should also be part of the ongoing responsibility of all those health service professionals who are in contact with the parents during this period.

Termination of Pregnancy

8.13 In some instances it may be advisable for the pregnancy to be terminated. It is not our intention to consider the Abortion Act 1967 except to draw attention to recent developments in the prenatal diagnosis of abnormalities in the fetus. If the early identification of fetal abnormality is followed by termination of pregnancy we may expect a reduction in the number of handicapped live-born infants. At present prenatal diagnosis is available for only a small number of mainly rare conditions and is mainly applicable to women who have either had an affected child or are known to be at risk because of genetic factors or advanced

117

maternal age. In such women prenatal investigation of the fetus has the great advantage that anxiety during pregnancy is greatly reduced when the tests prove normal. *For these reasons we advocate continued research and development in prenatal diagnosis and the careful planning of the specialised facilities required.*

Monitoring of Fetal Wellbeing

8.14 We were greatly impressed by the evidence which shows the attention now given by obstetricians to the monitoring of fetal wellbeing during gestation. A number of technical advances in endocrinology, radiology and ultrasonics and other scientific disciplines have contributed to the precision with which this can now be done. An important advantage of accurate determination of fetal growth and development lies in the better selection of women for delivery in maternity units which offer specialised perinatal care. *Further research in fetal monitoring should be encouraged particularly into methods which may be routinely applied and do not cause pain, discomfort or stress to the pregnant woman.*

The Perinatal Period

Care in Childbirth

8.15 The recommended pattern for the maternity services in England and Wales has been set out in the Report of the Peel Committee.([1]) Both this report and that of the Expert Group on Special Care([2]) emphasised the disadvantages of small maternity units and stressed the importance of cooperation between the obstetric and paediatric services for the attainment of an optimal service for the mother and her baby.

8.16 Statistics have been collected both nationally and internationally about mortality associated with childbirth and the tendency has been to concentrate on these as the primary indicators of the quality of the maternity services.

8.17 Maternal deaths due to pregnancy and childbirth are however now uncommon and few women fear that they will not survive labour and delivery of the infant. In part the reduction of maternal mortality is due to the greater safety of childbirth in hospital and this remains a strong argument for the retention of the policy which made it possible for over 90% of births in England and Wales to take place in hospital during 1975.

8.18 However, because childbirth is now a process carried out nearly always in hospital and closely supervised by doctors and midwives, there is an obligation on those concerned with the organisation of the hospital and the clinical care of the mothers and babies not only to exert their skills in the prevention and treatment of disease but also to ensure that the event is satisfying to the mother and her family. To do so makes good clinical sense because partnership between the mother and her attendants is likely to facilitate labour and create conditions in which attachment between mother and her baby is fostered.

8.19 The evidence we received however left us in no doubt that a number

([2]) Report of the Expert Group on Special Care for Babies. Department of Health and Social Security Reports on Public Health and Medical Subjects, No 127, 1971. HMSO, London.

118

of women were not satisfied with some aspects of maternity care in relation to themselves and to their babies. They felt that modern, institutional obstetric practice, while intended only to ensure maximal safety for mother and baby, and to reduce the pain, discomfort and complication of long and difficult labour, nevertheless deprived them of that element of personal choice and control over a natural process, which is vital for the satisfactory completion of childbirth and commencement of motherhood.

8.20 We believe that there may be a conflict at times between the treatment prescribed by the doctor or midwife and the wishes of the patient, and this can occur more readily when the "patient" is a healthy person who is performing a natural function. The conflict is not confined to the maternity services but may exist whenever medical interference, while thought desirable, is not solicited by the patient. It occurs more readily in institutional settings and is more intense when strong feelings and high expectations are involved. We hope that our report will serve to draw to the attention of those working in the maternity services the concern that some mothers feel on this matter. We would add that we are ourselves concerned that when new obstetric techniques are introduced, such as induction, the effects on both mother and baby should be fully evaluated before they are put to widespread use. We recognise however that minor adverse effects and in particular subtle long-term effects are difficult to ascertain with presently available research methods.

Early Contact between Mother and Baby
8.21 The majority of infants in England and Wales spend their first few days in hospital. The duration of stay varies from a few hours to a week or more and there has been little investigation of the merits of varying lengths of stay which fully take into account the interests of the child rather than those of the services or the mother. About 80% of babies born in hospital are nursed in the routine nurseries, where practices vary in regard to "rooming-in". Overall, about 16% of live babies are admitted to special care baby units, and the British Births Survey[3] gives information about the minority of babies who are moved from place to place without their mothers during the first week of life.

8.22 There are good reasons for regarding the mother and her baby as a dyad which should not be separated during the early weeks of life unless there are compelling grounds for so doing. Frequent close contact between mother and baby including early opportunities for suckling is believed to be important for the establishment of successful breast-feeding and continuity of feeding practice seems desirable if bottle-feeding is the adopted method.[4] Recent research[5,6] suggests that the opportunity to initiate and practise mothering which is attended by early close contact is helpful in fostering good parental care while separation may have adverse effects. The evidence we received left

---

(3) Chamberlain, R *et al* (1975). *British Births 1970*. Heinemann, London.

(4) Present Day Practice in Infant Feeding: Report of the Working Party of the Panel on Child Nutrition, 1974. DHSS.

(5) Leiderman, P H, and Seashore, M J (1975). Mother, infant neonatal separation: and some delayed consequences in parent infant interaction: in *CIBA Foundation Symposium No 33* (New Series). Associate Scientific Publishers.

(6) Klaus, M, and Kennell, J (1970). Mothers separated from their newborn infants. *Ped.I.A.J.Clin. N. America*. 17, 1015.

119

us in no doubt that there is a strong desire on the part of mothers to play a major part in the care of their infants during their stay in the maternity departments. It is important that there should be opportunities for "rooming-in" in the post-natal ward and also that where a baby has to be taken into special or intensive care or where the mother is confined to bed particular efforts be made to give the mother access to and contact with her child.

8.23 The British Births Survey showed that on the day of birth 39% of babies were nursed at their mother's bedside in hospital or were at home, 47% were in ward nurseries and 11% were in special care nurseries. Only about a quarter of babies were offered the breast on the first day of life and about a third were receiving breast milk on the third day.

Arrangements for Discharge
8.24 It is felt by some that domiciliary confinement is conducive to the promotion of an ideal relationship between the mother and baby and provides a more satisfying experience for the mother. An alternative to domiciliary confinement is hospital delivery with planned early discharge. We hesitate to advocate any major changes and do not believe that hard and fast rules should obtain. We were impressed by the findings of the British Births Survey which confirmed our experience of the prevalence of illness, mainly minor, in newly born babies, and which indicates that about one third have symptoms or signs such as jaundice, feeding problems, fits and hypothermia which require close surveillance, investigation or treatment. It is clear from this that the newborn baby whether in hospital or at home should be subject to close professional scrutiny. We would however emphasise that the decision on length of stay should always be taken in the light of individual circumstances, and that regard should be had to the mother's own preference as well as to clinical needs. *Moreover when it is necessary for mother and baby to stay in hospital, the maternity and neonatal department of the hospital should be sensitive to their social and psychological needs.*

Perinatal Mortality and Morbidity
8.25 In spite of increasing precision in the identification of the medical, biological and social factors which point to an unsatisfactory outcome of pregnancy it is not yet possible in every individual to predict it with accuracy, or to prevent its occurrence. Moreover any mother and baby during the period of childbirth may show sudden and unexpected signs of illness which may rapidly reach grave dimensions. Minor symptoms and signs may herald severe disease and the importance of minor deviations from the normal may not be appreciated by the unskilled or inexperienced. As Chapter 2 indicates the perinatal mortality rate in England and Wales is considerably higher, and the rate of decline slower than in other countries; facts which we view with considerable concern. About half of the perinatal mortality is accounted for by stillbirths which in about a quarter of instances in one sample(3) was associated with intra-uterine anoxia as the primary cause. Intensive monitoring of fetal well-being during labour is essential for the management of high risk deliveries.

8.26 In Chapter 2 we also drew attention to the significance of low birthweight as a cause of perinatal death. Not surprisingly it is the babies of the lowest birthweight who are almost always immature and have the least chance of survival. Unfortunately the likelihood of premature birth cannot be predicted with certainty nor can premature labour be stopped in the majority of cases. Since death is most likely to occur immediately after birth or during the first 24 hours of life, medical intervention to be effective must be available at the place of birth as well as subsequently in the newborn nursery so that the need for special care or treatment can be identified at the earliest opportunity.

Clinical Examination of the Newborn

8.27 The Peel Committee recommended that every infant should receive "a full clinical examination by a doctor trained and experienced in the detection of deviation from normal development." We understand that representatives of the Royal Colleges of Physicians, Obstetricians and Gynaecologists, and General Practitioners, and of the British Paediatric Association have considered certain of the implications of this recommendation and *we endorse the jointly agreed views of the representatives of these professional bodies that*

"(a) there is a need for every newborn baby to be evaluated immediately after delivery in order to (i) assess the need for active resuscitation, (ii) determine whether special care or urgent treatment is required, and (iii) exclude obvious disorders of growth and fetal development.

(b) it is desirable for every newborn infant, as part of routine post-natal care to be fully examined between the age of 6–10 days. This is the most suitable time for a full clinical examination which would elicit or exclude several conditions which might be of importance to the subsequent progress of the infant."

8.28 We also share the view of the representatives of these professional bodies that "all professional personnel responsible for attending deliveries should be trained and experienced in the immediate post-natal evaluation of the condition of the baby (8.27(a) above), and should be skilled in carrying out procedures such as resuscitation, and that responsibility for the organisation of this procedure should rest:

in consultant units with either the consultant obstetrician or the consultant paediatrician (the procedure to be adopted must be agreed by both paediatric and obstetric teams);

in general practice maternity units or where the baby is delivered at home with the doctor undertaking maternity care of the mother and baby."

We attach particular importance to the need for satisfactory arrangements to be made for the immediate resuscitation of the newly born whether delivery takes place at home or in hospital. Not only must the appropriate equipment be available but it must be regularly serviced and staff trained in its use. We know that the Standing Maternity and Midwifery Committee has already given advice to general practitioners on this subject(7) and we endorse their views.

8.29 With regard to the formal post-natal examination (8.27(b)) it was the view of the representatives of the professional bodies that this should be carried out by a doctor trained and experienced in neonatal paediatrics or working directly under the supervision of a consultant paediatrician. We share this view. We are

(7) Memorandum on Maternal Care by General Practitioners: Schedules to General Practitioners' Guide to Good Practice.

of the opinion that this post-natal examination should include not only a physical examination but a full assessment of any factors which will call for special medical or social intervention or might indicate the need for special surveillance subsequently. Ideally the parents should be present at this examination and the occasion should provide a further opportunity to develop their confidence in their ability to cope. The examining doctor should always communicate his findings in person to the mother of the child or other adult responsible for his care, and the details of the examination should be recorded and made available to the primary health care services. Where there are factors which call for social intervention, the hospital-based social workers should be involved at the earliest opportunity and the appropriate information made available to the social services department. We recognise that it may take some time before a full post-natal examination can be carried out by an appropriately trained doctor on every newborn infant. Meanwhile we consider it essential that all newborn babies continue to be tested for the presence of congenital malformation including congenital dislocation of the hip and phenylketonuria between the 6th and 14th days.

8.30 In Chapter 9 we consider in detail a programme of surveillance for young children. The period immediately after birth provides an opportunity for the medical examination of every child which does not recur until school entry. We therefore see the post-natal screening examination at 6–10 days as serving the purpose of closing the obstetric record insofar as the child is concerned and initiating the future health record on which the child's subsequent progress will be charted. *We therefore recommend that the formal post-natal examination of the newborn child between the 6th and 10th days should form the basis of the programme of serial examinations which will follow.*

8.31 At present persons notifying a birth are asked to report on the notification form the presence of congenital malformations observed at this time. We regard this procedure as of some value for epidemiological purposes in spite of the wide variations in the comprehensiveness of ascertainment and in the definition of many congenital malformations, and we think it should continue as it probably provides an effective means of noting an emergence or rapid increase in major defects hitherto rare or unrecognised, although it is of no clinical benefit to the individual child. On the other hand we hope that the result of the child's full post-natal examination, which includes details of any congenital abnormalities, will in future form the basis for the child health record.

Intensive and Special Care

8.32 In recent years it has been shown that intensive care of the immature and very ill infant not only succeeds in saving life but also in reducing the damaging sequelae of neonatal illness[8,9]. Such care can only be given in units which are specifically equipped and have adequate resources of trained medical and nursing manpower supported by specialised facilities for investigation and treatment. The proportion of live births requiring intensive care is about 1–2 per

---

[8] Rawlings, G, Reynolds, E O R, Stewart, A L, and Strang, L B (1971). Changing prognosis for infants of very low birthweight. *Lancet*, 1, 156.

[9] Stewart, A L, and Reynolds, E O R (1974). Improved prognosis for infants of very low birthweight. *Pediatrics*, 54, 274.

cent. Ideally all mothers expected to deliver high risk infants should be delivered in maternity units which can provide a high standard of intra-partum and post-natal care, and which are adjacent to an intensive care nursery. As this is not always possible it will be necessary at times to transfer seriously ill babies to intensive care nurseries from other hospitals *and it is important that adequate transport facilities exist for this, and the present arrangements should be reviewed.*

8.33 A regional centre for neonatal intensive care would have about 1,000 admissions annually, a volume of work which would justify the cost, enable the staff to maintain and develop skills, and utilise fully the equipment required. Such a centre would serve a limited special care function for the local district maternity department and an intensive care function for the region, and be the centre at which doctors and nurses would receive training in neonatal medicine.

8.34 Although centralisation of intensive neonatal care is a desirable aim it is not a realistic objective because the present pattern of maternity services is one of decentralisation and predominantly small, often isolated units. *We recommend that as far as possible neonatal intensive care should be provided in units containing 25 cots and preferably 40, which are staffed and equipped according to the recommendations of the Expert Group on Special Care for Babies.*[2] *Each Region should have at least one centre for neonatal intensive care directed by a consultant paediatrician who is exclusively or mainly concerned with neonatal medicine, and there should be a substantial proportion of trained nursing staff who have satisfactorily completed Joint Board of Clinical Nursing Studies courses in the special and intensive care of babies.*

8.35 Although only about 1–2% of newly born infants require intensive care a much larger proportion need a greater amount of medical and nursing super-vision or care than is usually found in the routine lying-in wards or at home. Many of these babies require special care for only a short time, usually im-mediately after birth and for only a few hours or days. There is little factual information about the criteria for admission to special care units. The question is an important one because newborn babies should not be deprived of any medical or nursing care which may be needed, nor should they be unnecessarily separated from their mothers.

8.36 Overall there would seem to be no shortage of special and intensive care cots for babies although they are assembled into units which are generally smaller in size than the 24 cots hitherto recommended. In 1973, 106,000 babies were admitted to special care in England representing some 16% of all live births. A similar proportion of babies admitted was reported in the British Births Survey, and a rather larger one in two Thames Regions by Alberman and her colleagues.[10] The latter report refers to a census of 41 units providing both special and intensive care and showed that while many units were deficient in staff and equipment the workload consisted largely of observation and com-paratively simple management of neonatal problems, often transitory in nature.

8.37 We are agreed that provision needs to be made for the high standard of surveillance and care required by the 15–30%[3] of babies whose post-natal state

---

(10) Personal Communication.

is not entirely normal. In view of the low occupancies (average 64% in England in 1974) of many units there may be grounds for lowering the present provision for special and intensive care of 6 cots per 1,000 live births and for reducing the number of units by the closure of small maternity units. The provision of paediatric medical and nursing cover throughout the 24 hours is a considerable strain on manpower and is made much more difficult when the special care nursery is in a hospital or building not adjacent to the main children's department.

8.38 Economies in staffing and probably a higher standard of care is achieved when neonatal care (other than intensive care) is shared by paediatric and obstetric junior staff. It is essential that adequate nurse staffing should be provided within special care baby units if they are to offer a higher standard of observation and care than that given by the routine nursery.

8.39 We were glad to note that the Consultative Document on Priorities for Health and Personal Social Services in England recognises the urgent need to improve the level of special care for the newborn and to learn that the Department of Health has now issued a circular commending to health authorities the report of the working party on the Prevention of Early Neonatal Mortality and Morbidity,([11]) and asking them to carry out a review of their services for the newborn. We regard this as a high priority. We remain however seriously concerned at the continuing marked variation in perinatal mortality and morbidity rates both between regions and social classes. The precise reasons for these variations are not easy to understand, and only when they are understood will it be possible to make positive recommendations as to the best way of using resources to help those apparently most at risk. *We therefore recommend that further research should be carried out to identify the reasons for these variations, particularly those apparently related to social class.* We understand that the Children's Research Liaison Group at the Department of Health and Social Security (see Chapter 21) has recently set up a working party "to consider infant and perinatal mortality and morbidity and to advise on priorities for research". It may be that this group will already have in mind the need for research on this particular aspect.

The Baby with Congenital Defects

8.40 About 1 in 50 babies is born with an obvious abnormality or one which is found on examination. Serious congenital defects such as myelo-meningocele (spina bifida), intestinal obstruction, and some types of congenital heart disease require immediate specialised medical or surgical care of the kind available only in large children's departments. Less severe defects may be managed successfully in the special care and maternity department or the children's department of the district general hospital. In some cases special intervention is not immediately required but a plan of future action has to be discussed with the parents.

8.41 *We are in no doubt that parents are entitled to a full and sympathetically given description of any abnormalities or deviations from the normal which have*

([11]) DHSS circular, No HC(76)40.

been discovered in their child, and that this should be given as soon as the diagnosis is certain. The task of conveying the diagnosis, providing an explanation for the occurrence and outlining future management and prognosis should not be delegated to inexperienced doctors or members of the nursing and midwifery staff. In consultant units it should be the responsibility of the consultant paediatrician or an experienced member of the paediatric department; in general practitioner units the general practitioner should do so only after consultation with a specialist. Some parents may have difficulty in accepting the diagnosis and in planning for the future and may need the help of a social worker experienced in the field of handicap. The birth of a child with an inherited or congenital abnormality whether anatomical, eg spina bifida, cleft lip and palate, or metabolic, eg phenylketonuria, glactosaemia, will almost always mean that the parents will benefit from genetic counselling. In some cases the paediatrician or obstetrician is competent to provide genetic counselling and as clinical genetic counselling services expand, (see also Chapter 18), they should increasingly be able to provide training for these doctors which will increase their competence in this difficult field. In other cases, however, where the problem is more complex, referral to a genetic counselling centre will be necessary.

8.42 Where it is likely that the child has or may develop a disability or handicap the district handicap team should be involved at an early stage, and the parents should be aware of a network of people and services ready to help. We were interested to learn of a local scheme whereby shortly after a baby with Down's disease was born the health service staff offered the parents the opportunity, at this early stage, to meet a self-help group of parents with similarly handicapped children, and no doubt an arrangement of this kind can be of considerable practical and psychological help.

Links between Hospital and the Community

8.43 The medical care of the fetus and newly born baby is linked closely with that of the mother and as such is shared between the hospital-based maternity service which includes obstetricians, midwives and paediatricians and the primary health care team in the community. For the primary health care team the occurrence of a pregnancy is an episode, albeit an important one, in the continuous responsibility which it holds for the health care of a family. On the other hand the responsibilities of the obstetrician and midwife are discharged when mother and baby no longer need the specialised service which they provide. The paediatrician in the hospital has a special concern for the health of the neonate but will only have a continuing responsibility for babies which require expert supervision or supportive care. Within the primary care team the midwife has a special responsibility for the expectant mother during the antenatal period and for both mother and baby for a time after delivery, at which point the health visitor takes on the advisory and supportive rôle.

8.44 Integration of the hospital and community maternity services has achieved a considerable measure of success and within those hospitals which contain both maternity and children's departments there is generally an advanced degree of collaboration between the obstetric and paediatric services.

Difficulties arise when the departments are separated and paediatric cover has to be provided from another hospital and these should lessen with the phasing out of isolated maternity units.

8.45 Nevertheless we are not completely satisfied that the infant on discharge from hospital always receives the standard of medical and nursing care which is needed during a period in which he is particularly vulnerable and his acceptance within the family may still be fragile. Special efforts need to be made to maintain contact and offer continued support to mothers who may have difficulty in coping for any reason with motherhood and whose children may be at risk of deprivation or non-accidental injury. Evidence we received emphasises the importance given by mothers to continuity of care, the availability of expert support, and the avoidance of contradictory or confusing advice at the time of return home with the new baby and the first few weeks thereafter. We also recognise that the mother's physical and mental health should be carefully checked post-partum and any medical problems treated. The post-partum examination provides an excellent opportunity for discussion regarding family planning and family spacing with advice about methods of contraception which take into account lactation and other factors which have altered since the mother's pregnancy.

8.46 Improvement in communication between those who share responsibility for the care of mothers and young infants is desirable particularly when observations have been made by hospital staff which point to a need for a special effort to be made by the community services to give surveillance, support or care. Good communication is also essential at the time when the midwife hands over to the health visitor and as much attention needs to be given to social and emotional problems as to those of a physical nature. The unification of the hospital-based social work services with the local authority services should improve the communication and care necessary for those families who present particular social problems and risks.

8.47 We were impressed by evidence which emphasised the advantages of the health visitor having contact with the expectant mother during the pregnancy and in the first days of the baby's post-natal life. We think that this should be encouraged and *recommend that this should become an accepted responsibility for the child health visitor in addition to retention of her duty to visit the family following the notification of birth.*

8.48 Our proposals relating to the establishment of a GPP and for the restructuring of primary and supporting care for children have implications for the maternity services which will require discussion and wide consultation. At present general practitioners undertaking maternal care are expected to provide in relation to the child, preventive antenatal care, anticipatory advice to the mother, immediate examination and care of the child at birth, a clinical examination at about the 7th day, and medical care for the mother and child for a period of 14 days after delivery.[7]

8.49 It is particularly important that there is continuity of care following the birth of a child. In many instances this is provided by the general practitioner who not only undertakes the care of the mother during the antenatal period, but also continues the care of both mother and child thereafter. If our proposals are accepted the situation may occur where a general practitioner with a special interest in obstetrics undertakes the care of the mother during the antenatal period and that the care of the child and mother may, after delivery, be transferred to a general practitioner with a special interest in paediatrics. If the special needs of mother and child for medical care are to be met satisfactorily it is essential that in these circumstances there are well-defined plans for the management of the transfer of responsibility. The GPP should be involved at an early stage after delivery and the mother should be clear as to who is responsible for her and her baby at each stage. These arrangements will need to be worked out locally, but when the GPP scheme has been in operation for some years, it should be possible to establish, in the light of local experience, the most effective allocation of responsibility.

Training

8.50 We agree with the views expressed by representatives of the Royal Colleges and the BPA (see paragraph 8.27) that undergraduate training should continue to provide the student with an understanding of the principles of the care of the newborn (preventive and curative) and with the handling and examination of babies. In the postgraduate training of obstetricians, paediatricians and general practitioners undertaking maternity care or becoming GPPs, greater emphasis should be placed on the acquisition of knowledge, skills and clinical judgment in neonatal paediatrics. *In addition we propose that neonatal paediatrics should be recognised as a specialty and that training programmes should be set up so as to provide at least one consultant in neonatal paediatrics in each Region.*

8.51 We were impressed by the evidence which indicated that increasing recognition was now being given during midwifery training to the care of the fetus and the newborn, and to the social and emotional aspects of childbirth. We think that this should be encouraged.

8.52 We recognise that the nursing of infants requiring special and intensive care calls for the exercise of knowledge, skills and attitudes which are additional to those included in the basic training of midwives and paediatric nurses. The post certificate courses in the subject organised by the Joint Board of Clinical Nursing Studies fulfil the requirements as at present ascertained and *nurses occupying a position of responsibility in special and intensive care units should be required to have successfully completed the appropriate course.*

Research

8.53 A heavy burden of care rests upon the child health and social services because of the personal and family needs of children with chronic physical and mental handicap. The extent to which this is reducible through genetic counselling, termination of pregnancy and selective management of severely deformed live-born infants is a matter of social as much as medical policy.

8.54 Nevertheless some of the conditions which cause or pre-dispose to handicap are preventible and their incidence could be reduced by application of present knowledge, and the sharing of that knowledge with the public. However there are many conditions for which the cause is not known and research is required to elicit the cause. We believe that *priority should be given to research into the aetiology of handicapping conditions.*

8.55 Many of the procedures practised in obstetrics and neonatal paediatrics have not been fully evaluated. Examples are the use of induction of labour, the effects of drugs on the fetus and the newborn. We advocate further work on the evaluation of these procedures and the inclusion in such studies of the emotional and social effects on the mother before these procedures are applied as part of routine obstetric care.

Postscript: Family Planning

8.56 It is believed that the majority of people who use reliable methods of family planning obtain their advice and supplies through the NHS family planning service although a large number of men obtain sheaths from retail outlets or by mail order. Since 1 April 1974 family planning advice, treatment and supplies have been available free of charge to all who need them regardless of age, sex or marital status from NHS family planning clinics; in most areas domiciliary services are provided for people who for personal and social reasons have difficulty in attending clinics regularly. Similarly free family planning services (including male and female sterilisation) are available to all in hospitals. These services are provided and staffed by area health authorities although in some areas, clinics and domiciliary services are still provided by the Family Planning Association, a voluntary organisation which was one of the pioneers of a free service. They are at present made available to the area health authority on an agency basis but are due to be taken over by area health authorities by October 1976. Advice may be given by any suitably trained health service professional staff. Currently doctors are responsible for prescriptions for oral contraceptives but nurses issue non-medical supplies and in some circumstances fit devices. In addition advice and treatment for women only have since 1 July 1975 been available free from most general practitioners. Family planning supplies for women prescribed by general practitioners are dispensed free of charge in chemist shops. Services are coordinated at area level and liaison maintained with the social services department to ensure full knowledge of the varying social conditions in the area and to aid cooperation between health and social services workers in identifying and helping those most in need.

8.57 During recent years there has been a considerable fall in the birth rate and a comparable decline in the proportion of very large families. There has also been a marked rise in the use of efficient methods of contraception[1], yet the situation regarding family planning remains most unsatisfactory on several different counts. Firstly there has been no drop in the proportion of unintended and unwanted pregnancies. Secondly there is usually a delay of several years between the time of beginning to have sexual intercourse and the time of first using efficient methods of contraception. Thirdly a high proportion of women are already pregnant when they marry (about one quarter in those under 20

---

[1] Cartwright, A (1976). *How Many Children?* Routledge and Kegan Paul, London.

years of age). Fourthly the illegitimacy ratio has continued to rise. Fifthly the number of abortions has also increased each year up to 1974. Furthermore, it is clear that many of the people having sexual relationships and not using birth control are aware of contraceptive techniques, have no religious objections to their usage and do not wish to become pregnant. This pattern is found in all sections of the community but is particularly common among sexually active young people before marriage and in socially disadvantaged groups.[1,2,3] There are many reasons why people who do not wish to become pregnant nevertheless fail to use contraception. These include conflicts over sexuality, socio-cultural attitudes (including a male antagonism to female autonomy), lack of foresight and (especially in socially disadvantaged groups) a pervasive feeling of hopelessness and inevitability. Our particular concern over this matter stems from the knowledge that unwanted and illegitimate children have a much increased risk for a variety of medical, educational and social troubles[4,5] and from the fact that teenagers constitute one of the groups most liable to produce unwanted pregnancies although the numbers of occurrences in the single under 20 age group are beginning to show signs of dropping.

8.58 The remedy does not lie simply in the free provision of family planning services, both because the failure to use contraception is sometimes part of a much wider pattern of attitudes and behaviour involving a lack of foresight and planning, and because some of the groups which fail to use contraception tend not to avail themselves of official services, despite their scale and diversity.

8.59 We recommend that several steps be taken to reduce the number of unwanted babies. First, more extensive and better education on family planning is needed. At present information is provided at national level by the Family Planning Association and the Health Education Council (both financed from Government funds) and at local level by the area health education service. At the end of 1975 and the beginning of 1976, the Health Education Council undertook a cinema family planning campaign directed at the young. But more needs to be done. Greater use should be made of informal and formal publicity through the press, TV and other sources of communication.[6] Discussions in schools and talks to groups (eg youth clubs, young wives groups, homeless families' units, etc.) can also be of value. However, information on methods of birth control is not enough in itself. Young people need to have the opportunity to discuss sexual matters in the context of personal relationships and a sense of responsibility towards reproduction. Health visitors and other health professionals are often invited to participate in the work of school health education and area health authorities have been advised to consider establishing counselling services for the young as an adjunct to family planning services. Counselling for the young is also available from local authority and voluntary services.

[2] Askham, J (1975). *Fertility and deprivation.* Cambridge University Press, London.

[3] Schofield, M (1973). *The Sexual Behaviour of Young Adults.* Allen Lane, London.

[4] Crellin, E, Pringle, M L K, and West, P (1971). *Born Illegitimate: social and educational implications.* NFER, Slough.

[5] Forssman, H, and Thuwe, I (1966). One hundred and twenty children born after application for therapeutic abortion refused. *Acta Psychiat. Scand.* 42, 71–99.

[6] Allen, I (1974). *Birth control in Runcorn and Coalville: a study of the FPA campaign.* PEP Broadsheet 549. PEP, London.

8.60 Second, community workers need to be well informed on family planning services and the kinds of help they provide. Child health clinics, health visiting, social work contacts and school counselling all involve interactions in which family planning issues often arise and the DHSS is encouraging professional workers other than doctors to play a greater rôle in family planning by providing funds for training nurses, health visitors, midwives and social workers in family planning. This is of particular importance since there are several disadvantages in basing the service predominantly on doctors. From the users' point of view, the identification of contraception with "becoming a patient" may well be counter-productive to the greater usage of family planning methods. From the service point of view, we feel that it is an expensive and inappropriate use of highly trained doctors since the medical skills involved are readily taught to nurses and other professionals, and do not require a complete medical training. A working group, set up at the invitation of the Secretaries of State for Social Services and for Wales by the Central Health Services Council, the Medicines Commission and the Committee on Safety of Medicines is looking at the question of extending the availability of oral contraceptives and whether any changes would be desirable. At present oral contraceptives are available only on prescription by a registered medical practitioner, mainly to ensure that women who are more liable to suffer complications are identified. However it seems likely that in the past, general practitioners often did not conduct an examination at the time of prescribing oral contraceptives[7] and that most of the general practitioners then providing family planning services had not been specifically trained for this work. Developments during the past few years have been rapid and short training programmes have been extensively organised as a result of the general practitioner's greater participation in family planning services since July 1975. We were encouraged to learn that demand has far exceeded supply in places on training courses recognised by the Joint Committee of the RCOG and the RCGP. It is as yet too early to assess the effects of these measures.

8.61 Third, more active steps need to be taken to bring family planning services to particularly needy groups. Domiciliary family planning services, local information centres, and "grapevine" contacts all have an important part to play in this connection. Finally there is a need for greater cooperation between different groups of professional workers concerned with family planning, both within and without the NHS. The district management team has a special responsibility for the planning and management of family planning services at district level. It is advised by a working group which should initially consist of representatives of the hospital service; gp services; the clinic service; nurses and midwives; pharmaceutical services; health education; social services in the District; and voluntary services.

---

(7) Cartwright, A (1970). *Parents and Family Planning Services*. Routledge and Kegan Paul.

130

CHAPTER 9

HEALTH AND DEVELOPMENT IN THE EARLY YEARS

Child Development and Parental Needs

9.1 Early childhood is a time of rapid growth and development; the time when a child begins to walk and talk and become a person. That most children achieve such skills without major difficulty should not blunt our awareness of either the complexity or the hazards of the transformation from helpless newborn infant to active toddler.

9.2 The main responsibility for bringing up children lies with their parents. Most parents are concerned for their children's health and development, and successfully provide for them; they find it a satisfying experience, remembered later with pleasure if not always with accuracy. But the complexity of growth and development are such that all parents at times become discouraged and even exhausted, uncertain of the significance of a problem and what to do about it. At such times they need re-assurance, when this can be given, and advice and guidance on the care and management of their normal child.

9.3 It is not unreasonable that parents should have these anxieties, for at this young age rapid development and danger are intimately related. The bright picture for most children today deepens the shadows for those with defective development, recurrent illness or social disadvantage (Chapters 1 and 2). More children die in infancy than in all the remaining years up to adult life, and mortality is only the tip of the iceberg of illness and disability. The risk of death and serious disease is much nearer to many children than it should be. The harmful effect of social disadvantage on survival, growth, health and the ability to learn in the pre-school years is well known. Even with our present incomplete knowledge much of the death, illness and injury in early childhood is avoidable.

9.4 The fact of growth and development and that this natural process is at the same time complex and hazardous determines the nature of the preventive child health services. The objectives are to provide:

   (i) comprehensive coverage of all children in order to identify those with health care needs that are not being adequately met;

   (ii) a service to parents of sound, professional advice and support, that is readily available.

9.5 Preventive child health services have existed for many years and we have already discussed their strengths and weaknesses. The question arises, however, as to how effective they have been in preventing avoidable illness and injury, achieving early recognition of developmental disorders and handicaps, and supporting parents. With the exception of the well-documented impact of infectious disease prophylaxis [1,2] firm evidence does not exist one way or the

---

[1] *Infants at Risk: An historical and international comparison* (1964). Office of Economics London.

[2] Department of Health and Social Security (1976). *Prevention and Health: everybody's business*. HMSO, London.

131

other, and *more attention should be given to operational and evaluative research in this field*.[3] We share the general views of others before us [4,5] of the value of these services. The use that parents make of the health visiting services and child health clinics speaks for itself, and if these services were improved in the ways we shall suggest more families would use them. In this chapter we outline the principal measures that need to be undertaken by professional health staff to promote young children's health and development; consider how this work can be strengthened and integrated as an essential component of both primary and supporting care; and examine certain practical issues arising from this.

Health Surveillance

Objectives and Professional Responsibilities

9.6 There are five principal professional activities required of health care staff who work in child health preventive services. These are:

oversight of health and physical growth of all children;
monitoring the developmental progress of all children;
providing advice and support to parents, and treatment and referral of the child;
providing a programme of effective infectious disease prophylaxis;
participation in health education and training in parenthood.

Although we shall describe these separately, in practice they overlap and it is both convenient and helpful to describe this whole aspect of health care as *health surveillance*.

9.7 First, *oversight of health and physical growth of all children*. An evaluation of a child's state of health and pattern of growth requires a medical history, paediatric clinical examination and serial measurements of weight, height and head circumference suitably recorded on standardised charts giving centile norms rated for children of this country. It also includes the application of certain screening tests for specific disorders (eg PKU, congenital dislocation of the hip).

9.8 Second, *monitoring the developmental progress of all children*. An evaluation of a child's developmental progress requires a developmental and family history and the observation of, as well as the assessment of, maturity of the child's sensory-motor skills, speech and language, and social and emotional development. It also includes the application of certain screening tests for impairment of vision and hearing. Monitoring developmental progress has frequently been referred to as developmental screening, not least by many experts in this field whose work [6,7] has both convinced us of the value of the

(3) Hutchison, J H (1973). An experiment in developmental screening of pre-school children. *Health Bulletin,* Scottish Home and Health Department. HMSO, London.

(4) Central Health Services Council, Standing Medical Advisory Committee: Report of a sub-committee on Child Welfare Centres (Chairman: Sir Wilfred Sheldon) (1967). Ministry of Health. HMSO, London.

(5) *Paediatrics in the Seventies: Developing the child health services* (1972). Ed. Court, D, and Jackson, A. Oxford University Press, London.

(6) Sheridan, M (1968). *Monthly Bulletin of the Ministry of Health.* 21, 238.

(7) Egan, D F, Illingworth, R S, and MacKeith, R C (1969). *Developmental Screening 0–5 years.* Heinemann, London.

clinical oversight of development and also helped us to appreciate some of the disadvantages of equating such oversight with screening. We have avoided the use of the term "developmental screening" because we firmly reject the notion of a developmental screening programme for children in favour of a programme of health surveillance, although we accept the usefulness of certain developmental screening tests applied to individual children in the course of such surveillance.

9.9 Third, *providing advice and support to parents, and when necessary arranging treatment or referral of the child.* The purpose of oversight of health and physical growth and the monitoring of developmental progress is two-fold: to provide an expert opinion that growth and development are normal with advice on how the parents might deal with problems relating to the management of the child (eg as regards feeding, sleeping, the avoidance of infection and injury, and social adaptation); to detect significant deviations from the normal in health or development (bearing in mind the wide range of normality seen among young children in their rate and overall pattern of development), so that the child and parents can be offered further investigation and appropriate and appropriately timed help. The second of these objectives has tended to receive more attention than the first. Although we do not wish to minimise the importance of the early recognition of handicaps, there are important practical reasons for redressing the balance.

9.10 Children are developing persons and serious training in child development must be the basis of the skills of all professional staff concerned with their care. Also, an understanding of normality is an essential prerequisite for the safe recognition of abnormality. Parents need to feel assured that staff involved in health surveillance have been as carefully and appropriately trained as staff in other branches of paediatrics and paediatric nursing, and are as conversant with the promotion of health and development as they are in the detection of unsuspected abnormality. It is possible, but not always easy, to adopt a positive attitude in health surveillance without exaggerating professional interest into a "healthier-than-healthy" approach.

9.11 The primary prevention of handicaps is now an increasing possibility; the methods are more fully discussed in Chapters 8 and 14. Emphasis on early recognition has been criticised on the grounds that while it can lead to earlier treatment there is little evidence that this improves the outlook. We agree that a more critical appraisal of early treatment over a sufficient period of time is necessary. However, in our concern for improvement in the condition we must not forget the problems and the burden of those who have the day to day care of a handicapped child—a point on which evidence presented to us was distressingly insistent. The handicapped life must be lived; and while treatment should be evaluated advice and support for the parents should be sustained.

9.12 Proffering advice in the course of professional health surveillance is not quite as straightforward as it may appear. Preventive practice reverses the customary situation in which the patient seeks medical advice and initiates the contact with the medical services. Because preventive services have had (and still do have) a responsibility for promoting the health and preventing the ill-health of all children in a defined population, it has usually been health care

133

staff who have taken the initiative in inviting parents to bring their children for periodic health surveillance. Under these circumstances they have been offering unsolicited services and there has always been the danger that their advice, though offered with the best intentions, could be misconstrued as interference. This has been especially likely to happen when liaison between clinical medical officers and general practitioners has been insufficient and parents have been given conflicting advice or unnecessary cause for concern when a defect is suspected in their child. In the past, a further difficulty has arisen when, as a result of health surveillance, clinical medical officers have found or suspected significant deviations from normal in health, growth or development and thought it desirable that professional advice to the parents be accompanied by professional care of the child. Such care may include the prescription of medicines and remedial therapy as well as referral for consultant opinion and treatment. Clinical medical officers have not been expected to undertake treatment and have not been in a position to provide free treatment; nor have they had a duty to provide a 24-hour service, even in respect of advisory services to parents.

9.13 These problems have to date governed the continued separation in the organisation and staffing of preventive and therapeutic services but it has become our conviction that the preventive and therapeutic care of children are not incompatible but on the contrary inextricable. In the interests of the child, good clinical practice requires that a request by parents for treatment from primary and supporting care services should be seen as an opportunity to offer advice on health promotion and the prevention of illness and injury; similarly, in the course of observing and monitoring health and development the opportunity should be taken to offer any advice and treatment thought necessary on the management of deviations from accepted norms. *Health surveillance is, in practice, essentially a function of primary health care;* and one of the objects of integrating the former local authority pre-school and school health services with the general medical services provided by general practitioners is *to ensure that one and the same health care team has clinical responsibility for both the promotion of a child's health and the treatment of any ill-health or developmental disorder or handicap,* no matter under what circumstances contact between child and professional staff is first made. In a number of small studies evaluating the "developmental screening" of pre-school children in general practice, different investigators independently commented upon the opportunity presented by such encounters for "health education" of parents about their children.[8,9] The introduction of the GPP will overcome both of the difficulties to which we have referred in the previous paragraph. We anticipate that as a result of his training and experience in comprehensive child health care, he will not overlook the need for unsolicited services and be able to provide them without arousing unnecessary anxiety in the minds of the parents.

9.14 Fourth, *providing a programme of effective infectious disease prophylaxis.* These procedures are usually carried out according to a schedule advised and monitored by the Joint Committee on Vaccination and Immunisation of the

[8] Starte, G D (1974). Developmental assessment of the young child in general practice. *Practitioner.* 213, 823.

[9] Bain, D J G (1974). The results of developmental screening in general practice. *Health Bulletin of the Scottish Home and Health Department.* HMSO, London.

Department of Health and Social Security. At present, immunisation against tetanus, diphtheria, pertussis (whooping cough) and poliomyelitis is recommended for young children. BCG vaccination against tuberculosis is usually offered to susceptible secondary school children and vaccination against rubella (german measles) is now available for pre-adolescent girls. Vaccination against smallpox is no longer recommended as a routine. While there are no grounds for complacency, statistics showing the uptake of immunisation procedures by children reveal a fairly satisfactory situation at least up to 1974. (Statistical Appendix, Table E3.) However, we are concerned at the variations in uptake reported in different regions and often associated with adverse socio-economic circumstances. Every effort should be made to reduce these.

9.15 The practical, professional and ethical problems that arise in so doing must be faced. In spite of every attempt to ensure complete safety, the hazards which an immunising agent may hold for a very small number of children are only discovered with time. The success of the immunisation programmes has resulted in a whole generation of both parents and doctors who have not witnessed the effects of unchecked epidemic diseases upon children and it is disturbing that this success should be tarnished by a disproportionate emotional reaction to the unfortunate, but rare, side-effects in a tiny minority of children.

9.16 We also recognise that the doctor responsible for carrying out immunisation may feel himself to be in a position of professional conflict in advising parents. This may arise from his personal views as to the potential advantages and dangers of the procedures being at variance with the policy advocated by the Joint Committee. It may also arise from his dual responsibility, on the one hand to the community for maintaining adequately high levels of immunity in the population, and on the other hand to individual children for their personal well-being, bearing in mind particularly that at present no compensation is payable if the child is injured as a result of immunisation agreed to by the parents in the interest of the community.

9.17 *We think it is important that parents should be fully informed of the risks as well as the benefits associated with immunisation of their child prior to any request for their consent, which should immediately precede immunisation. We further suggest that the DHSS keep all doctors informed of the current state of infectious disease and immunisation policies.*

9.18 Fifth, *participation in health education and training in parenthood.* We have referred to this work in Chapters 8 and 10. Here, we wish to emphasise that health education is not the prerogative of health care staff; they should nonetheless use every professional contact with a child and his parents as an opportunity to inform them about health care.

A Basic Programme of Health Surveillance
9.19 *We suggest in the schedule below a basic programme of interviews between health care staff and a child and his parents which will enable both parties to participate in health surveillance.* Such a programme should be offered to all children. Three points need to be emphasised. First the schedule represents a framework around which health surveillance can be practised: the schedule

SCHEDULE FOR BASIC SURVEILLANCE PROGRAMME

Note: The term "clinic" is used here to cover health surveillance in group practices, health centres or child health clinics.

Age (approx)	By whom	Where	Aims and Comments
1. At birth	To be organised, where baby born in consultant unit by consultant obstetrician or consultant paediatrician; in general practice maternity unit or at home by doctor providing maternity care. (see paragraph 8.28)	Maternity Unit or at home	Immediate evaluation to assess need for resuscitation and special care, and identify obvious disorders.
Between 6–10 days	Doctor trained in neonatal paediatrics or working under supervision of consultant paediatrician.	Maternity Unit or at home	Full post-natal examination: start of ongoing child health record (including relevant pre- and perinatal data). Arrangements for achieving this examination in association with policies of early discharge from hospital need to take into account the time factor and the later onset of cardiac and other important physical signs. These examinations should ensure prompt recognition and explanation of apparent defects, reassurance to mother of a normal infant. Mothers require positive advice, and mere absence of adverse comment is always insufficient.
2. 6 weeks	GPP, CHP, or consultant paediatrician ————————— Child health visitor*		Introduction to the "clinic" premises, facilities and staff: opportunity for professionals to listen and advise on infant management and family problems and to give sympathetic support (and, where necessary, to initiate treatment or referral) to mothers experiencing fatigue, isolation and possibly depression. Unless for any reason the neonatal examination was not carried out, there will be a relatively low emphasis at this stage upon detection of handicaps.

* for "non-attenders"

No.	Age	Professional	Location	Review
3.	7–8 months	Child health visitor	"clinic" or home	Review of development, especially hearing and vision. The timing of this contact is important; 6 months is not a rewarding age to check motor development, while 9–10 months is often too late for the first routine hearing test.
4.	18 months	Child health visitor	"clinic" or home	Review of development, eg mobility, manipulative skills, hearing and early language, social relationships: opportunity to discuss growth and behaviour.
5.	2½–3 years	GPP or CHP	"clinic"	Review of development: opportunity to discuss behaviour: language: appropriate vision testing and cover test for squint.
6.	4½–5 years (immediately prior to school entry)	GPP or CHP acting as school doctor	"clinic" or school	Summing up of early health and development in relation to imminent entry to school: early warning to teachers of potential or established difficulties (eg speech, behaviour) which could affect child's response to school: appropriate testing of vision (including cover test for squint) and hearing. This examination, which should apply to all children should form the basis of a subsequent selective (ie non-routine) approach to ongoing oversight of the health and behaviour of children in school.

itself does not constitute surveillance. Second the programme is to be regarded as a minimum number of interviews. Some children will need more (see paragraph 9.23), and parents will have their own reasons for seeking advice from health care staff in clinics at more frequent intervals. Thirdly a framework needs to be flexible, and our comments on the rationale of each interview are in no way intended to lay down how these opportunities for health surveillance should necessarily be used. Their timing has been suggested to allow for checks on important parameters of development, especially vision, hearing and language, and to anticipate the most likely needs for advice to meet "normal" development problems.

9.20 A particular difficulty arises because the recommended schedule of immunisation does not match with a helpful schedule of health surveillance in respect of growth and development. There are obvious reasons for encouraging young minds to dissociate the relatively less pleasant encounters with experience of injections from what should be the relaxed and interesting experience of developmental monitoring. On the other hand, the more often mothers of young children are asked to attend appointments (often a major organisational and physical effort) the more appointments tend not to be kept, to the detriment of both the immunisation and health surveillance of the child. We believe the relative efficiency of computer-linked immunisation recording and computer-assisted appointment schemes (which can be made directly available for immunisation sessions on GP premises) have done much to overcome this problem and have contributed to the high level of uptake of immunisation in many areas. We understand that computers available to local authorities at March 1974 provided these facilities for about 58% of the population, and *we welcome steps that are being taken by the DHSS to extend their use, nationally*.

Cover for All Children

9.21 Ensuring that contact is made with every child born in or entering a given neighbourhood, and then maintained, raises many practical problems. Birth notification is already required and this provides the information health visitors need to carry out their first visit to mother and child in their own home. Education is compulsory from the age of 5 and virtually all children attend a school. During the intervening years of rapid development when children are particularly vulnerable to adverse physical and social factors, it is much less easy to achieve and maintain effective contact with families. We believe it could be helped in the following ways:

   (i) *Nursing Officers (child health visiting) should have an explicit responsibility for arranging that CHVs who are members of primary health care teams are also assigned a geographically defined community with which they should ensure that the child health services keep in touch.*

  (ii) *Parents should be required to declare a change of address when they claim family allowances; AHAs should be notified of such changes so that CHVs may be informed and arrange to visit.*

 (iii) *An effective system should be devised of recording "transfers in" (ie families moving into the neighbourhood) and of "transfers out", and for passing such information to receiving health authorities.* This would require nationally agreed procedures.

(iv) If adopted, better record systems and more rigorous follow up procedures should help to identify families where surveillance services are not being taken up. In such cases, or where there is suspicion of serious ill-health for which medical help is not being sought, the child health visitor should initially seek access to the child by persuasion but in the event of failure, she should have the right to apply for a legally enforceable medical examination. (Chapter 16, paragraph 6.)

Children in Special Need

9.22 We have stressed the need for flexibility in any basic programme of health surveillance. Staff and facilities must be available to meet the needs that the majority of families at times have for advice and support. These needs vary according to family structure, social circumstances, and many other factors, including the occurrence of crises within the family. Any of the interviews in the suggested schedule, and any other contact between health care staff and the child, may indicate the need of some children for more intensive oversight of health and the monitoring of developmental progress.

9.23 *We regard the arrangements for the additional surveillance of such children as one of the most important dimensions of the health surveillance concept.* Experienced professionals may have a shrewd idea of which children these might be from the presence of certain features in their personal, developmental and medical history and from the social and environmental circumstances of their families. These include a history of low birthweight, neonatal illness and paediatric concern during the neonatal period for other reasons, congenital malformation and the occurrence in other members of the family of hereditary disorders and markedly abnormal behaviour. We have already referred (in Chapter 1) to disadvantageous social conditions that tend to be associated with special health service needs: for example, living in substandard houses or overcrowded households, or living in families that are constantly on the move or heavily dependent on supplementary benefits and social services, or in which there are adult members with chronic physical or mental illness.

9.24 We have wished to avoid a categorisation of children "at risk" on account of selected social factors, similar to registers of children kept by health departments of children "at risk" on account of medical and other factors in their history. This might limit concern inappropriately to certain groups of children at the expense of others among whom there might still be individual children in need of special health surveillance. Health Department "At Risk" Registers were in fact intended as an economical substitute for total child population screening, the expectation being that children with handicaps would be found principally among those in whom certain high-risk factors could be demonstrated. In practice, "At Risk" Registers (as presently understood) have not proved satisfactory. Not only do we reject an extension of their use in relation to the health surveillance of children who experience social disadvantage; *we endorse the view of a Working Party* [10] *on Risk Registers that health departments should cease to use them.* (In Appendix F we quote the arguments against their retention that were set out in the Working Party's Report.) What is more

---

[10] Report of the Working Party on Risk Registers (Chairman: Professor Thomas Oppé) (1972). Unpublished report of the Department of Health and Social Security.

important is that in their health surveillance of all children, health care staff should recognise in the case of each child any factor that should alert them to a greater than average risk of ill-health, developmental disorder or handicap occurring in that child.

The Rôles of the GPP and CHV

9.25 The schedule of interviews suggested above indicates how the responsibility for carrying out a basic programme of health surveillance might be shared between CHV and GPP.

9.26 The child health visitor is the key person in this partnership; she has a crucial rôle in the discovery of all young children living in her neighbourhood and she is responsible for initially visiting their families and subsequently maintaining contact with them either in their homes or in child health clinics. In her new rôle (outlined in Chapter 7) she will be able to provide more complete health care than in the past by providing nursing care in illness treated at home. Yet as a child health visitor she will have more time than health visitors have at present to concentrate on health surveillance of children. As a result of her special training and subsequent experience we anticipate that she will be able to bring to health surveillance the necessary skill in monitoring child development and the quality of counselling and expertise in guiding and supporting parents that the work requires.

9.27 *As a member of the primary health care team the child health visitor should herself undertake some developmental examinations.* Fears have been expressed that these could not be properly carried out by health visitors because they are skilled assessment procedures for which medical training is necessary. We think this may be true in respect of some children and these would be the ones that the child health visitor would refer to the GPP but we do not think this is true of the majority, given that child health visitors are properly trained for their tasks. The basic surveillance programme provides ample safeguards since it is proposed that the GPP should himself carry out some examinations; and since the two are working together, mutual consultation will follow. Health visitors are already sharing these examinations in a number of surveillance programmes, some of which are being carefully studied. Evidence so far indicates that health visitors may be as discriminating as doctors in recognising children who need full investigation of health or development, just as they may be in reaching decisions regarding the urgency of treatment and management advice.[11]

9.28 If the child health visitor is to spearhead integrated child health care in this way her case-loads will need re-adjusting from those currently recommended. Allowance must also be made for the special needs of particular populations eg those in disadvantaged neighbourhoods. There will consequently be a need for a considerable increase in the total health visiting staff in some districts. The organisational implications of this are taken up in Chapter 17.

9.29 In addition to carrying out medical assessment at two key periods during a child's first five years, the GPP will provide primary medical support to CHVs,

[11] Moore, M F, Barber, J H, Robinson, E T, and Taylor, T R (1973). First contact decisions in general practice. *Lancet.* 1, 817–822.

either through consultation or the referral of individual children. Between them, the GPP and CHV undertaking health surveillance must have the professional capability of dealing with any query raised about the health and development of children. This means that they must receive training of appropriate breadth and depth for their respective rôles and also that they establish close links with staff in the supporting services and especially those in the district handicap team.

9.30 As we have explained in paragraph 9.13 the introduction of the GPP will allow one primary care doctor to provide both preventive and therapeutic health care to many more children than at present. The importance of this unitary approach to child health care is such that *we think any doctor who undertakes the serial observation of health and physical growth and the monitoring of developmental progress of children should also be in a position to prescribe for a child any medical treatment that he may consider necessary and to seek consultant opinion if he so desires.* This has important implications for the organisation of services and the training of clinical medical officers who become child health practitioners (CHPs) during the transition period. These we discuss in detail in Chapters 19 and 20, respectively.

Essentials in the Setting and Approach

Home Visiting

9.31 The CHV's rôle as a child and family nurse in health and illness, and her access to the child in his home, give her unique and essential opportunities to observe young children in their natural environment. In present general practice, the tendency towards fewer home visits by GPs makes this contribution to a continuing relationship between the primary health care team and the family even more important. Home visiting is relatively expensive in time but it often provides more effective help and yields more pertinent information than visits by the mother and child to a clinic or surgery. It is essential for contact with clinic non-attenders. *We are convinced that home visiting has an indispensable and increasing place in the future child health services.*

Clinics

9.32 We use the word "clinics" to imply a service rather than a building. They have a very important rôle in enabling and educating mothers to care for their children. We are concerned, therefore, at the continued fall-off in attendance after the early months following birth. *We recommend that a national study be made of the reasons why mothers do not attend clinics regularly.* In the meantime, there are certain ways in which it seems to us these services might be made more effective.

9.33 Many mothers nowadays cannot attend clinics held during conventional working hours; clinics therefore need to be organised in a more flexible manner. This means that some clinics should be provided in the evenings and on Saturdays. We realise that all CHVs, like GPs, will find that a proportion of the families need services at times outside their normal working hours but *when, if the needs of the children and parents are to be acceptably met, a substantial part of the work has to be carried out at unusual hours they should receive additional payment, and compensatory time off-duty.*

9.34 Many mothers will not attend clinics if they have to travel any distance to reach them. A distance that appears reasonable to a car-driving professional or child-free user of public transport does not feel the same when a mother has several children with her, especially if her normal daily routine is lived within a very small geographical radius. *More experiments should therefore be made in providing clinics in mobile units.* They might be combined with other travelling services, such as toy libraries and play buses, that are known to have been successful and to have modified previous patterns of apathy or even hostility to the services concerned.

9.35 An effective clinic can be arranged in special "clinic" premises, in health centres, GPs' surgeries and hired premises such as church halls, provided they are *appropriately designed or adapted for clinic use.* Many hired premises and GP surgeries are not. It is important that clinics should be sited close to other services and amenities, and there would be advantages if places with which mothers are already familiar such as GP surgeries could be so adapted that health surveillance could be carried out there, under good conditions. The premises need to be made as attractive as possible. The design and décor should be child-oriented. Rooms should be sufficiently large, ventilated and illuminated; they need to be cheerful and informal. The areas used for clinical assessments should be adequately insulated, be large enough for assessment of vision and hearing, and part of the floor at least should be carpeted. Nursery furniture and equipment is essential. It is also desirable that clinics should serve a social function, such as 1 o'clock clubs, mother and baby clubs, toy libraries and book clubs.

9.36 In some places social workers do sessional work in conjunction with child health clinics and handle particular problems brought to them by health visitors or by mothers who already see the clinic as a source of help. We would like to see the potential value of these sessions more fully realised. The relief of the isolated mother of a new baby meeting in a group where others are experiencing similar physical, mental and emotional stresses is enormous; the value of this group for giving her support, informal advice and time with other mothers is insufficiently recognised. Some clinics do run regular mothers' groups which are topic centred but there is also a need for more unstructured groups which look at the problems of early parent/child relationships and enable mothers to gain support and understanding from one another without the loss of self-respect that is often attendant upon seeking individual help from a professional worker. If groups of this kind were more generally accepted, specific groups could be provided for parents at particular risk, for example the parent at risk of battering, or the parents of a handicapped child. There was frequent testimony in the evidence submitted to us which showed the loneliness and tension of parents particularly mothers with problems they felt no one could share. The running of such groups for parents may require the additional skills of a social worker experienced in group work and *we suggest that part-time sessional work of this kind should be given serious consideration* in spite of the shortage of trained social workers.

9.37 The CHV is the key person at the clinic but as much GPP time as possible should be available thereby saving time for families as well as staff. The

142

organisation of the clinic will require a judicious blend of the appointment system and "open door" access: the former to ensure efficient whole-population surveillance, the latter to allow crises and emergencies to be dealt with without delay.

Links with Social Services

9.38 Social Services departments provide many services for children under five, including day nurseries, day centres and play groups. They are used by families with a wide range of social problems. Children from such families also attend nursery schools and private play groups. There is considerable overlap in the functions of these services and parents tend to use what is available. For this reason there should be the maximum coordination of the facilities and liaison between the professional staff; *we think the CHV should have a continuing involvement in the health surveillance of children placed in these settings.*

Records

9.39 Good records do not themselves constitute good practice but they may do much to encourage it: the converse is also true. There would be considerable advantage for the child and for the efficiency of the integrated child health services if a system of record keeping were devised which included information concerning both health surveillance and illness. The record should be continuously maintained from birth until school leaving age and possibly later. This is a complex matter which has to be considered in the context of NHS record systems as a whole. *We therefore recommend that a national system of child health records be considered by appropriate experts.*

CHAPTER 10

HEALTH FOR EDUCATION

Educational Medicine Defined

10.1 The extent to which a child is able to benefit from education is directly related to how far his health and normal development have been promoted. Growth and learning are of necessity connected. The child health and education services must see themselves as engaged to a large extent upon different aspects of a common task and our proposals urge and require the closest cooperation between them.

10.2 We have tried to frame our proposals for the educational health services of the future in a way that will recognise and be in harmony with the deep-seated trends in educational philosophy which have been represented to us. Increasingly in the future schools are likely to place at the centre of their thinking a concern for the effectiveness of the learning system taken as a whole—curriculum content, styles of learning, personal relationships and the day to day school organisation—and the relationship of all this to the world experienced by the children outside school.

10.3 In nursery education this will be characterised by a closer relationship with the family and other caring services and particularly the social services. The family is recognised as the most important influence on the young child. A prerequisite of successful "pre-school" services is that the family should feel supported, and not be made to feel inadequate. The objectives of teachers, child health visitors and child doctors must be to increase both parents' understanding of their child's needs and their skills.

10.4 We have been impressed by what we have learned of the determination of primary and secondary schools to continue to move away from providing education solely through "direct teaching" towards creating of the school a learning community. At the nub of this philosophy is the realisation that children are at least as much affected by the value system and implicit assumptions of the school (sometimes called the "hidden curriculum") as by its advertised mores. Values of hard work, self-discipline, caring for others and working cooperatively as well as competitively can only thrive if the school is organised and the pupils, teachers and parents actually relate to one another according to the principles advocated. Such an educational philosophy makes new and, we believe, welcome demands on health service staff if they are to work with the schools appropriately.

10.5 The physical health of children has improved immeasurably this century. At the same time there is still a substantial amount of acute illness and injury in school children, and there are many pupils with physical and mental handicap and developmental and learning disorders. Teachers may at any time need help with these children in school.

10.6 Behavioural problems of children, especially in secondary schools, are causing considerable concern to teachers and parents. Some of these arise from the experience of failure at school—not only of academic failure, of which reading retardation is a prominent sign—but equally of a growing sense in the adolescent of being out of touch with the things and values held to be important by the adults in the school and the "successful" among his peers. The inevitable reaction of these children is to scorn the teachers and contemporaries who value things they themselves cannot get to grips with. An emotional wedge may thus be driven between ourselves and our children and, perhaps worse still, between child and child. It is to be hoped that by adapting curricula, methods and above all the ethos of the school more Heads and their staffs will find ways of reducing what has been called "induction into the culture of failure". But it will never be entirely removed and in any case there are other and often less manageable sources of emotional disturbance in shool children, ranging from the personal experience of adolescence through social and cultural deprivation to pathology. These are considered in more detail in Chapter 15. Yet the distinction between normal and abnormal behaviour during puberty and adolescence is often difficult and teachers also need help in these matters.

10.7 Although there are shortcomings in the existing school health services and unacceptable regional differences, the total body of knowledge and commitment that has been created since they were founded in 1907 is of inestimable value and must not be squandered. School doctors and nurses have based their work not only on symptoms of disorder but upon an understanding of the whole functioning of the developing and dependent individual. And they have appreciated that the child is not only an individual but also, especially in the processes of learning, a member of many inter-relating groups. It is these insights and this methodology that will be required in the future, especially as the health services for children turn more and more to preventive measures now that many diseases and disorders have been brought under control. The momentum must not be lost.

10.8 Surveying the educational scene as a whole we are convinced that there is an urgent and proven need for the new, unified child health service which we have proposed to build upon existing foundations in providing a more comprehensive health care for children in school. *There is a body of knowledge and practice, both preventive and therapeutic, which can be recognised as educational medicine.* A simple definition might be:

"Educational medicine is the study and practice of child health and paediatrics in relation to the processes of learning. It requires an understanding of child development, the educational environment, the child's response to schooling, the disorders which interfere with a child's capacity to learn, and the special needs of the handicapped. Its practitioners need to work cooperatively with the teachers, psychologists and others who may be involved with the child and to understand the influences of family and social environment".

10.9 The primary objectives of the child health service in relation to the education of children and support of the schools and the LEA are:

(i) to promote the understanding and practice of child health and paediatrics in relation to the process of learning;

146

(ii) to provide a continuing service of health surveillance and medical protection throughout the years of childhood and adolescence;

(iii) to recognise, and ensure the proper management of what may broadly be described as medical, surgical and neurodevelopmental disorders insofar as they may influence, directly or indirectly, the child's learning and social development, particularly in school but also at home;

(iv) to ensure that parents and teachers are aware of the presence of such disorders and of their significance for the child's education and care;

(v) to give advice and services to the LEA as required in the Education Act and the NHS Reorganisation Act.

The Work of Doctors and Nurses in Schools

10.10 For these objectives to be achieved, doctors and nurses are required who will work with teachers and others in the schools as partners in a joint enterprise with the parents. *Every school needs to have a doctor and nurse nominated as their school doctor and school nurse who are suitably qualified and knowledgeable about educational medicine and nursing,* and have sufficient time to get to know their schools and to meet the teachers regularly.

10.11 Between them, the doctor and nurse need to carry out a programme of health surveillance, and if necessary immunisation, on each child in the school; to acquaint teachers, psychologists and parents of any condition which might affect a child's educational progress and to advise and discuss with them the implications for teaching and the care of the child in school; to provide or ensure treatment for those children who need it, especially handicapped pupils; to maintain liaison between the school and other primary care and hospital staff; to participate in the advisory and counselling arrangements for boys and girls, and in health and social education programmes, in school; and to concern themselves with the environmental health of the school, the standards of hygiene especially in relation to school meals, and in the prevention and control of outbreaks of infectious diseases in the school.

10.12 The school doctor will need to undertake further medical examinations of some children at varying intervals. He will also have to advise which children for medical reasons need free milk from the age of seven, special transport to school, or special education. He will need to examine children who wish to seek employment out of school hours, and advise careers officers and the Employment Medical Advisory Service regarding medical conditions that might affect the employment of school leavers, especially those with handicaps. He should provide help for teachers in the management of pupil's emotional and behaviour problems in school, and involve the child psychiatric service in the more difficult cases. He should be alert to signs that might indicate child abuse and the need to obtain advice from social workers and he should take part in discussions with social workers and teachers about the welfare and future of school children who are in the care of the local authority. The school doctor should contribute to community-based district activities such as epidemiological studies and research in educational medicine.

10.13 The rôle of the nurse in relation to education is of the utmost importance and in the past it has tended to be overlooked and under-valued. The school

147

nurse is required to be the representative of health in the everyday life of the school. It is she who mainly provides health surveillance of school children through her annual hygiene interviews, and she is indispensable in the early recognition of sensory and other disorders. The school nurse will frequently be the first point of contact in the school on most health service matters, and she will be the person most concerned in maintaining continuous direct and regular contract with teachers over relevant health and family problems of individual children and in maintaining liaison between the home and the school on matters of health. She should be concerned particularly with the health of those children who may be inadequately cared for at home. She has a special contribution to make in the curriculum planning and provision of health education in the school, and in individual health teaching and counselling of pupils.

10.14 For the objectives of the child health service in schools to be achieved there is a further need for primary health care and education staff to have support and advice from various specialised services, particularly from consultant community paediatricians and child psychiatric staff, and from speech therapists and physiotherapists. This support and treatment of the child also needs at times to be provided actually in the school. Most special schools need regular consultant services, including those of allied specialists, such as medical audiologists and orthopaedic surgeons.

The Function of Specialists in Community Medicine and Nursing

10.15 The position of the Local Education Authority needs special attention. The LEA needs to be able to plan its services in the light amongst other things of full and continuing advice from the Area Health Authority. The NHS Reorganisation Act made AHAs responsible for providing health staff and services the LEA might need in carrying out its duty to provide special education for handicapped pupils and to perform certain miscellaneous functions for pupils involving medical advice or action. DHSS Circular HRC(74)5 and Welsh Office Circular WHRC(74)7 set out the various responsibilities of AHAs and required them to appoint a Specialist in Community Medicine (Child Health), a Senior Nursing Officer and a Senior Dental Officer to discharge them. We discuss in Chapter 21 certain features of the organisation of health services in support of LEAs and the functions of the staff mentioned above, but we wish to stress from the outset that our recommendations in this present chapter recognise this general duty towards the LEA which is laid upon the AHA.

Proposed Programme of Health Surveillance

10.16 *The pattern of health surveillance for school children that we propose below should be seen as a continuation of that suggested for children in the years before school.*

During pre-school years

| At 6–10 days | examination by doctor trained in neonatal paediatrics. |
| At 6 weeks | examination by GPP, CHP or consultant paediatrician, or in the case of non-attenders by CHV. |

148

At 7–8 months ⎱ 18 months ⎰	review of development by CHV.
At 2½–3 years	review of development as appropriate and vision testing by GPP or CHP: dental examination by a dentist.
At school entry: 4½–5 years	review of health and development by GPP or CHP acting as school doctor: dental examination by a dentist.

During school years

Annually up to the age of 13–14 years	health care interview with a school nurse, including a vision test and measurement of height and weight; dental examination by a dentist.
Twice during primary education	hearing test by school nurse.
At approximately 13 years	interview with the school doctor.

There are two crucial periods in relation to education when every child would be seen by a doctor: on entering school and at about the period of puberty.

Primary School Period

10.17 We have been convinced of the value of a medical assessment of every child before he goes full-time to school. The purpose of such a pre-entry examination is two-fold: to review the child's state of growth and development, with special reference to sensory and neurological development, before he starts school in order to make sure that he does not have conditions for which treatment has been overlooked or neglected; and to consider what is collectively known about the child by child health staff so that, in the light of his present state and for the benefit of his education, teachers may be informed and advised about his special needs in school. Every effort has to be made to arrange this examination so that the parent(s) can be present for their contribution is vital. The child health visitor should also be present not only because of her special rôle in the child's health surveillance during pre-school years but also to maintain the primary health care team approach to educational medicine. Following this assessment, teachers should learn directly from the doctor and nurse about conditions which require their informed response and understanding. In this way they would acquire greater insight into the pupils in their charge and feel more secure and adequate in teaching those with special needs. Once the child has entered school the observations of teachers will be added to what is known about him and in some cases there will be the need for further discussion with health service staff. Entry to school is a significant experience for the child and may be harmful if it goes wrong; it is in the tradition of the school health service wherever possible to prevent difficulties and disorders from arising. The importance of this examination and the opportunity that compulsory attendance at school present for introducing total health care cover for all children, are such that *we recommend the "entrant" examination should again be statutory.*

10.18 An entrant examination of the kind we have outlined takes 20–30 minutes to perform. Three further medical examinations, even of shorter duration, of every child during his school life could place an intolerable burden on medical manpower. However, we are satisfied that these *further routine examinations are not necessary and should be discontinued* (see paragraph 10.24). We believe a more efficient and rewarding system of health surveillance would be one based upon a network of serial screening of vision, hearing and growth and of annual health care interviews by the school nurse, with increasing encouragement to children as they get older to refer themselves to the school doctor or nurse; on vigilance by teachers who in future would be better trained to recognise children who are ill or in difficulties; and on regular meetings between doctors, nurses, teachers and psychologists. If at any time during school life the pupil seemed to be failing to thrive, his teacher would know that the school doctor would welcome being brought into consultation. This we regard as the most important safeguard of all—a trust and understanding between teachers and nurses and doctors based on regular discussion and shared in-service training.

10.19 An annual test of vision is desirable up to and through the pubertal phase of growth; and during the primary school years a child's hearing should be tested at least twice. Such a schedule of sensory screening is already standard practice in many authorities and should become universal. We are aware that serial measurement of children's height and weight has gone out of fashion, possibly because they were not recorded on standardised charts giving the normal range and so the evidence of growth delay or decline was missed. Nevertheless, these measurements are among the few well standardised procedures available to health workers and we believe they are valuable as a screening device to help alert staff to nutritional and growth deficiency which may, after all, be a danger signal to a wider variety of deleterious circumstances. *These three serial screening procedures would best be included in the annual health care interview between school nurse and child.* This would allow a trained person to cast an eye (and ear) over the general health and development of each child once a year; we regard this as essential for proper health surveillance.

Secondary School Period

10.20 Throughout the child's secondary school life, surveillance by the school nurse needs to continue with the school doctor being available at any time on referral of the child by the nurse, the teachers or the parents. In addition, however, *every boy and girl at about the age of* 13 *should have a private interview with the school doctor.* The purpose of this would be to allow the pupil to discuss general matters concerning health and development and especially to establish a link with a doctor for reasons other than sickness. We think this would help to create a basis for continuing confidence on the part of the growing individual (the parent of the future) in the positive and helpful attitude of health workers and the opportunities that exist to make use of health services. It is not suggested that it should be a conventional medical examination. The doctor would so approach the situation that the pupil would be given the opportunity to identify himself as a young person with or without problems of a physical, emotional or academic nature with which he required help. The timing of the interview is related to the onset of puberty and early adolescence for many pupils and also to the need to make decisions at about the age of 13–14 on appropriate educational courses. If the records have been adequately maintained the doctor and teachers would already know of any areas of difficulty being experienced by the child or noted by his teachers and parents. It would be at this point that the value of the services available to young people could be made clear and encouragement given to further discussion, with or without the parent being present. The parents would always be informed of the 13-year interview usually in the same way as they would be informed of the child's academic progress, careers interviews and other important stages in school life. However, the value of treating the pupil as a young adult would be lost if it were a requirement that a parent should be present at the first stage of the interview. Should further medical examination or treatment prove to be necessary the parent would be fully involved subsequently. Parents should in any case know that at any time they can ask to meet the doctor or nurse to discuss their child's health and development.

10.21 In most cases the 13-year interview would reassure the pupil that all was well. In others it might permit adult intervention at a time when for some neither school nor home is an acceptable authority, and might help to prevent the all too frequent breakdown of relations between the young person and the adults with whom he is in daily contact. It can be anticipated that these interviews will reveal some problems which may more appropriately be dealt with by other professionals, and an adequate system of liaison needs especially to be built up with social workers and others who are able to provide specialised services for adolescents.

10.22 The 13-year interview would be an integral part of the counselling services and programme of social education provided by the school, for the problems of adolescence are not only physical but also emotional, social, moral and economic. Secondary schools have responded in a variety of ways to the need to create personal counselling services. We have studied a number of these and noted differences of philosophy in their approach. Their common feature is the desire of teachers to build up good relationships with children, especially those who have problems, and maintain a positive link between school and home. It is essential for health care staff to be able to participate in this work, not only because the youngster's health may be involved but also because a relationship built up solely on a teacher/counsellor/pupil basis cannot readily be taken into the adult world and indeed cannot easily be continued outside the school.

10.23 For this reason, and because social, health and development problems requiring help do not necessarily commence or provoke referral by the age of 13, there needs to be a health advisory service continually available in the school, and which pupils should be encouraged to use. The school nurse will more often provide this than the school doctor, because of her more frequent sessions in school, but *the school doctor also needs to have a regular clinic in school which adolescent pupils should be able to attend,* if they choose, independently and in confidence. The need for such advisory services extends beyond the school, and these are discussed more fully in Chapter 15. Some counselling services already exist outside the school, and school doctors and nurses and the teachers, need to be fully aware of what is available.

10.24 We know that in the past some local education authorities have carried out a series of medical examinations of pupils at pre-determined ages during school life, and others have found it helpful to arrange selective medical examinations of older pupils as a result of questionnaires to their parents and teachers.

Both periodic and selective examinations unavoidably mean that the examination is carried out at an arbitrary stage in the pupil's life decided by the authority and not by the individual. They also occupy a great deal of time of doctors and nurses and we are not convinced that either pattern of health surveillance is any longer justified by the benefits to the children or to their parents and teachers. This is why we are advocating a more flexible pattern, that allows for individual needs at the time they arise.

10.25 Having explained our proposed health service for primary and secondary schools we wish to make a recommendation which we believe would greatly assist the health services to provide for children who may require additional health care but who are failing in the ordinary way to receive it. Because of the importance of medical opinion on certain rare occasions when the health and perhaps the safety of a child may be at stake (as in suspected cases of non-accidental injury) we believe it should be within the power of a head teacher to request and consent to the medical examination of that child. For all school children therefore *we recommend that the school doctor should have the right to examine a child, if necessary without the consent of the parents, if there is in the opinion of the head teacher reasonable grounds for concern.* If this requires a change in the law, then we recommend the necessary change should be made. We would not wish to modify a child's present legal position in regard to permitting medical examination of himself. As we see it, our recommendation is fully compatible with the rôle of the teacher acting in loco parentis in respect of a pupil's health, as of other matters.

Education for Health

10.26 Education for health has become of greater significance because, individual behaviour has a greater effect on individual health than was apparent a generation ago. It is now within the power of an individual in our kind of society to improve his own life prospects and those of his children by his own behaviour. This is indeed part of the general shift in our lifetime towards a greater control over the environment—with all the connected problems of man's tendency to behave irrationally. Improved health education may therefore be the most promising opportunity to extend preventive medicine now available to us. Its goal is to strengthen individual "health behaviour". The question is how it can be effectively pursued.

10.27 Epidemiological studies may establish causal relationships between certain behaviour and certain illness (eg smoking and lung cancer). But the behaviour in question is not only individual but also social and, in its origin, may have nothing to do with the individual's perception of health or illness. A rational approach which merely demonstrates cause and effect is unlikely to be successful—especially with vulnerable groups or individuals who are especially prey to advertising, poor social conditions, or stress. Indeed there is an unavoidable conflict, even for a rationalist, between, for example, risking cancer in the future and finding relief from stress in smoking now. In other words a solely factual and objective approach to health education by itself is unlikely to be satisfactory.

10.28 Changes in society's attitude to behaviour are also fundamental to much that is subsumed within health education. Attitudes to divorce, contraception, abortion and religious belief for example, have to be clarified before immature boys and girls can be helped towards personal decisions on morals and conduct which may affect their health and that of others. The question presses in: are the "experts" (doctors and teachers for example) to be left to make these decisions about the thought-context of health education or is there a will within a wider community to take this responsibility?

10.29 Within the more limited field of health education in the school curriculum it mus' be recognised that the schools themselves have widened their objectives and enlarged their methodology in the past generation. Relations between pupil and teacher have become less formal; there is more emphasis on curricula with direct relevance to the lives of the pupils and their future; and more encouragement to the pupils to think for themselves. There is a willingness to make a contribution from the school to the community; but less willingness to accept unjustified social structures or status relationships. In short the good school tries to come clean with its pupils about both its aims and its methods. A health education programme that was not equally honest would have a hollow ring in such a community. We also think that improved relationships between teachers and the health services and a better perception by the boys and girls of the efforts being made to keep their own health under surveillance would have a marked effect on the efficancy of health education.

10.30 If our recommendations for health surveillance were accepted the child's awareness and understanding of the care provided for him by the health service would develop as he progressed from dependency to independence. In parallel with this he should acquire a knowledge of normal growth and development and the part the individual himself can play in the process needed for healthy living.

10.31 We warmly welcome the tendency, especially in secondary schools, for the nexus of topics connected with health education to be taken as a serious subject of study and discussion by senior teachers whose experience of life is as important to their success as their mastery of fact. We have been impressed by the quality of the teaching materials created by the Schools Council project on Health Education for children aged 5–13. We also welcome the increased involvement of health service staff in health education in schools. But we urge that society should not leave the job solely to the schools and that where necessary the same degree of thought should now be applied to the other programmes of health education mounted within the community through, for example, child health clinics, health visitors, general practice, TV and press advertising.

10.32 We find the DHSS circular on Health Education (HRC(74)27) disappointing in many respects and hope that the low priority proposed for health education in it will not prevent authorities from creating an impetus.

Education for Parenthood

10.33 Within the general topic of education for health there is, for those concerned with child health, the specially important area of education for parenthood. We began our consideration of this in CHAPTER 8. There is a strong desire to find ways of improving the general quality of "parenting" and the schools and other educational agencies are expected to contribute to this programme. While acknowledging that the duty exists and ought to be fulfilled as far as possible, it is important not to advocate naive solutions.

10.34 Being a "good parent" is not simply a matter of having the right knowledge, or even the right skills. So much also depends on the personal characteristics of the child (and other children) and parents involved; their social and economic condition; their ability to cope with stress; their relationships with one another; their sensibility to the aspirations and needs of others. Thus, even if there were an agreed body of knowledge about parenting to be transmitted (and there is not) and one could work on the assumption that knowledge always changes behaviour (which one cannot), it would still be necessary to bear in mind how much the inter-personal relationships and integrity of the parents affect their ability to be successful. So many previous well-meaning programmes aimed at changing behaviour for the benefit of health have fallen short of their objectives that we urge that any programme of education for parenthood should be based on principles rather than prescriptions.

10.35 Attention to improving an individual's general ability to cope with life is the chief issue and should in any case be a primary objective of schools. To the extent that it is achieved it will help pupils to cope better in the future as parents. Emphasis should be placed on skills in inter-personal relationships, in communication and in helping children to understand themselves and the world around them. There is a place for the teaching of normal child development and about the psychological needs of children. But old heads cannot be put onto young shoulders and in any case the limits of what we know should be emphasised so that the feeling that they are not "experts" does not undermine another generation of parents who would probably cope very well if they trusted a trained commonsense. This training should emphasise that there is no single answer to a general problem such as aggressive behaviour in a child. Such behaviour may stem from one of a number of causes and parents must be helped to understand that appropriate response depends on understanding the cause not the symptom. They also have to appreciate that children affect their parents; the process is not all one-way. The larger the family the more subtle and teasing this influence probably becomes. If this is the approach to education for parenthood which seems most intelligent in the present state of our knowledge, then two things are clear. The programme within the school curriculum cannot be just a "course" or even a thread running through several courses; it must be concerned with the whole development of the pupil's personality and concerned to promote knowledge of certain principles at appropriate stages. Nor can it be confined to the period the "parents" spend at school; opportunities must be found to improve understanding of these principles when the parents are actually meeting the problems and the pleasures of having to bring up a child and when there will be a reality to what they learn. The health centre, the nursery class, the child health visitor, educational visitor and adult education service, are only some of the more obvious agencies that should be orchestrated in this work within the community.

Special Education for Handicapped Children

10.36 The interdependence of the health and education services is nowhere more marked or necessary than in the education of handicapped children. The 1944 Education Act placed a duty upon every LEA to "ascertain" which children in their area required "special educational treatment" and subsequently defined various "categories" of handicapped pupils as a guide to the provision of appropriate special schools.

10.37 Since then, a sea-change has come over the special educational scene leaving no aspect the same. Formal ascertainment procedures have been widely discarded as unnecessary and undesirable. Sharp categories of handicap have been softened following appreciation of the extent to which handicaps overlap and are inter-related. Special education is now seen not as one thing but a continuum of specially contrived educational provision extending from the ordinary school without special help (except for visiting advisory staff) to special class, special day school, boarding school, hospital school, remedial centre, child guidance centre, or home tuition, according to the needs of the child. The Education Act 1970 formally recognised the obligation on the part of local education authorities to provide special education for severely mentally handicapped children who were formerly considered to be "unsuitable for education in school" —which for most of them had meant in practice "ineducable". There is an increasing desire to include the handicapped child within the normal school as far as possible and to provide his special education as part of his individual curriculum. For the child who needs to attend a special school special education is now regarded as a bridge leading or returning the child to his local school. There is a will to start earlier, to know more of the general field of education and to pay more heed to the life the child will have to live after school.

10.38 These changes have brought into sharper focus three features of the scene that affect the contribution of the professions principally concerned. First, the needs of many handicapped children are apparent from the earliest stages of life. The point at which the education service should make a contribution to assessment and management of the child cannot be related solely to chronological age. *We therefore recommend that the present legal limitation upon the power of LEAs to make this contribution before the age of two years (already ignored in the best services) should be removed.*

10.39 Second, the real cause of educational failure may lie in the individual's psyche or physical health or in the environment of home, school or society. To disentangle the strands is beyond any single expertise. Medical, social and psychological advice have therefore to be available if the child is to receive the best education that can be offered, and a full team approach with the teacher will sometimes be essential.

155

10.40 Third, the distribution of handicapped children between ordinary and special schools and the balance of the special school population has been strikingly altered both in the type and severity of handicap. More children with serious physical handicap now remain in their own schools whilst children in special schools are more likely to be severely handicapped in more ways than one. This is especially the case with severely mentally handicapped children; now a quarter of all the special schools are for these pupils who constitute 20% of the special school population. These changes call for a larger contribution from doctors and nurses in ordinary schools and a stronger and more regular health service in special schools in order to supervise the health of these children, support the school staff in their management, and to link up with the surveillance and support being given in the home by health and social services staff.

The PROPOSED ORGANISATION of Health Services to Schools

10.41 Since re-organisation the NHS, through Area Health Authorities, has been responsible for meeting all the requirements of the educational health service. Day to day organisation and methodology have remained much as they were in 1974 awaiting this Committee's report and the decisions that must flow from it. We have presented a critique of past practice in this chapter and in CHAPTER 4. Essentially, we do not consider that the separation between therapy on the one hand and health surveillance, health promotion and the assessment of handicapped pupils on the other that has underlain the organisation of the school health service has been beneficial to either the pupils or the service. It is a measure of the failure to appreciate the clinical nature of the educational and child health services that doctors who undertake this work are still regarded as generalists in public health, are not required to be trained in either clinical child health or paediatric practice, or to have knowledge of child development and education. Our proposals for the educational health services, with certain stipulations, offer a new pattern of medical and nursing services. They are based on the general proposition put forward in this report, that there should be a single child health service which integrates preventive and therapeutic medicine, and hospital and community services, and accepts fully its responsibility to search for and extend health care support to those children whose parents do not or cannot seek it for them.

Primary Medical Care
10.42 Primary medical care is to be centred upon the general practitioner and the GPP and *we propose that the latter should also be the school doctor for one or more schools in the vicinity.* This would provide the service the schools need, subject to the following conditions being met:

i. The GPP would be trained in the educational component of child medicine;

ii. The GPP would be in contract directly with the AHA to act as school doctor to certain nominated primary and/or secondary schools. In these schools he would be responsible for the educational health service for all the children registered at the school whether they were on his general practice list or not. (The contractual arrangements are considered in Chapter 17.)

iii. The GPP would have to accept that in some essential aspects of his work he would be part of a managed service. Without this it would not be possible for the SCM(CH) to ensure that the necessary level of service was being maintained. The aspects of his work in the child health services to which this would principally apply are:

providing cover for all children in school

participation in training courses for other health, education and social work staff

undertaking necessary inservice training

the maintenance, updating, interpretation and application of epidemiological data.

For these aspects which relate to the management of the service (as distinct from clinical aspects) the GPP through the "school doctor contract", would be directly responsible to the SCM(CH) thereby making it feasible for the latter to discharge his responsibilities to both LEA and AHA.

10.43 To satisfy the needs of ordinary schools, *we expect two sessions (7 hours) of doctor time to be spent per week of the school year in a larger secondary school (c 1,000 students), and one session per fortnight in a primary school (c 240 children)*. This would allow time for the medical examinations of children prior to their entry to school, the 13 year old interviews in secondary schools and the various other elements of educational medicine that we have described (paras. 10.12 to 10.14). We would also expect some GPPs to wish to take a special interest in the adolescent and therefore work as school doctor to a secondary school and others to concentrate on work with younger children in primary schools.

Supporting Medical Care

10.44 From time to time problems in educational medicine of a more profound nature arise in children in ordinary schools and these require the opinion and advice of staff working in the supporting services. These are most likely to be needed in the case of children with complex handicaps and severe learning disorders. We see it as an important function of the consultant community paediatrician to provide a consultant service in respect of such children referred by GPPs from ordinary schools. We hope such collaboration will take place in schools more often than it has done, so that teachers may take part in subsequent assessment and discussion with the child and his parents. Children with severe behaviour disorders also create serious problems for teachers in ordinary schools. We recognise the need for health care staff and other professionals to be involved in the management of these children but this is a difficult field. The GPP and the school nurse though better trained than school doctors and nurses in the past, will need to be guided through consultations with the staff of child psychiatric services. These matters are discussed more fully in Chapter 15.

10.45 The level and continuity of medical care required by children who attend special schools is also usually of a kind that needs to be provided not as part of primary care by the GPP but by supporting care staff. *We therefore propose that a consultant community paediatrician should be nominated as school doctor to the special schools in his district,* whether these be day or residential. Other consultant specialists, such as orthopaedic surgeons, ophthalmologists, may also need to pay regular visits to certain special schools.

10.46 Appointment to a post of consultant community paediatrician will be made, as to all other consultant posts, by the RHA, or AHA(T); and it will be conditional upon the applicant having had the necessary training and experience in a wide range of paediatrics including educational medicine and the care of handicapped children (see CHAPTER 20). The consultant community paediatrician's contract would need to stipulate that he would be required to act as a school doctor to named special schools in his district and to provide, as necessary, consultant services in educational medicine in respect of children in ordinary schools. As for the GPP so for the consultant community paediatrician, for such aspects of his work that relate to the management of the child health service (as distinct from clinical aspects) he would be directly responsible to the SCM(CH).

Nursing Care
10.47 The nursing needs of children at school should be met by a coordinated service within the global responsibility of the child health visiting service. The scale of organisation of nursing services in schools must be small enough to provide opportunities for continuing and regular contact between teachers and nurses, *and each school should have its nominated school nurse.* The school nurse must be employed by the health authority and kept in touch with the mainstream of her profession.

10.48 We estimate that *each primary school (c240 children) requires 6 hours of nurse time per week and each secondary school (c1,000 pupils) 15 hours during term time.*

10.49 We see the day to day nursing in ordinary schools being carried out by specially trained school nurses rather than by child health visitors themselves, although the latter will retain overall responsibility for the nursing service provided in the schools. Nevertheless, *the school nurse should be an integral member of the primary health care team.*

10.50 The precise pattern of staffing in any district would vary according to the number and location of schools in relation to the practices in which the GPPs work. This is discussed in more detail in Chapter 17. Typically, two child health visitors might be working in primary health care teams with two GPPs and thus be responsible for organising the educational nursing services to 5 primary schools and one secondary school for which the GPPs were the nominated school doctors. Each child health visitor might then supervise one school nurse serving a secondary and two primary schools, or three primary schools, and undertaking duties at special clinics held for school children. The time spent in the schools would be a matter for agreement between the head teacher and the nurses but it would need to be sufficient to include counselling and health education. Both school nurse and child health visitor need to be known to the heads.

10.51 In the larger secondary schools from which we have received reports it is clear that the appointment of a full-time nurse brings considerable advantage. She can provide clinical services required by a community of 1,000–2,000 adolescents and contribute to the planning and teaching of the health education and allied programmes in the school. Besides this, the addition to the adult team of a mature person from a discipline other than education is seen to be desirable by both teachers and pupils. The good nurse, in this situation, becomes one of those adults to whom adolescents may turn with more than their " health " problems. We have received convincing evidence to this effect from both nurses and heads. We recognise the crux that if all large secondary schools were to have a full-time nurse other equally or more important services might go short. Experience so far suggests, however, that the employment of full-time nurses in secondary schools is not predatory upon other parts of the health service because, in the main, the women who seek these appointments are temporarily out of the main stream of the profession and bringing up a family. They are able to take up employment in a school because the working hours of the day and the pattern of school holidays allow them also to meet their family responsibilities. *We recommend, therefore, that AHAs and LEAs should, wherever possible, approve the appointment of a full-time nurse in the larger secondary schools.*

10.52 In special schools the nursing load will vary considerably according to the principal category of handicapped pupil for which the school caters, and to whether the children are resident in the school or only attend daily. *We recommend that a sufficient number of nurses be appointed to each special school to meet its individual requirements, taking account not only of the actual nursing involved but also of the need for the nurses to participate in assessment and counselling.*

Transitional Arrangements
10.53 We realise that the proposed pattern of staffing may take some time to materialise in many parts of the country and that immediate and practicable plans to cover the interim stage are required. They must make the best possible use of the doctors experienced in child health who are now available and must be a help rather than a hindrance to moving towards the preferred pattern. It is especially urgent that the expertise and understanding of the essential relationships between health, education and social services that has been built up over 70 years in the best of the School Health Services should not be lost, and that the health services in schools that are so essential should not be run down.

10.54 These transitional arrangements are discussed in detail in Chapter 19. In short we expect that some of the existing clinical medical officers will become eligible for appointment as GPPs, on a full-time or part-time basis. Where however there is no GPP available to act as school doctor, a child health practitioner would be appointed by the AHA to be school doctor and carry out the full range of duties described in this chapter; he could if necessary also undertake the health surveillance of pre-school children. Wherever possible, the child health practitioner should be attached to one or more general practices; alternatively, he would be based on a local health centre or clinic. Any of these systems would be maintained, with new appointments being made and initial and in-service training provided, until the proposed system based on the GPP could be introduced.

10.55 Similarly, where it is not possible immediately to appoint a consultant community paediatrician in the district, a clinical specialist in paediatrics† would provide an advisory service in educational medicine and the health care of handicapped children for children in ordinary schools, and be nominated as school doctor to special schools in the district.

Training of School Doctors and Nurses

10.56 The most important single need in the child health services within which educational medical and school nursing are to be practised, is a proper training for the GPPs, the consultant community paediatricians, and the school nurses. *We regard training in educational medicine and nursing as essential and it should therefore be mandatory.* The general fields in which training would be required include:

normal growth and development in children;

disorders and diseases that may interfere with a child's capacity to learn;

relevant aspects of child and family psychiatry;

relevant aspects of audiology, speech therapy and physiotherapy;

the education system, its objectives and methods, and the facilities provided for special education;

the functions of teachers, social workers, educational psychologists, speech therapists, physiotherapists and others and viewed as relative and related to those of health workers.

Inter-Professional Collaboration

10.57 We stress the need for both doctors' and nurses' training to give greater understanding of the aims of education and the experience of teachers, and of the rôle of social workers, and to pay more attention to inter-professional collaboration. These are required initially and again during post-graduate training. Joint in-service training of medical, nursing, teaching and social work staff should be arranged by AHAs, LEAs and LASSDs.

10.58 The Committee was not empowered to consider the provision of social work services to schools. Nevertheless our recommendations concerning health services in schools presuppose a comparable development of social work services. We have been at pains throughout our report to emphasise the inter-relationship of health, educational and social factors in a child's development. The length of time that the majority of children spend at school makes it a unique setting in which preventive and remedial work may be

---

† See chapter 19, paragraph 22 et seq.

carried out. Hence it is crucial that the balance between a child's health needs and his educational and social needs be understood, and effective cooperation between the three authorities and between their professional staff be established. Continuity of association as equals seems to us to be the surest method of obtaining this.

10.59 For the doctors and nurses in the child health services, this means that as far as possible they be appointed to provide services to specified communities of children defined with due regard to the schools and other institutions they may attend, and that they assume a more personal professional responsibility than has been customary for seeing that the necessary services reach "their" children. This thinking informs both the proposal for the GPP to have a special contract as school doctor to certain nominated schools in the vicinity of his practice and for the consultant community paediatrician to be under contract to provide supporting services in educational medicine to schools within his district. *We recommend that such direct responsibility for a school or schools within a district be adopted as a matter of principle in the staffing and organisation of educational health services.* Organisational obligations of this kind can only ensure that opportunities are created for inter-professional cooperation. We believe our proposals for the initial and in-service training of staff in general, and of health service staff specifically, will ensure that such opportunities are not ignored. (Training is further discussed in CHAPTER 20.)

Records

10.60 The LEA have a duty to maintain records about children, and the Area Health Authority through the child health service workers must assist appropriately. Our recommendations will be set at nought unless appropriate health records are maintained for individual pupils and the relevant information made available to the education service. Considerable attention has already been given by the DES and DHSS to devising suitable records for both normal and handicapped pupils. We hope these efforts be sustained with a view to the use of standardised records throughout the child health services (see Chapter 21).

Conclusions

10.61 Our references to educational health services and the emphasis we have placed on the need for each school to have its own doctor and nurse might seem to imply that we visualise the continuation of a discrete school health service. This is not our intention, for it would be to depart from our central conviction that continuity of health care for school children no less than other children requires that their health services be based upon primary care by specially trained doctors centred in general practice, with close professional support from consultant paediatricians and allied specialists. This leads rationally to the primary medical component of educational health care being provided by GPPs.

10.62 We believe our recommendations would give the schools and the education authority a service that would incorporate the very best features of the school health service as it has developed since 1908 and allow necessary new developments in both primary and supporting care to take place as part of a new, integrated and much better trained child health service. Every school would have in first line support a school nurse and a school doctor both of whom would be appropriately trained, with time to maintain an interest in educational health care, the learning process and the aims of the education service, and both of whom would have the opportunity to assume a more personal professional responsibility than has been customary for seeing that the necessary services reach "their" children. Every special school would have as their school doctor a consultant paediatrician experienced and skilled in the total health care of handicapped children; and that paediatrician would have the duty to provide consultant services in educational medicine throughout his district. Every LEA would continue to have the advice and expertise of the Area Specialist in Community Medicine (Child Health) and the Area Nurse (Child Health) who would be responsible for planning and ensuring the quality of the services.

10.63 The general change in climate of opinion regarding the rôle of parents in effective education needs to extend to the educational health service so that parents feel more able to understand and make use of the services and feel more supported and needed by them. We believe that our recommendations for the school entrance medical examination, regular health surveillance during school life and better training of and communication between doctors, teachers and parents should facilitate this change of climate.

10.64 Children are seldom asked for their views about services. And yet those who work with children know that they often see things less myopically than adults. We arranged a small enquiry, by questionnaire and group discussion, of Vth and VIth formers. Their opinions and experience of health services (not only the school health service) proved interesting and chastening; they are summarised in Appendix G. We believe that our recommendations for health surveillance could do much to interest children in health services and show how and when they may be helpful and called upon.

CHAPTER 11

ADOLESCENTS

Introduction

11.1 Our terms of reference were to "review the provision made for health services for children up to and through school life . . ." and in preceding chapters we have tried to relate the needs of the unborn, the newborn, infants and children to this provision. We cannot however ignore the maturation of the child to the adult which will generally in its physical aspect occur during school years and in its social aspect be denoted by the transition from school to work or further education. *In recent years it has become increasingly evident that adolescents have needs and problems sufficiently distinguishable from those on the one hand of children and on the other of adults to warrant consideration as a distinct group for health care provision.*

11.2 The period of adolescence is defined by development rather than age. Its chief characteristics are a dramatic acceleration of physical development accompanied by emotional and social changes to all of which the adolescent must learn to adjust. The growth spurt normally takes place in girls between 10½ and 13 and in boys between 12½ and 15 but both the age of onset and the extent of growth are subject to considerable individual variation. Closely allied to this is the development of the reproductive system and the rate of growth and puberty may well be affected by genetic control, nutrition, socio-economic class, illness, exercise and even season of the year. At ages 10–15, there is within any group of boys and girls a range of development from pre-puberty to complete physical maturity. This fact alone raises social and educational problems and may be a contributory factor to the psychological maladjustments seen in some adolescents.

11.3 Once the physical changes of puberty are passed, the dominant aspects of development are social and behavioural, marked by self-discovery and an increasing assertion of independence of family and institutions. The final step to greater autonomy comes with the transition from school to either employment or further education. In this process of growth and transition, health, educational, behavioural, social and employment problems overlap and inter-relate to present complex situations to the statutory and voluntary services.

Physical Disorder and Injury

11.4 In total, adolescents make far less demand than younger children on health services for acute physical disorder. They consult general practitioners less and are less frequently admitted to hospital although for many conditions, they spend longer there once admitted. Of the major causes of admission of 0–19 year olds, respiratory and infectious diseases are largely left behind in early childhood and congenital abnormalities have been remedied to the extent possible or have taken their course. However injuries and musculo-skeletal disease occur with increased frequency in adolescence, as do diseases of the digestive system, particularly appendicitis. Existing conditions such as diabetes or asthma may present fresh difficulties and certain disorders such as genital or menstrual abnormalities and acne arise newly.

163

Accidents

11.5 Accidental injury is the commonest cause of death among adolescents. In 1973 in the 10–19 years age group, there were over 1,500 such deaths of which approximately 1,100 were due to road traffic accidents. For the 15–19 year old, the rate of road traffic accidents is almost twice the rate for the total population. The reasons for this alarmingly high incidence are not entirely clear but in part are no doubt due to the increasing use by older adolescents of mopeds, fast motorcycles and "old bangers" of doubtful mechanical efficiency; to the adolescent's desire for excitement and speed and to his lack of caution; and to the ever increasing volume of traffic on our roads. This is by no means a problem confined to Great Britain alone and on general 1974 figures this country does not compare unfavourably with its European neighbours. Even so, the figures for injury and death due to road traffic accidents are too high for complacency. *We welcome current proposals for the compulsory wearing of seat belts and a more rigorous driving test, though we feel this latter might well be extended to mopeds.* This recommendation stems from the sharp rise in fatal and serious casualties among the 16 year old riders of mopeds following the 1971 regulations precluding them from riding virtually all motorcycles and scooters.

TABLE 1

Fatal and Serious Casualties among Riders of 2-wheeled Motor Vehicles: Great Britain 1971–74

Year	Age			
	16			17
	Motorcycles and Scooters	Mopeds	All	
1971	2,265	95	2,360	2,170
1972	855	280	1,135	2,020
1973	290	690	980	2,500
1974	400	930	1,330	2,740

Source: Department of the Environment.

Although much work has already been done, *we feel strongly that further preventive measures need to be planned, executed and evaluated with urgency by either voluntary or statutory bodies.* These might include vehicle safety, protective clothing and most importantly, appropriate education. As in the case of all accidents, a prompt ambulance service and skilled accident and emergency services should be readily available.

11.6 Because of their exceptional participation in physical exercise, adolescents are also particularly prone to athletic injuries. Teachers of physical education receive special training in the prevention of such injuries insofar as this involves seeing that children are at minimum risk when engaging in sport. They might however look to the GPP/school doctor as a source of further advice on hazards in sport and handling of minor injuries and also for advice on the consequences of physical exercise in children and adolescents who had health problems. The outcome of any injury, the degree of recovery and the extent of permanent handicapping conditions depends not only on the nature of the injury itself but also on the action taken at the time of the injury as well as on subsequent treatment, convalescent care and counselling. The management of minor injuries would generally in the first instance be a matter for the school nurse. Cases of more serious injury would normally be taken straight to the hospital accident and emergency department. The specialised management of specific athletic injuries is still a new and developing area and we welcome the activities of the Association of Sports Medicine which is beginning to fill this gap.

Illness

11.7 Although accidents are the most common cause of death in adolescence, the leading medical cause of death is malignancy. The management of an adolescent who, at the spring of life, becomes the victim of a malignant disorder calls for the highest skills the physician can command in offering support, treatment and information. Other disorders, non-malignant but chronic, will also demand skilled counselling for the adolescent and often for his family to ameliorate adjustment to adulthood. For example, in the past a high fatality rate in infancy and early childhood confined cystic fibrosis to the paediatric age groups but with improved treatment, it is now found with increasing frequency among adolescents and young adults. This raises problems of over-protection and participation in normal teenage life, often necessitating general family counselling as well as genetic counselling. Adolescence also poses particular problems for the diabetic. For some, there may be temporary disturbances in diabetes both at menarche and during menstruation and for many the discipline of a fixed régime is difficult to accept when faced with the increasing and irregular demands of teenage social activities. Difficulties in selecting and obtaining suitable employment are a concomitant of several chronic conditions and the afflicted adolescent will need advice from his medical supervisor as well as sympathetic assistance from his employment counsellor.

Developmental Disorders

11.8 Sexual development may also bring problems with genital or, rather more commonly, menstrual disorders. Irregular menstruation, hypomenorrhoea and dysmenorrhoea are among the most common conditions in this age group for which advice is sought. The onset of menstruation is the overt manifestation of approaching womanhood and ability to reproduce; such irregularities are therefore a cause of much concern and apprehension to adolescent girls and of anxiety to their parents. During this period, physical appearance assumes greater importance and disorders such as acne or irregularities in breast development can give rise to very real emotional difficulties. Obesity likewise can often create special problems since the gradual onset during early childhood may well become exaggerated during the pre-pubertal period when increase in fat is common to girls and sometimes occurs in boys. All these disorders pose both psychological and emotional problems which require particularly sensitive handling by those involved in treatment.

Services

11.9 Both at primary and supporting care levels, adolescents have needs unique to themselves for which improved services should be provided. In the past, insufficient attention has been paid to the training of doctors in understanding their development and problems. *While we do not feel that there is need for specialisation in adolescent medicine, it is inherent in our concept of the GPP that his training should provide him with special skills to meet adolescents' needs and in chapter 10: Health for Education, we have recognised that as school doctor he may develop an interest in one or other end of the age spectrum.* Throughout adolescence the key medical practitioners at primary care level will therefore be the GP or the GPP and since adolescence should be seen as a continuum extending after entry into employment, they should have adequate links with services such as the Employment Medical Advisory Service and the Careers Advisory Service. At hospital level, the services available for the treatment of illness and injury in adolescence are generally those provided for children or for adults. However mature adolescents have little in common with the average child on a children's ward and the ward's routine may be inappropriate for them. Conversely an immature adolescent of 14 or more is often unsuited to the environment of an adults' ward. We feel that there is need for the establishment of more appropriate in-patient facilities in acute hospitals. A special unit for adolescent patients in Manchester is proving successful; patients prefer separate accommodation, bed occupancy is high and medical and nursing staff approve the arrangements. *We therefore recommend that consideration be given to the provision of small adolescent units or failing that, of a partitioned 'adolescent area' in a children's ward.* Decisions on placement should be made on biological rather than chronological grounds and all rigid age limits for admission to children's wards should be abolished. Close collaboration between paediatricians and colleagues in surgical specialties and in adult medicine should be maintained to ensure proper attention to adolescents' needs.

Facilities for Physical Recreation

11.10 In an earlier chapter (2.39) we proclaimed our concern "not only with the prevention of children's illness and death, but with laying the foundations of health in adulthood". In this context we recognise that while appropriate physical activity should be part and parcel of a healthy and balanced way of life at every age, it has perhaps particular relevance for the adolescent. At this stage, not only are there present and future benefits to physical structure and function, but opportunity is afforded for the harmless release of energy and aggression, for the expression of adventurousness and the urge for excitement, and for companionship. Incentives toward physical fitness and away from smoking and other addictions are established, and a framework is provided in which young people can develop a rewarding relationship with concerned but disinterested adults. Most school children take part in some kind of physical activity, but the end of school all too often signals the end of even a nominal involvement in games and sports. The reasons for this sudden and massive drop-out are no doubt basically cultural, but it is only too apparent that lack of facilities and the limitations of official support are crucial. Many countries of differing philosophies have

166

thought it a wise investment enormously to expand the provision for their young people to take part in swimming, athletics, gymnastics, and the many other activities in the vast repertoire of physical recreation. We would emphasise here our conviction of the value of physical activity in enhancing the present and future health of our young people and would urge that special consideration be given to promoting the continued involvement in active games and sports of school leavers in particular.

Social and Behavioural Development

11.11 In the culminating phase of development to adulthood, the dominant aspects are social and behavioural rather than physical. The worst difficulties of congenital abnormalities, of growth and of the repeated infections of childhood are over and the signs of degenerative disease have not yet begun to develop. The adolescent's main problems are therefore not those of ill-health but of emotional adjustment to the adult world, particularly with regard to education and work, sex and integration into the community as an individual. Although this may be a period of emotional and intellectual ferment, most adolescents will make the voyage to self-discovery and independence without the need of professional intervention. For some, however, self-discovery can be painful and the bid for independence hazardous if it outstrips knowledge and maturity. The difficulties have perhaps increased as the earlier onset of puberty reduces the age at which problems have to be faced and the permissiveness of our times demands that the individual exercise greater personal responsibility. That there are casualties is shown by the prevalence in adolescence of psychiatric disorder, unwanted pregnancies, abortions, sexually transmitted diseases and drug and alcohol abuse. Not the least of the problems of this age group are the "runaway children" whose difficulties are exacerbated by their homelessness. Many of these problems have similar implications for the provision of services and in the following paragraphs we outline the main areas of need.

Pregnancy
11.12 The steady decline in the age of menarche and changing social attitudes have led to earlier sexual activity. A study in 1973[1] found that sexual intercourse before marriage is quite common among young people and in recent years, there has been growing concern about the number of pregnancies occurring in young girls, particularly in those under 16 years of age. This number has increased steadily up to 1974 (Statistical Appendix, Tables A15 and A16). It seems likely that substantial numbers of young people are sexually active for several years before seeking advice on contraception though the reasons—whether ignorance, fear or deliberate choice—are unclear. *We feel that this demonstrates the need for better counselling which should be available in different forms from a variety of sources.* Home, school, the health services and voluntary groups have each a part to play; there can be no overall prescription. Since many parents seem unable or unwilling to undertake the sexual education of their children, it is important that the education services should take a more positive part in this work. Within the future integrated health service, the school nurse and

[1] Schofield, M (1973). The Sexual Behaviour of Young Adults. Allen Lane.

the school doctor will be an important source of advice on health matters including sex education and family planning. In addition to more formal teaching there should also be scope for counselling by other staff on a one to one basis as and when their advice is required by individual pupils. We feel this work should be encouraged and extended through the close collaboration of the headteacher, counsellors, the school nurse and the school doctor. This is working well in an increasing number of schools, and particularly so in one that we visited.

11.13 However adolescents spend only a limited time at school and many will in any event be reluctant to turn to school staff of any kind for help or advice. In a memorandum of May 1974, the DHSS asked area health authorities and local authorities jointly to consider providing facilities for counselling the young as an adjunct of contraceptive services. These should cover not only sexual matters but a wide range of health and social problems which young people might wish to discuss with doctors, nurses and social workers. Voluntary groups can be very helpful as can organisations such as Grapevine which are specifically designed to impart information to teenagers. The main need is for counselling services which take account of the adolescent's desire to do his own thing and which are based in a variety of settings which he will find acceptable and be prepared to use. If they are to be successful, they will need to recognise that for some young people sex is an activity undertaken in its own right and not seen in the context of family life or preparation for parenthood.

Abortion

11.14 The majority of pregnant girls are very vulnerable. Their situation is often complicated by educational, financial and other social problems in addition to the psychological repercussions. *When abortion is under consideration, skilled counselling and the opportunity for discussion and advice should be made available before any decision is taken.* This should be undertaken in the manner advocated in the Lane Committee Report([2]) and the DHSS draft paper on arrangements for the counselling of patients seeking abortion—informally, without hurry, in pleasant and private surroundings. Wherever possible and appropriate, the whole family and particularly the boyfriend should be encouraged to participate in counselling sessions though some part of the interview should be undertaken with the pregnant girl alone. We endorse the view of the Lane Committee that pregnant girls in care raise special difficulties in respect of abortion and if they so desire, they should be given the opportunity of discussion with someone not administratively concerned with their care. Also we agree that there is great need for further research into the psychological and sociological characteristics of these girls and their male partners; of the physical effects of abortion upon young girls; and of the psychological and social effects of abortion or of failing to obtain it upon the girl herself and her family.

([2]) Report of the Committee on the Working of the Abortion Act (Chairman: Hon Mrs Justice Lane, DBE) (1974). Department of Health and Social Security, HMSO, London.

Sexually Transmitted Diseases

11.15 Freer sexual activity amongst teenagers is also reflected in the general increase in sexually transmitted diseases since 1970. (Statistical Appendix, Table D14). Sharp increases in 1973 in adolescents have however been followed by a decrease in the occurrence of gonorrhoea during 1974 though syphilis (except in 16–17 year old boys) continued to increase steadily. Its increased incidence in girls during 1974 suggests a trend towards more heterosexual transmission whereas male homosexuals had in recent years been the group at highest risk. Although modern methods of treating gonorrhoea and early syphilis are generally effective, there are many obstacles to checking their transmission. Principal amongst these are the lack of an effective vaccine; the absence of satisfactory serologic screening tests for gonorrhoea; the short incubation period of gonorrhoea and problems of speedy contact tracing; the existence of asymptomatic carriers (possibly 50% of females with gonorrhoea) and the lack of immunity to gonorrhoea conferred by previous infection.

11.16 These problems inevitably mean that at present the only means of control are health education, treatment and contact tracing all of which are particularly difficult to effect among homeless and rootless young people. Moreover we are concerned to note the findings of the *Lambeth and Wandsworth project (1972–1974) that although a high level of knowledge about gonorrhoea amongst at-risk groups encouraged them to seek treatment, it was not effective as a deterrent. Nonetheless for lack of any more effective alternative, *we recommend that all sex education for young people— but particularly that in schools—should include information on the transmission and detection of venereal disease and that publicity campaigns should be concentrated on the at-risk groups.* Health education and counselling services should be freely available in all clinics for the treatment of adolescents with sexually transmitted diseases.

Drug Abuse

11.17 Many of those addicted to or misusing drugs are young people with a variety of problems and often a history of emotional deprivation, disturbance and separation in the family and sometimes institutionalism.[3] The notification system for narcotic addicts has identified only the tip of the iceberg of drug misuse.[4] Although the number of "under-20" narcotic addicts known to the Home Office fell steadily from 1970 to 1974 (Table 2, below), the total number of misusers of drugs for which notification is not mandatory is difficult to estimate.

---

* Undertaken by the Health Education Council in conjunction with St Thomas' Hospital.

[3] Department of Health and Social Security (1975). Better Services for the Mentally Ill. Cmnd 6233, HMSO, London.

[4] Department of Health and Social Security, Annual Report 1974. Cmnd 6150, HMSO, London.

TABLE 2
Number of Under-20 Addicts known to the Home Office: by Age

Year	Under 15 Years	15 Years	16 Years	17 Years	18 Years	19 Years	Total
1970	—	1	1	18	30	92	142
1971	—	—	2	13	34	69	118
1972	—	—	3	13	24	56	96
1973	—	—	2	9	24	49	84
1974	—	—	1	7	15	41	64

It is clear from known notifications that for many addicts the taking of drugs began at an early stage. In one study,[5] 24% of males and 18% of females began taking hard drugs—an opiate or methadone or cocaine—under the age of 17. Only 7% and 9% respectively began taking them when they were aged 25 or over. Misuse of soft drugs, especially of barbiturates, amongst young people appears to be increasing and gives cause for concern.

11.18 Drug misuse differs from other forms of addiction (eg alcohol and smoking) in that it is an offence to be in illegal possession of certain drugs subject to misuse. This fact added to the personal and social problems which may have led to the addiction, and the legal problems caused by it, sometimes explains why these adolescents conceal the need for help. Physical ill-health caused by drugs and exacerbated for some by a homeless and rootless way of life is superimposed on their emotional problems. The Advisory Committee on the Misuse of Drugs has recently recommended that a steering group of doctors direct a campaign aimed at persuading both doctors to reduce their prescribing of barbiturates and members of the public to rely less on hypnotics. As a result the CURB campaign to reduce the prescription and use of such drugs is now well under way and is having encouraging results. The disturbing trend towards multiple drug misuse by young people, particularly the injection intravenously of drugs such as barbiturates not prepared for this form of administration, has led to the proposal that this small but highly disturbed and unstable group of young people could perhaps be helped initially if there was a special residential centre for them which could see how they could be helped. Voluntary agencies in the drugs field, in conjunction with the London Boroughs Association and the health authority are planning to set up such a centre in central London.

11.19 The prevention of misuse, and also the treatment and rehabilitation of addicts, involve a wide range of services both official and voluntary. To be effective close cooperation is necessary between them, particularly health, education, social services and law enforcement authorities. Many of the young persons addicted or misusing drugs are attracted to the activities of voluntary bodies which have a less rigid approach than official organisations. *Prevention can be attempted by better health education and by the*

---

[5] Bransby, E R (1971). A study of patients notified by hospitals as addicted to drugs. Health Trends, November 1971. Department of Health and Social Security.

control of the availability of drugs. In the longer term, health education dealing with health issues in the wider context of young people's problems including their personal relationships, may be the best approach. There have been several experiments in providing general advice and counselling services for young people. It is hoped that these will show whether this approach can contribute to the prevention of drug misuse.

Alcohol Abuse

11.20 While the prevalence of drinking among adolescents is difficult to estimate accurately, it seems likely that it is increasing. As a corollary, there are indications of increases in alcohol-related offences amongst young people. A legal drinking age of 18 means in practice that the actual drinking age may be as low as 15 or 16 because of deceptive appearances, and increased amounts of pocket money have brought alcohol within the teenagers' reach. The effects of alcoholism are deleterious, leading to physical and psychiatric problems in the patient and social problems affecting the patient, his family and society itself. A 1970 study[6] suggested that the prognosis for young alcoholics is particularly poor. Given the general acceptance of alcohol consumption amongst adults, *we feel it unreasonable to demand abstinence of adolescents but would encourage all those involved in health education to promote moderate and controlled drinking habits.* In the past some alcohol advertisements have been directed at the young and we note with approval the recommendations in the Advertising Standards Authority Code of Advertising that advertisements should not be directed at young people nor in any way encourage them to start drinking. So far as we are aware, there are no services designed specifically to help adolescents with drinking problems, though services for alcoholics in general and counselling services for the young undoubtedly offer assistance when it is needed. We understand that the Alcoholism Advisory Committee, set up last year to advise Health Ministers on services for alcoholics and related matters, has studied the available evidence that the consumption of alcohol is increasing among the young and is keeping the matter under review.

Services

11.21 None of these problems is unique to the adolescent and none offers an easy solution. They derive largely from general societal attitudes in which the views of the family, peers and the media have more relevance than the health services.[7] Nonetheless it seems self-evident that the uncertainties and ignorance of his age render the adolescent especially vulnerable and in need of an exceptional measure of support and assistance. Within the school, adolescents are a captive population, thus providing the first and possibly most important opportunity to identify their problems, to advise and help them or to see that they are referred to the appropriate agencies for help. In CHAPTER 10 we have recommended that all 13 year olds be offered an interview with the school doctor. This should define the need for further selective contacts and may establish the foundations for willing self-referral.

[6] Ritson, B and Hassell, C (1970). The Management of Alcoholism. Livingstone, Edinburgh and London.

[7] Millar, H E C (1975). Approaches to Adolescent Health Care in the 1970s. US Dept. of Health, Education and Welfare. Publication No (HSA) 75–5014.

Subsequently *reliance should be placed on informal vigilance by all who come into contact with the adolescents, notably teachers. This is very much the present de facto system but if it is to be effective, it must be improved by training the teachers themselves and by the availability to teachers of expert advice from doctors, nurses, psychologists and social workers.* As in the more physically dominated period of child development, there is likely to be value in intervening at an early stage before a problem can distort the course of development. Hence the need for vigilance, despite many adolescents' resistance to conventionally presented or unsolicited services.

11.22 *In addition to such informal supervision, there should be every opportunity for self-referral by the adolescents themselves to school doctors and nurses.* If such a policy is to succeed, those offering assistance must be not only acceptable in approach and attitude but also readily available and we have recommended elsewhere the regular and frequent commitment of professional staff to particular schools. However the image of authority and the known liaison between school and parents may deter adolescents from seeking individual help from this quarter or from any other general practitioner who is already identified with the family. In such cases, the need for informality, easy access and privacy can perhaps best be met by "walk-in" advice centres. These can be particularly valuable in areas in which homeless, rootless young people congregate since they are particularly likely to shun an organisation which smacks of authority. During our consideration some members of the Committee visited one well-established "open" centre with good professional services and effective contact with local schools. Such self-referral centres are beginning to develop but, as yet, their funding remains dependent on a variety of sources and their policy and organisation variable. We believe that there are strong grounds of principle for believing that if knowledge and advice were available in an acceptable form, much illness and distress might be prevented. We recognise however that this has yet to be clearly demonstrated and *we therefore recommend both further epidemiological study of the pathology of adolescence and the scientific evaluation of a demonstration pilot "walk-in counselling service" (on the lines of the student health service) before resources are invested in the wider development of such services.* Given a successful outcome the provision and responsibilities of such walk-in facilities might be planned in a co-ordinated manner and integrated within the existing statutory services without sacrificing those features such as treatment without appointment which render the centres attractive to adolescents. Since the problems of personal relationships with family, school and peer groups, and sexual relationships are at this age so closely allied, such an advisory service should ideally be able to offer advice, support, prevention, diagnosis and treatment over a wide range of difficulties. These would include contraception, pregnancy testing, screening for sexually transmitted disease, facilities for abortion and counselling of many forms. This approach is widely supported by the teachers and members of youth services we have met.

Smoking
11.23 Finally we should like to add our voice to the current call from many professional quarters for a reduction in cigarette smoking, particularly

172

amongst youngsters. The deleterious effects of smoking have been promulgated only relatively recently and it may be that the impact has yet to be felt fully. Studies([8]) of 5,000 young people in 1961, 1968 and 1971/72 do seem to indicate a slight downward trend in the prevalence of smoking by almost all groups of young men although, in line with figures for all ages, the percentage of female smokers has risen. Even so, the percentage of smokers at 15 and 16 is still unacceptably high. Like alcohol consumption, cigarette smoking is closely related to prevailing social attitudes. Health education directed at young people is unlikely to achieve dramatic results if adults—parents and teachers in particular—are not seen to practise what they preach. In these difficult areas, the Health Education Officer and his staff and facilities can give valuable assistance to Education and Social Services personnel and directly to young people in schools, clubs and other meeting places.

Psychiatric Disorder

11.24 This subject is largely covered for adolescents as well as for children in Chapter 15: Psychiatric Disorder and will not therefore be considered in detail here. Below we outline only the main areas of need.

11.25 As we have said, adolescence is a time of growth, of change, sometimes of anxiety over scholastic achievement and parental expectations. The majority adjust but for a minority, the result is new disturbed behaviour or the exacerbation of earlier problems. A rise in depressive disorders is reflected in the rising incidence of suicide, and attempted suicide among young people as well as in the number seeking help from the Samaritans. Suicide rates as one of the more common causes of death in this age group and it has been estimated that for every successful suicide, there are 50 attempted suicides among adolescents. Additionally conduct disorders ranging from nuisance behaviour to delinquency and criminality appear to be increasing, along with truancy and violence in schools. Another predominantly adolescent disorder in anorexia nervosa, characterised by a preoccupation about weight and food, associated with an inability to eat.

11.26 Despite the suggestions that the prevalence of psychiatric disorder rises in adolescence, many adolescents are wary of the services available, particularly if these cater also for children or involve parents. The psychiatric problems of older adolescents, who may have left school and be financially and otherwise independent of their families, often have more in common with adult disorders. Nevertheless there remains a great amount of adolescent disorder for which a range of wholly separate facilities embracing schools, hostels and hospital units is required. The greater need exists among adolescents whose chronic socially disruptive behaviour renders them unsuited to hospital care but for whom a clear alternative mode of treatment in a secure setting has yet to be identified. The implications for services include the need for greater facilities for counselling over a range of problems; for the provision of psychiatric help or walk-in clinics; for collaboration between child and adolescent psychiatrists and "adult" colleagues in the treatment of older adolescents; for an increase in the facilities for

([8]) Statistics of Smoking in the United Kingdom, ed Todd, G. F. Tobacco Research Council Research Paper I. Sixth edition.

residential care and treatment; and for the evaluation of treatment of the chronically socially disruptive adolescent. Detailed consideration of these recommendations is given in paragraphs 55 to 59 of CHAPTER 15: Psychiatric Disorder.

Handicap

11.27 The aim of this chapter is to consider problems specific to adolescence; those which are common to handicapped children and adolescents in general are discussed in Chapter 14: Handicap below. Here we discuss briefly the problems associated with continuing handicap in adolescents with chronic disorders.

11.28 By adolescence, most serious handicapping conditions have been manifest for some years and the opportunity and need for prevention are past. However physical and mental handicaps predispose children to psychiatric disorder and in this and other ways may aggravate and prolong the developmental problems facing all adolescents. The constraints to living imposed by handicap affect the adolescent's life at home, at school, in employment and in society. Additionally he is subject to all the stresses of accelerated physical, sexual and emotional development and to the prospect of change in environment and occupation. For the handicapped, adolescence is a period of crisis yet at the moment of leaving school, there is the danger that they are less supported than at any time hitherto.

11.29 Permanent handicapping conditions in many who now survive to adulthood are making increasing demands on economic, medical, nursing, educational, social and family resources. With adolescence may come an increase in and increased awareness of physical disability and the power of parents to cope at home may be strained as they themselves become older and their adolescent child heavier and more difficult to manage. This is particularly true in the case of mental handicap: often during the period of adolescence, the family finds the burden of caring increasingly difficult and sometimes impossible. Additional support and relief may be needed at this time together with sympathetic understanding of the problems involved. If it becomes necessary for the adolescent to leave home, the family should have the assurance that suitable residential care is available.

11.30 In the adolescent, an increasing awareness of the permanence of his handicap and of his physical and financial dependence on his family may contribute to a degree of emotional distress. The handicapped adolescent will feel more keenly the restrictions, and often the isolation, of his daily life. The lack of opportunity to take part in normal teenage activities may result in an inability to adapt to normal society, in lack of confidence and motivation. Simultaneously sexual awareness becomes more pronounced and disfigured adolescents may become conscious of their own physical unattractiveness, particularly to members of the opposite sex. *We recommend that much wider recognition should be given to the handicapped adolescent's need of psychiatric, genetic and psycho-sexual counselling to prepare him for adulthood. Such services should be available through school and hospital and as with healthy adolescents, there should be scope for self-referral independent of parents.*

11.31 We would envisage that throughout adolescence the district handicap team would provide specialist paediatric support, with system specialist advice and involvement as necessary. GPPs and CHVs, with their basic training in child health and handicapped children supplemented by some training in child and adolescent psychiatry, would provide continuity of primary clinical care for handicapped children attending ordinary schools. The district handicap team, especially the consultant community paediatrician, would provide health services to special schools, the primary care team providing services to the children when at home. *Like all other adolescents, the handicapped should be able and encouraged to seek help and guidance on their own initiative. They must therefore have direct access to professional people involved in their treatment and management, and this means the district handicap team as well as the GPP.* We do not fear heavy and unnecessary demands on the district team where the GPP is meeting primary health care needs. It would offer adolescents an additional safeguard when they were not receiving sufficient help, for example as a consequence of attending a residential special school.

11.32 The transfer of health care and surveillance from the child-oriented to adult services is a cause of much concern. It would be neither possible nor desirable to set rigid demarcation lines and as in the case of psychiatric disorder, we recognise the need for flexibility and for ascertaining the adolescent's own wishes. In some cases the paediatrician should continue to care for children with chronic handicap into late adolescence whereas in others, an early transfer to adult physicians or surgeons would be more appropriate. What is essential is that close liaison should be maintained between child and adult oriented services and that the responsibility for overall care should at all times be clear. It is important to appreciate the vital rôle of the general practitioner in coordinating the activities of different specialties and consequently the need to keep him informed. The passage from school to work is currently being considered in detail by the Warnock Committee of Enquiry into Special Education. Without wishing to pre-empt their decisions in any way, we should like to record our view that the responsibilities of services supporting young people and their parents during this period of transition should be clearly defined. At present facilities for individual preparation for work are very limited although the needs are substantial. We feel that school doctors would be well placed to provide continuing liaison with welfare and employment agencies and the Employment Medical Advisory Service after the adolescent has left school. Local education authorities already have powers and duties in relation to the provision of careers services for young people[9] and we recommend that they should keep in close touch with the employment status and career of handicapped young people for at least 2 years after they leave school to give any help necessary and to collect information on their needs.

---

[9] Employment and Training Act 1973, Section 8. The Careers Service: Guidance to Local Education Authorities in England and Wales (1975). Department of Employment. HMSO, London.

CHAPTER 12

ILLNESS

The Nature of Childhood Illness

12.1 Chapter 2 presented a general survey of childhood ill-health today and showed clearly that, while the children of this country are healthier than they have ever been, they still experience a wide range of illness. Certain aspects which present particularly testing problems both of management and prevention we have considered separately in Chapter 8 (the Unborn and Newborn Baby), Chapter 13 (Dental Health) and Chapter 15 (Psychiatric Disorder). In this chapter we are concerned with illness in general, including accidental and non-accidental injury, and the way in which services should be organised to meet the needs which arise from it. We have not repeated in this chapter the epidemiological data on ill-health which is to be found in Chapter 2; rather we start from the general conclusions which can be drawn from that data for the organisation of services.

12.2 Firstly, much ill-health in children is preventible. This has already been demonstrated, for example in the case of many infectious diseases. But obvious challenges remain, notably accidents which are now the main cause of death between 1 and 15 years. In future those involved in treatment should give increasing attention to prevention and health education. This means in turn that they must have adequate understanding of what can be done with present knowledge and where further research and evaluation of accepted procedures are necessary. Secondly there have been major advances in the understanding and treatment both of common childhood disorders such as asthma, as well as in the more rare and complex conditions. If children are to have the full benefit of these advances, then it is essential that doctors providing primary care have up-to-date knowledge of them and are able to work closely with their consultant colleagues, with the latter increasingly providing advice on children's illness in group practices and health centres. Thirdly, we have noted the social and familial dimension of ill-health and the extent to which environmental factors affect prevalence. Effective treatment often requires an understanding of the child's family circumstances and overall development, and the health services may need to work closely with the staff of the local authority social services department. Fourthly our analysis showed the extent to which recurrent and chronic illness, physical and mental handicap and psycho-social disorders have overtaken acute episodic illness among the dominant features of childhood ill-health. The training of doctors and nurses must reflect these changes, increasingly emphasising for example that their concern is not simply with an infected respiratory tract but with an unhappy child, whose family is exhausted and whose schooling is interrupted, and that cooperation with teachers, and other members of the health and social service professions is important if the effects of continued ill-health on overall development are to be minimised. We hope to see an increasing appreciation of what parents can and do contribute, in particular to the care of the chronically ill child and of the practical implications of this for the organisation of services and for communication between doctors and other professional staff and parents.

176

Finally we would emphasise the importance of teamwork. The successful management of ill-health is now rarely the task of one person alone. It requires the application of the relevant professional knowledge at every stage. Respiratory disease provides an illuminating example since it is the commonest illness in children with which general practitioners and paediatricians have to deal, and is responsible for 2000 child deaths a year of which 3 out of 4 are in infants and almost half occur at home. The needs are for advice to parents about prevention from health visitors and midwives; a prompt response from practitioners when called to any affected infant and admission to hospital where this is necessary; and rapid diagnosis and treatment in hospital using every requisite clinical, laboratory and technical resource. The whole exercise must be carried out as a concerted effort by parents, health visitors, general practitioners, radiologists, laboratory technicians and paediatricians.

12.3 The need to provide an effective service for the care and treatment of sick children and their parents, particularly at the primary level, which reflects these general principles has played a major part in our fundamental recommendations for structural changes in the pattern of services, and to that extent this chapter should be read in conjunction, not only with Chapter 2, but also with Chapters 4 and 5 in Part I. In this chapter we examine the way in which illness is treated at present and the way in which our proposed changes in the services might lead to more effective care.

Assessing the Scale of the Problem

12.4 Illness can be an acute isolated experience, a series of recurring episodes, or an established state; it is characteristically a dynamic process whose evolution can generally be modified and sometimes controlled by standard medical techniques. Episodes range from a trivial inconvenience for which no medical help is sought, to a life-threatening disorder requiring all the resources of a children's hospital or regional centre. At national level particularly there are considerable difficulties in obtaining a comprehensive statistical picture of illness. Unlike death, illness is not a precise, definable occurrence. While therefore mortality data can provide a pointer to the incidence of life-threatening illness, for information on less severe conditions we are heavily dependent, as section D of the Statistical Appendix shows, on statistics relating to reported contacts with the health services. Such data have many short-comings as a measure of the scale and nature of childhood ill-health. Firstly there is the risk of duplication, since a patient may be treated by more than one part of the services for the same condition. Secondly the reported contact may only indicate for example the hospital department attended and not the reason. Thirdly such data by definition tell us nothing of the illness which is not brought to the attention of health services. A study of illness in a Northern English city over the 15 years from 1947 to 1962[1,2] presented a portrait in depth of illness in an urban

[1] Miller, F J W, Court, S D M Walton, W S, and Knox, E G (1960). Growing up in Newcastle on Tyne. Oxford University Press, London.
[2] Miller, F J W, Court, S D M, Knox, E G and Brandon, S (1974). The School Years in Newcastle on Tyne. Oxford University Press, London.

locality. This showed the reality, submerged in national data, of illness as a family problem, to be resolved perhaps by parental care alone, or by a consultation with the chemist, as well as the conditions for which the help of health visitor, general practitioner or casualty department was sought. The portrait is fifteen years old and the details no longer wholly representative, but we have yet no corresponding up-to-date replacement.

12.5 At the same time, the standard categories of illness fail to reveal the adverse social factors, family stress or disruption and the delayed development or educational failure in the child which may lie behind the diagnostic label and contribute significantly to the management and outcome of the illness. Informed interpretation of the official categories suggests that much of the illness coming to primary care has a strong psycho-social element. The limitations of treating illness without regard to the child's family environment are increasingly recognised but these factors are not revealed in standard classifications. The urban study referred to above clearly established the need for family diagnosis and for simple, measurable categories of family function. Although it is a difficult task, illness can be defined and measured and important local and national studies have been made. The problem is that epidemiological machinery and resources have been insufficient to produce morbidity data suitable for local planning and which together would provide an ongoing national picture of childhood illness. Comprehensive, meaningful statistics are easier to obtain on a local basis than at national level and we believe that the machinery of the reorganised NHS provides new opportunities for doing so, and hence for planning services to take account of local variations in morbidity. We have new and valuable information on regional variations in mortality but there is little evidence about the corresponding variations in morbidity. We feel certain these exist, due to the different socio-economic patterns in different populations, and the unequal provision of services. *We recommend that further studies should be carried out aimed at supplementing national and regional statistics with more local data which are "patient" and "disease" oriented.*

Illness for which Treatment is not Sought

12.6 Although there is still a large amount of illness in children, not all of it needs professional attention. Many illnesses are treated by parents with the advice of relatives, neighbours, friends or the local pharmacist. Self-help is to be encouraged provided it is well informed and parents have sufficient understanding of illness in their children to make a proper assessment of the need to call in professional help. *We see it as an important function of the primary care team, and in particular of the child health visitor to give advice to parents on symptoms of illness in their children which call for straightforward measures by them or a prompt call to the doctor* and to help them to use the health services available. We see this as a natural extension of the health visitor's rôle as adviser on the care and development of the young child. With the integration of primary preventive and therapeutic services based on general practice, the danger of conflicting and confusing advice from two separate sources, the child health clinic and the general practice, should disappear and the practice team should be able to provide ongoing and consistent advice to the families in their care. This means that there must be sufficient child health visitors to know all the families in a locality and with time to visit and teach. In the school years, education for health should of course come from teachers, school nurses and school doctors working together with the children.

12.7 We are however concerned that there are other reasons why illness —which may not be trivial—never reaches the doctor. Such illness may be concentrated in unsettled mobile families living in the decaying areas of large cities who are not registered with a general practitioner. There are however individual disadvantaged families, with a greater incidence of childhood illness, in every community and there are limited inarticulate families who fail to use the services. The educated too are sometimes reluctant to call the doctor; outwardly because "he is so busy", but inwardly because of previous experience of unsympathetic response from a receptionist or from the doctor himself.

Doctor and Patient Relationships

12.8 The establishment of good working relationships between general practitoners and parents, particularly in areas of disadvantage, where doctors may be overworked and parents under stress of many kinds is not easy. It requires skills in communication on the part of doctors and time to build up trust and confidence. *Doctors must recognise the importance of involving parents in the health care of their children.* In spite of the pressure of time they should encourage them to ask questions and endeavour to provide them with information in ways which are appropriate to their level of understanding. *They should endeavour to ensure that their receptionists and other office staff adopt a sensitive approach to parents seeking help,* and that they hold some open surgeries as well as appointment sessions. Equally parents must recognise that doctors are only human and that for their general practitioner to adapt on every occasion to each individual parent's blend of interest, stamina and other qualities would require heroic resources of time, insight and empathy.

12.9 There are no easy answers, but the fact that in an integrated service general practice will undertake developmental oversight as well as treatment will help by providing more opportunities for regular contact between parents and members of the primary care team. The restoration of the health visitor's territorial responsibility, combined with her attachment to the practice team, should also play an important part in ensuring that all children are put in contact with the appropriate primary care team.

The Primary Care Team

12.10 Every year approximately three out of four children in the age range 0-14 years see their general practitioners, and on average they have four or five consultations each. The average varies from eight consultations in infancy to two a year for children aged 10 years or older.[3,4] In general,

---

[3] Fry, J (1966). Profiles of disease: a study in the natural history of common diseases. Livingstone.

[4] Morell, D C, Gage, H G and Robinson, M A (1970). Patterns of demand in general practice, *J. Roy. Coll. Gen. Pract.*, 19, 331.

work with children occupies from 25 to 30% of a practitioner's time and he will deal with 80 to 90% of their illness without help beyond the primary care team.

12.11 The second National Morbidity Study gave details of illness among children aged 0 to 15, and referred to 53 general practices, (Statistical Appendix, Table D15) but the General Household Survey in 1971 showed the degree of variation in referral rates that can occur both between and within regions. The information from this national survey and from the city study referred to in paragraph 12.4 above, illustrate both the amount and range of illness with which general practice is involved. Moreover, although the present child and school health services are essentially concerned with health surveillance, two recent studies have drawn attention to the amount of illness which is seen in the course of this work. (See tables 2 and 3 Appendix D.)

12.12 Primary care at professional level has a two-fold responsibility; the effective management of a large volume of common illness and the recognition within it of infrequent, often unfamiliar, but potentially serious conditions. What appears familiar and straightforward when first seen can change in a matter of hours to a severe and life-threatening condition. We have already referred to the need for increased training in paediatrics for general practitioners if they are to fulfil these responsibilities in a world of ever-advancing medical knowledge, and we welcome the steps in practice organisation and vocational training which are already being taken to bring this about. We hope that our own proposals for the development of the GPP will help to stimulate further improvement in the standard of therapeutic primary care. Many children will of course continue to be registered with doctors who are not themselves GPPs, but we envisage that within a group practice the GPP with his special training will provide his partners with a source of further advice within the practice on particular problems they encounter with their child patients. At the same time the fact that the GPP working with the child health visitor will also be responsible for ensuring the developmental surveillance of child patients within the practice, means that therapeutic primary care can be undertaken against the background of knowledge of the child's overall developmental progress.

12.13 Childhood illness occurs not simply in children but in families. This family dimension is the essence of good general practice and there is no reason why the development of greater paediatric skills in some general practitioners within the group should weaken it. Equally, the development of child health visitors will ensure that doctors are well informed about family needs, and will make possible an integrated primary medical service providing prevention, education and care.

12.14 *With both general practitioners and health visitors more skilled in the management of childhood illness and working closely together, a wide-ranging examination of their joint task could begin.* This review should include, for example, the development of care for those aspects of chronic or recurrent illness hitherto more associated with hospital patterns of management and will require general practitioners increasingly to accept the necessity for monitoring progress at predetermined intervals and taking positive steps to ensure that non-attendances are noted and investigated.

12.15 To be effective a primary care service must be readily available. The sick child's condition can change rapidly and we are concerned at the use of deputising services where the paediatric experience of doctors varies widely and is unknown to the parents, and at the difficulties which some parents experience in making contacts with doctors on call, and, where they feel the condition demands an immediate visit to the Accident and Emergency Department, in discovering quickly which is open. We have noted the comments made in 1975 in the Journal of the Royal College of General Practitioners: "Complaints about badly run appointment systems and principals who are habitually unavailable for emergency care after tea-time are too common for comfort".[5] Essentially responsibility for providing an adequate 24 hour service for the treatment of illness rests with the general practitioner. While not wishing to detract from this responsibility, we believe it would be foolish to ignore the difficulties which may sometimes face parents in trying to contact a doctor on call, particularly at night, and particularly if they have to make repeated calls from a public call box. *We recommend that health authorities should be asked to explore the possibility of providing a mechanism (we had in mind for example a published telephone number in each district) whereby a parent seeking help for a sick child could be put in touch with whoever is providing the service.* In some areas we suspect that for some time to come parents will continue to use Accident and Emergency Departments for treatment which could more appropriately be provided by general practice. The implications of this are referred to in paragraph 12.33 below.

12.16 We have already emphasised the need for the primary care service to be more closely concerned in prevention and in educating parents in the steps that need to be taken to protect their children's health. We also consider that in future they should be increasingly concerned wih the support of parents caring for sick children at home. At the root of our thinking on the services for ill children is the need to reorientate care wherever possible from hospital to home. While this is highly desirable in avoiding the stress of hospital admission for the child, it will place increased burdens on his parents. It is in this connection that we see the development of the child health visitor and the child health nurse as of particular importance. Health visitors have always had a primary concern for young children and have educated their parents in health protection and self-help in minor illness. The child health visitor will in addition be responsible for ensuring that parents have the necessary practical guidance on the management of childhood illness which can be treated at home, and for providing the necessary nursing support. This will require not only wider training in childhood illness but also the maintenance and indeed the advancement of their paediatric nursing skills. We suspect moreover that if the primary care services are strengthened and reach more families, more cases of need for

[5] Irvine, D (1975). 1984 The Quiet Revolution? *J. Roy. Coll. Gen. Pract.,* 25, 399.

this service will come to light. It is unrealistic to suppose that sufficient child health visitors could be recruited and trained to meet the potential increase in service requirements, nor would all the work require the level of skill and training of the child health visitor. *We have therefore proposed that the latter should have to support her qualified nurses with paediatric experience,—child health nurses—to carry out both clinical duties in connection with preventive and immunisation sessions and such tasks in the field of home nursing as the child health visitor felt she could appropriately delegate.* While it would properly be the child health visitor to whom families would turn for nursing advice and doctors direct their referrals, we envisage that the child health visitor would normally involve herself directly only in the more complex nursing cases, although the pattern of delegation to the child health nurse should in no way amount to a back-door method of perpetuating the separation of preventive and curative nursing. Nursing support for sick children in the community is currently an undeveloped area and in terms of its commitment to practical aid and education for parents of sick children, what we are proposing will be in many ways a new nursing service. *Such developments will need to be introduced with care and we recommend that they should be the subject of local research aimed at establishing what is the most efficient and economic deployment of nursing skills.*

Hospital Services

12.17 For more than two centuries hospitals have dominated the practice of medicine and the imagination of the public. Their contribution to medical care and knowledge is immense. Yet in addition to the changing pattern of illness in childhood there are other reasons why their rôle should be re-examined. Public appreciation though strong is not unqualified and in a period of financial restraint the size of their share of total expenditure makes re-examination an economic necessity.

12.18 During the last 15, and especially the last 5, years there has been a wealth of enquiry into the design and function of hospitals for children. Where the new knowledge has been applied it has strengthened internal development but not led to closer links with general practice and the community services. *The community is too often thought of as what happens outside the hospital; for us the hospital is one important activity in a community health service.*

12.19 If review is to lead to reform the guiding principles should be these:

Whenever the illness and circumstances allow a child will be cared for at home;

The doctors and nurses providing primary care, better trained in paediatrics, will manage the majority of these illnesses;

They will be supported by consultation with paediatricians and allied specialists in the consulting room or health centre and, hopefully, in the home. This should reduce referral to hospital and make it more selective;

Hospital services will be more varied than in the past providing not only outpatient consultation and admission but assessment and care for the handicapped, day attendance for investigation or treatment, admission to a 5 day or 7 day ward, paediatric and specialist attention in the accident and emergency department, and "intensive care" for severe illness and injury.

The District General Hospital

12.20 The district is the basic community in the reorganised health service and the district general hospital the main source of hospital care. The development of these hospitals has been one of the most significant contributions by the NHS to the care of children. Their intended structure and function in relation to children have been expressed with clarity and conviction in the Department of Health's memorandum (HM(71)22) and its explanatory annexe Hospital Facilities for Children. *We are in essential agreement with these recommendations and wish to see them fully implemented.* The central conclusion of the circular was this: *To make the most efficient and economic use of resources, the district services for acutely ill children should be centralised in one department, in one part of the main hospital, accommodating all children and providing paediatric and specialty services.* This also implies, for example, that in urban areas where closely adjacent district hospitals may each maintain a children's department, every effort must be made, without ignoring all the complex geographical, human and other factors, to concentrate the paediatric services in one hospital only. In this way alone can duplication of staff, accommodation and equipment be avoided, and families seem on the whole prepared to recognise that greater inconvenience for some may be the price that has to be paid to ensure better care for all.

12.21 Such principles apply equally to the special case of children with infectious disease, many of whom are still cared for in infectious diseases (ID) hospitals. Paediatric wards can deal with infective illness as part of childhood illness, and isolation facilities and barrier nursing techniques are an accepted part of ward design and practice. The range of illness in infectious disease hospitals has widened too, and what is more two-thirds of their patients are children. Everything we know about the nature and needs of children suggests that they should not be "isolated" unless it is absolutely necessary and then for the shortest possible time. Parents, paediatricians and the Department of Health want children to be cared for in a children's setting by doctors and nurses trained in their care. While general paediatric departments are making such long term adaptations as are necessary to provide appropriate care for children with infectious diseases, the ID hospitals should ensure that their paediatric facilities and accommodation are of an acceptable standard. Paediatric advice should be sought and given and paediatric nurses trained in infectious diseases should form part of the staff of children's wards in ID hospitals. Effective isolation facilities should be part of children's departments, the training of paediatric nurses in the nursing of infectious diseases improved, and all paediatricians, one especially in each regional centre, should have a wider training in the understanding and management of infective illness.

183

12.22 In almost every district there is a grim legacy of outmoded 19th century buildings which are a stubborn obstacle to creating single comprehensive children's departments. Ever receding recommendations for new hospitals are dispiriting for those destined to go on working in the old. Yet this need not mean that no improvement is possible. If district management teams will examine the scatter of children among the various hospitals they will find that with a measure of professional compromise they could gather some of them into more efficient units. In our visits we have seen remarkable adaptation of the most unpromising buildings. And although separation may not be entirely overcome the units can be linked through a common philosophy and shared staff. Yet whatever the difficulties *the comprehensive department caring for all children is central to the provision of a rational and humane district hospital service.*

Outpatient Services

12.23 With the changing emphasis from the child in hospital to the child at hospital, outpatient consultation grows in importance. There has been a steady increase in the provision of hospital outpatient services for children, greater in some regions than others. (Statistical Appendix, Table E24. The range of problems dealt with in a typical district general hospital outpatient department is shown in Table E30.) National figures show that both first and subsequent visits have increased, the second at a faster rate as each new patient is making more return visits. Even though the rise in new patient referrals might be interpreted in part as reflecting an improvement in hitherto inadequate services, such trends cannot be ignored. They are at odds with our professed aim of diverting the ongoing medical care of children as far as possible from hospital to general practice, and for families they mean greater inconvenience, more interrupted schooling, and added expense. The reasons are undoubtedly complex. To attribute the disproportionate increase in return visits entirely to a tendency for consultants to underestimate the capacities of their general practitioner colleagues would be an over simplification. Account has also to be taken of such factors as a change in the consultant's perception of his rôle and an increasing tendency to substitute a series of outpatient appointments for an extended stay in hospital. The implications are correspondingly uncertain and valid judgments could only be based on much broader data than is presently available.

12.24 If real need remains unmet a low rate of referral is not necessarily a sign of professional virtue. However it has been shown that with greater paediatric knowledge in primary care the need to refer children to hospital can be reduced. In group practices in Livingston the development of general practitioner paediatricians in our sense of the term, together with paediatric consultation in the practice by a visiting consultant has reduced the referral rate to hospital outpatients to 2%, a notable reduction from the 17% and 10% of previous surveys. We were impressed by this experiment and believe its approach could be effective in more conventional communities. We were encouraged too by what we saw at other centres and our impression is that particular features of the Livingston pattern are already more widely developed than is generally recognised. We consider that *consultant paediatricians should regard the maintenance of high standards of paediatric*

184

primary care as one of their main responsibilities, and we recommend that regular consultation clinics in group practice or health centre should be developed as an essential prerequisite of the more selective use of district and regional hospital facilities particularly in view of the decline in domiciliary consultations. The discrepancy in numbers between consultant paediatricians and group practices makes it clear however that, until there is a significant increase in paediatric manpower, only a few practices (and those, for cost efficiency reasons presumably the larger ones) will be able to take part in this exercise. Nevertheless the gradual development of paediatric competence in general practice should in time reduce the number of first and subsequent outpatient visits, and since the essence of outpatient consultation is time a selective reduction in numbers will improve its quality and usefulness.

12.25 The need to attend clinics in hospitals often places acute stress on mothers and their children. The non-medical support they receive at this time can be a crucial factor in their ability to cope successfully with the situation. A mother who has had to spend a prolonged waiting period trying to cope with her ill child and entertain his siblings will most likely not be able to ask sensible questions, or to assimilate information given during the short time she spends with the doctor. We have been concerned at the evidence of continued failure to recognise the mother's needs for assistance in these situations or to provide suitable facilities for children attending outpatient clinics. The most complete evidence came from Wales[6], but information from many sources confirmed that, leaving aside paediatrics and child psychiatry, child-oriented outpatient clinics are the exception among those specialties which deal with the majority of children who reach hospital.

TABLE 4

Welsh Hospital Board—Survey November 1971 to March 1972[6]
Main Outpatient Clinics: Total and % for Children only

Specialty	Outpatient Clinics		
	Total	Children Only	% Children Only
Ophthalmology	34	10	30
ENT	41	7	17
Orthopaedics	29	4	14
Dentistry	11	1	9
General Surgery	44	3	7
Respiratory Medicine	35	2	6
General Medicine	20	1	5
Dermatology	25	1	4
Psychiatry	10	7	70
Paediatrics	36	36	100

[6] *Children in Hospital in Wales*, (1972). Unpublished Report produced for the Welsh Hospital Board.

185

12.26 A total of 334 outpatient clinics were studied: 17 or 5% provided separate children's toilets; 50 (15%) small chairs; 120 (35%) pram space; 63 (18%) toys and comics; 244 (71%) comics only. Only one hospital reported a nappy changing room. Fifty-seven clinics provided none of these facilities. Of the 334, 80 (23%) provided separate accommodation for children; in 58 the waiting space was shared by adults attending other clinics, and 5 hospitals reported "only corridor waiting space" for their clinics. *The evidence is that in the majority of outpatient departments attended by children in Wales scant attention is paid to their personal needs.*

12.27 As similar conditions occur in many parts of England too we support the conclusions of the Welsh Working Party.

"The advantages of outpatient clinics held specifically for children are considerable. A waiting area may be set aside for their exclusive use, appropriate toys and books provided, and consulting rooms suitably set out. The staff can be child experienced at least for the period of the clinic. The objection has been made that busy consultants cannot afford the time to see children separately. We submit that it takes no longer to see 25 children in one morning than to see 5 children on each of 5 days along with adults. We therefore ask consultants, particularly those seeing more than 50 children a month, to set aside one session or half a session for children only. There should be sufficient waiting space (a subject which needs further investigation), furnished and equipped for both children and parents. The contribution of children's trained or experienced nursing staff will be increased by the presence of a play worker."

12.28 The Welsh survey and the submissions of women's and parents' associations brought home to us both the central importance and the many deficiencies of outpatient consultation in the total pattern of hospital care. Although local circumstances will affect local arrangements, *we recommend a comparable study by the Department of Health and Social Security, in association with professional and parent associations of outpatient clinics for children in England.* Moreover without delay, district planning teams and community health councils can measure their present facilities by the standards set out in the report on the Planning of Hospital Children's Departments.[7]

12.29 We note that the then Ministry of Health issued a circular commending a proper appointment system for outpatients in 1964, and we trust that health authorities will adhere to this advice. Block booking for hospital outpatient clinics for children inevitably increases waiting time and stress for parents and children.

Day Care
12.30 Day care, already well established for certain forms of surgery, is increasing in the investigation and treatment of illness. Children treated by day admission were first recorded separately in 1972, when more than 11,000 cases were reported (Statistical Appendix, Table E24). The recording of day cases is however confused by problems of definition and there is an urgent

---

[7] Report of British Paediatric Association Working Party (1974).

need for an agreed definition followed by the fullest possible recording and reporting by all disciplines dealing with children, so that the extent of the practice and local variations in its use may be known. We accept the definition of a day patient proposed by a professional working party,[8] as one, "attending as a non-resident patient for observation, investigation, therapeutic test, operative procedure or other treatment, and who requires some form of supervision, preparation, or period of recovery involving the provision of accommodation and services."

12.31 The present position and suggested development have been effectively reviewed in individual articles and in the report of the working party previously mentioned.[8] The advantages to child and family are clear, and we *believe that day care is desirable at all ages, but that it is especially important for young children. We believe it will prove one of the most useful extensions of the hospital service.* Reports from several centres indicate that over half the elective general surgery of children can be carried out by day admission. One estimate suggests that a paediatric day surgery session a week could save £12,000 a year. We understand that the Royal Sick Childrens Hospital, Glasgow, using a ward unit of 12 beds deals with 3,000 day admission a year. Day care is also particularly effective in the treatment of dental surgical problems in healthy children. When consistently practised by all disciplines dealing with children day care would have a significant effect on the number of admissions.

12.32 At the same time it is important that the implications for staff and facilities are properly understood and that there should be careful evaluation of children treated in this way. A decision to treat a child as a day patient should have regard not only to clinical considerations but also to the home facilities, and whether the mother is working or has other young children to care for. Appropriate facilities should be provided preferably as a separate unit, within a children's ward and as part of the children's department. The unit should have a distinct complement of nursing staff under the general supervision of the children's ward sister. (The staffing implications of this are considered in Chapter 18.) Safe and effective day care requires particularly close liaison with the primary health care team. Although parents are usually more than willing to share in the care of their child they may well lack confidence in their ability to take care of a child immediately after surgery. Where possible a nurse should call on the family after the child has reached home to check that all is well. The way in which this back-up service is provided will vary from one district to another. It can be provided direct by the nursing staff of the paediatric department, or alternatively by the child health visitor and her team. Whatever arrangements are made, it is essential that when the child leaves hospital the professional staff ensure that the parents are clear where to go for medical or nursing advice at any time during the convalescent period, and that they know how the child's condition is likely to progress and will therefore not call on professional staff unnecessarily.

[8] Day Care in Hospitals: Report of Working Party of the British Paediatric Association and British Association of Paediatric Surgeons (1975).

Accident and Emergency Departments

12.33 Regrettably there are no national statistics for the total number of children attending Accident and Emergency departments, although they are an essential element in hospital care. Their range of work with children is shown for three district general hospitals in Tables E27–29 in the Statistical Appendix. They illustrate the wide range of conditions reaching these departments, and in particular that these departments deal with a substantial amount of illness. There is also a considerable overlap between the conditions reaching outpatient departments and those presenting to Accident and Emergency departments. Figures from the Children's Hospital in Sheffield suggest that in inner urban areas some 20% of all children attend in the course of a year, and of this enormous total nearly one quarter are under 5 and one third under 3, and their numbers have more than doubled in 10 years. Analysis[9] of attendances at the Accident and Emergency Department of the Children's Hospital in Sheffield showed that in one year there were 21,000 new cases of which 12% were admitted. Analysis of these admissions showed that at least half the children had medical conditions and that social pathology was important in all categories.

12.34 Quantitatively the use of A and E departments is clearly very great. We need to know what proportion of their patient load might have been dealt with more appropriately by primary care or planned outpatient consultation, and why the children were not dealt with in this way. With this information it would be possible to define their true field of work and reduce the excessive and often capricious use of their services. *We therefore recommend that District Planning Teams for children, should as a high priority review the use of A and E departments by children and make recommendations for the development of a more rational working relationship between these departments and primary care and outpatient services.* In doing so we consider they should bear in mind the following general principles. When resources are severely limited it is the more important to deploy them with maximum efficiency. In towns or small or medium-sized cities this will usually mean that there should be no more than one A and E department dealing with children. In larger cities or conurbations, while the same general principle should apply wherever possible, it will not always be expedient for independently viable paediatric departments to share the services of a single common A and E department. Every department dealing with children should have the right facilities. (We have already referred in Chapter 4 to the absence of such facilities revealed by the review carried out in Wales by the Welsh Hospital Board.) Separate waiting and examination rooms should be available with equipment of the right size, acceptable furnishing and toys and books. The department must be appropriately staffed. We consider in Chapter 18 the numbers of children's nurses required to ensure that adequate cover is available. We would also stress the need for social workers to be readily available in the Accident and Emergency Departments in view of the social pathology affecting so many of the children who attend. In particular there may be the risk of non-accidental injury, or children from neglected homes requiring further care. We understand that

---

(9) Illingworth, C. Personal Communication.

an association of consultants responsible for such departments, the Casualty Surgeons' Association, has been formed. We welcome this and were glad to know that it includes several physicians and one paediatrician. We understand that a joint committee of the Royal Colleges of Physicians and Surgeons is considering the content of their training. In our view this should include experience of paediatrics as well as the surgery of children. Until this broader specialist training is established, we think it desirable that a consultant paediatrician should share responsibility for the department's policy on children, and that there should be a daily rota of paediatric residents on call. We hope too that the appointment of consultant paediatricians to A and E Departments in large children's hospitals and departments as in Sheffield, will increase.

12.35 In those areas—and we suspect they will be largely inner city districts—where, in the light of review it is considered inevitable that for the foreseeable future, the A and E department will continue to be used as a source of primary care this will have to be taken into account in staffing arrangements. It should however be the practice that once the immediate problem has been dealt with, every effort is made to ensure that the parents make contact with their child's general practitioner for further help, or if the child is not registered with a practitioner, that they are put in touch with an appropriate practice.

12.36 In many cases, however, parents will bring a child to hospital themselves for injuries which undoubtedly do require hospital treatment. Faced with an emergency the parents naturally go straight to hospital without waiting and calling an ambulance. *We believe that health authorities must provide for this situation by ensuring that adequate up-to-date information is available to the public on the opening hours of Accident and Emergency Departments in their areas.*

In-patient Services
12.37 Information about in-patients is available from the hospital in-patient enquiry and hospital activity analysis. Each year some 6% of children are admitted to hospital (excluding psychiatric hospitals). Their age distribution and the departments to which they are admitted are shown in Table E18 in the Statistical Appendix. Half the admissions are emergencies and nearly half require some form of surgery. There are big differences in the discharge rates of the various conditions within each age group. There is still a wide range of conditions for which admission to hospital is essential. The most severe will require "intensive care" and all will need "technical care" beyond the capacity of the primary care team. Inevitably there will still be some children admitted because the facilities of their home or the skill of their parents are inadequate for safe domiciliary management, but our proposals are consistently directed towards reducing the size of this group.

12.38 One day censuses suggested that between 1965 and 1970 available beds for children fell from 22,525 to 21,252, with a fall in occupancy from 72% to 66%. We note the trend but find little practical meaning in these overall figures. The hospital service has been changing for some time, but if the opportunity is taken to record all children admitted to all departments, the facts should be available on which policy can be soundly based. Adjustment may be necessary, but we have no firm grounds at present for suggesting a change in the Department of Health's estimate of 0.5 children's beds per 1,000 population "to provide for acute medical, surgical, and psychiatric conditions, for assessment of children with mental and or physical handicaps and for the long-stay care of all handicapped children requiring it. The greater part (0.37 beds per 1,000 total population) will be for children suffering from acute medical and surgical conditions" (HM(71)22).

12.39 During our visits and enquiries we have become increasingly concerned with the setting in which children are cared for, in particular the importance of recognising their special needs when they are in hospital, away from home. To some extent this is a matter of staffing. Children in hospital are under the clinical care of the appropriate consultant. It is essential that as far as possible and as quickly as possible they should be cared for in children's departments which are under the general oversight of a paediatrician and nursed by trained children's nurses. Such departments should have adequate support from social workers trained in child care. (We refer to the implications for staffing of services in more detail in Chapter 18). Essentially these conclusions were reached by the Platt Committee 17 years ago. Yet, whilst much progress has been made in some hospitals, a great deal of the evidence we received underlined that it is in the sphere of social understanding of their needs that children are least well cared for. Whilst this is particularly true of the long-stay hospitals our visits made it clear that the personal needs of children in acute hospitals were not always being met. Most of the staff are well aware of the difficulties, but tend to see them in terms of financial and manpower restraints. It is true that the current economic situation does place limits on what can be achieved, but at the same time we think it is important to recognise that whatever the financial position, progress will continue to depend most of all on the interest and initiative of those working within the individual hospital.

12.40 That hospital admission can be psychologically highly stressful for children is now widely known and accepted. But much more could be done in practice to reduce the risk that it will be so. For example, more hospitals could adopt the practice of inviting a child patient to visit the ward prior to admission, or admit a child initially to a play room. Booklets on hospital routine designed and illustrated for children are now widely used but should be standard practice. The personal facilities provided for children admitted to hospital were presented to us with facts and feeling. In a careful study made in 1972/73 the National Association for the Welfare of Children in Hospital viewed these in terms of a ward "as this is the unit replacing home as far as the child is concerned". We hope their submission to us will be made available to others. It is a picture of partial progress, varying in different hospitals in different departments within hospitals. It is 50 years since James Spence first admitted mothers with their children. Yet this facility was still not available in a third of the hospitals studied and only 1 in 10 had accommodation for 5 or more adults. Just over half the wards had unrestricted or generous visiting. We support the belief of NAWCH in the value of unrestricted visiting by parents, relatives, older brothers and sisters and school friends, and the need to have sufficient rooms able to accommodate a parent or other relative with simple domestic facilities nearby.

12.41 We suspect too that hospital staff often fail to realise that parents may have relatively little knowledge of how hospitals work or how to make their views heard. Many parents do not know to whom they should speak and are afraid to impose themselves on busy professionals. They may also be overawed by the size and strangeness of the place, and may fear to offend in case there are repercussions for their child. Nevertheless parents have a unique personal knowledge of their own child which should be used to form part of any consideration of a programme of treatment. Doctors and nurses therefore need to learn from the parents who in turn need to understand what is happening and learn how best to help their child by being more aware of the implications of treatment. Each has therefore something to offer to the care of the sick child and ideally they form a team in which each learns from the other. Once the immediate physical danger is removed, contact between professional and parent presents the opportunity for mutual explanation and advice which initial anxiety has limited. Unrestricted visiting gives the parents opportunities to witness many more tests and examinations than they would normally see during a shorter visit. Information about these, while time-consuming for the nurses, is vital for the parents. Whilst most of the anxieties of parents are naturally focused initially on the illness and medical condition of their child this may give way to concern about his general care and treatment. The hospital-based social worker has an important part to play as a member of the multi-disciplinary team responsible for assessing and developing policy relating to the total needs of the child. She will have a particular concern with the personal needs of the child and his family, including the maintenance of family links. We discuss in CHAPTER 16 (paragraphs 12–17) the need to ensure that the well-being and needs of children in long-stay hospitals are adequately reviewed at appropriate intervals and that particular attention is given to the risk of abandonment. On a more individual level the hospital-based social worker will also be involved in close consultation with ward staff, in helping parents to communicate their fears and anxieties. She will also mobilise any necessary practical services and ensure continuity of care with social workers in the community.

12.42 *The relevance of play for the effective care of children in hospital is now widely accepted by paediatricians,* radical and conservative alike, and the speed with which they have been converted is impressive. The reality of the need, the qualities needed for the work, the sources of recruits, the content of training and the complementary roles of professional and voluntary worker have been carefully examined by an expert committee.[10] The ambivalent response of the Department of Health to their progressive report took us by surprise. Doubts about the feasibility of creating another category of hospital staff at this time of restricted resources are well understood; we believe the correct approach is first to decide whether the case for change is

[10] Play for Children in Hospital. DHSS Circular HC(76)5.

strong and then its priority among other claims. At a time when the provision of children's nurses in many hospitals is insufficient for basic nursing it is evasive to suggest that they can meet the need for play. We would ask the Department to think again, and invite experienced play workers to suggest possible ways forward. We believe that in time play may be seen as part of the educational provision for the ward and financed accordingly. In the meantime voluntary help and voluntary funds should be used to the full.

12.43 Admission of a child to hospital, particularly to a distant regional centre, will have considerable repercussions for the parents, and for other children in the family. There will be the expense of fares, an ever-rising burden, and the possible need to find overnight accommodation near to the hospital if the hospital does not provide it. Arrangements may need to be made for other children or elderly relatives to be looked after, while the mother is away. We consider that the GP and his colleagues in the primary care team should make themselves responsible for making the family aware of the help that they might receive not only from the health service but also from the Social Services Department perhaps by way of material assistance, home help or day care for other children. Similarly they should inform the social worker of any family who appears to need help so that prompt action may be taken.

12.44 Changes in the pattern of childhood illness which have been a recurrent theme in our report make it more necessary than ever that discharge, like admission should be planned to take account not only of the clinical considerations but also of home circumstances. Paediatric doctors and nurses are very conscious of this and of the need to ensure that general practitioners and health visitors are kept fully informed. In many cases the hospital-based social workers will also be involved and where there is major social pathology will provide an invaluable link with the area social services department. In all cases the maximum amount of notice should be given to parents and an opportunity provided for the doctor or nurse who has been looking after the child to give the parents clear advice on their children's condition and future care.

12.45 Up to this point we have been considering certain aspects of the provision of hospital services at district level. Before the Committee began its work it was encouraged by a distinguished medical journal to go out from the committee room and discover "models of clinical excellence". We have made our journeys and found district hospitals in all parts of the country fulfilling that ideal more impressively than they realise, and in spite of the stubborn difficulties we have described. The principles and practices which impressed us and which we felt pointed the way forward were these:

In a complete or in a functional sense a children's department had been created caring for all children, with a child and family centred philosophy of care widely shared by the staff.

There was a better understanding and closer collaboration with specialist colleagues in hospital and with doctors in the child and school health services.

The trained involvement of paediatric secretaries, as the open line of first contact and on-going information and support has been fostered.

The centre of the department's life was a combined outpatient clinic and child development centre with nurses, therapists and play worker providing a setting in which child and parents felt at home and clinical, developmental and social assessment was possible.

There was increasing use of day care.

When admission was necessary, mothers were able to come in with a young child, and to share as fully as possible in his care; for all the other children there was unrestricted visiting, and both were supplemented by substitute mothers or grannies drawn from a rota of "friends of the ward".

There was a sense of belonging to the local community: paediatricians knowing colleagues in general practice and consulting in group practices; therapists and social workers in working contact with local play groups, opportunity groups and day nurseries.

There was mutual professional involvement in particular local needs, such as children and families with special problems or differing cultural backgrounds.

No single department had all these virtues! Some were in new purpose-built hospitals, but the majority had transformed unpromising separate buildings into a connected department. We believe the persistent critics of the Health Service would reach a more balanced judgement if they sometimes looked at its achievements as well as its deficiencies, especially if they were able to remember the position before 1948.

Regional Children's Centres

12.46 General figures drawn from all hospitals admitting children fail to illustrate the special types of illness reaching regional centres and major children's hospitals. These are shown for one University Department working in 5 hospitals and for a major children's hospital in Table E23 in the Statistical Appendix. The need to maintain a strong service and academic centre was recognised in 1964. "There is the need for at least one large unit in a region preferably as part of a teaching group. Such an arrangement can preserve the advantages of association with all the other specialties while allowing the needed concentration on the problems of children by specially trained medical, nursing and other staff".[11] Seven years later, when excellent guidance was offered to district hospitals, this was omitted. The omission has now been repaired.[12] But if the future well-being of regional children's centres is to be secure, we must understand why they were overlooked in 1971, and why they are essential to our proposals today. The omission was due essentially to the assumption that the district general hospital could provide for every form of childhood illness or injury. The effects have been damaging to long term planning and to professional confidence. *Our hope is that with the principle of their necessity re-established the regional children's centres can develop their specialist service.*

[11] Report of the Chief Medical Officer on the State of the Public Health 1964. Ministry of Health, HMSO, London.

[12] Facilities for children: Paper by the Department of Health presented to Regional Medical Officers, October 1975.

12.47 The case for the regional children's centre can be stated quite simply. There are a small number of children with very serious conditions which require expert management and the skills of specialists which can only be provided on a regional as distinct from a district basis. The choice lies therefore between providing children's wards within regional centres organised on a system or specialty basis, and providing regional children's centres which bring together the various specialties and deal solely with children. We believe that the balance of advantage lies strongly in favour of the latter, because these children, just as much as those whose conditions can be treated within the district service, need to have the overall paediatric oversight associated with a comprehensive children's department. In view of the variety of illness reaching them and the range of services they are expected to provide it is necessary to define exactly what their contribution should be in future. These would seem the essentials:

To be a centre to which patients from districts within the region can be referred for:

Outpatient and inpatient services from the paediatric specialties, accepting that for some conditions this will need to be provided at supra-regional centres;

Intensive care for severe illness and injury;

An experienced multi-professional service for children with complex and multiple handicaps (see CHAPTER 14);

Outpatient and inpatient services from the allied specialties;

To give an exemplary clinical service for their surrounding district or districts.

12.48 Advances in resuscitation and in maintaining vital bodily functions have radically altered the outlook for the seriously ill child. Conditions previously regarded as incompatible with life can now be treated successfully. This has made it necessary to create units for "intensive care" where highly trained medical and nursing staff and the necessary facilities are readily available. A large children's hospital or department will need several of these, for very severe illness, major accidents, complex surgery especially in the newborn and for severe burns. To achieve concentration of resources and flexibility of use the units should ideally be grouped together in one area. The number of cots and beds in each will depend on size of hospital, types of illness admitted and the extent and character of referrals from the region. There should be a high staffing level of nurses in the units, at least one per child throughout the 24 hours with a high proportion children trained. Intensive care is not restricted to regional centres. We realise that it will not be possible for many district hospitals to maintain separate units, and children will be nursed in intensive care units for adults. In these circumstances, the close cooperation of consultant paediatrician and the consultant in charge of the unit, secondment of children's nurses to work with the unit nurses, and the maximum isolation of the child from adult patients compatible with continuous observation are necessary for the best results.

12.49 We decided in relation to district hospitals that we had insufficient information to recommend a change in the number of beds from the figure of 0.37 per 1,000 total population suggested in HM(71)22. The size of the regional children's centre would therefore be based on the size of the district or districts for which it would provide "district hospital" care plus a figure for referrals from paediatricians, allied specialists and general practitioners in the region. In one centre, over a number of years, between 35 and 40% of the beds were occupied by regional referrals. *Our analysis of the activities which are collectively called a hospital will have made it clear that we think in terms of services rather than size. Although fewer beds may be required in future, inpatient services will still be necessary and if the concentration of all children in one hospital proceeds as it should, regional centres will need from 150 to 350 cots and beds.* (We consider further in CHAPTER 18 some of the staffing implications of these centres for medical and nursing manpower.)

Planning for the Future

12.50 Since there is likely to be little new hopsital building in the next few years, District Planning Teams will have time to estimate how many children are in hospital, whether they are in the right hospital, and whether they could have been dealt with as day patients or by primary care had the facilities for these been adequate. We are not suggesting the return of isolated specialist hospitals, but we wonder from where the administrative distrust of children's hospitals has come. It is shared by none of our European neighbours, nor by Canada, Australia or the United States. We can only suppose that administrators in the United Kingdom are largely unfamiliar with the quality of care children's hospitals in other countries provide. We have not overlooked the international standing of the Hospital for Sick Children London, the Royal Sick Children's Hospital, Glasgow, and the children's hospitals in Birmingham, Sheffield, Manchester and Liverpool but many University and Regional Centres in England and Wales are seriously handicapped in comparison with our European neighbours.

12.51 In 1974 the Department of Health put forward the concept of the Community Hospital. The document which describes their purpose[13] suggests that they are essentially for adults. However, this is not absolute since it is suggested that "occasionally a child with a short term illness which a family doctor would normally treat at home might be admitted to a community hospital because of lack of the usual facilities at home". We cannot accept this view. There will be too few children in such a hospital to warrant the quality of staff and facilities we consider essential; and unhappy incidents in the past have demonstrated the risks run by ill children in small isolated units. In 1975 the Department put forward proposals for "Nucleus Hospitals". They raise again the question of the right ratio of acute beds to population for contemporary needs. We feel that for children the facts are not available on which a reliable answer can be reached. *The prior need is to discover in each district hospital and regional centre how many children are coming through every door, and what services they receive,* and we have already emphasised the need for local patient oriented statistics. Until the

[13] Community Hospitals: Their Rôle and Development in the National Health Service. Annex to DHSS Circular HSC(IS)75.

standard of paediatric primary care is raised in the way we propose, the use of hospitals will continue to be greater than we would wish. Nucleus Hospitals are also viewed in economic terms; building what you can afford when you can afford it, and extending if necessary when resources are available. We understand the economic necessity for this approach, but are concerned that a multiplicity of small hospitals caring for children will lead to coninuing inefficiency and waste of our present fragmented system of child care.

Postscript: The Care of the Dying Child

12.52 Sadly doctors and their colleagues both in hospital and in the primary care services sometimes have to face with parents the prospect of caring for a dying child. Nowadays the death of a child is relatively rare and this means that its impact and the demands which it makes both on the professional staff concerned and on the parents are all the more severe. Some contemporary treatment trying to break through to cure, may make the experience more protracted. The inner strength of children and parents varies, but all need considerable support from the professional they feel closest to—general practitioner, ward sister, resident doctor, social worker or consultant. Doctors and nurses need to develop greater sensitivity and skill through sharing the experience with each other, with child psychiatrists and experienced social workers. Nor should it be forgotten that parents who have experienced the loss of a child can offer very great support to others in similar circumstances and indeed to professional staff as well. Since life must be as full as possible for as long as possible, children with terminal illness should remain with other children in the ward, but, as soon as the need arises, privacy for child and parents should be available. Support will also be needed for some time after the child's death, and again the professional closest to the parents should, if possible, accept this ongoing responsibility. Where this is the general practitioner, the hospital must make sure that he is informed and involved as soon as the eventual outcome is known. At the same time it may be helpful for parents to be put in touch with voluntary organisations who can also offer help at this time.

CHAPTER 13
THE PATH TO DENTAL HEALTH

Dental Disease and the Child

13.1 Dental decay is the most prevalent disease in our society and children are more susceptible than adults. Because they are growing they are exposed to the cumulative effect of dental disorders throughout childhood and adolescence. In addition to dental caries, these include irregularities of oral and dental growth, and periodontal disease involving the gums and structures supporting the teeth. Dental health is an integral part of general health, and our aim should be to bring up children free from dental disease with sound teeth in good occlusion and with healthy supporting tissues.

13.2 Despite extensive and increasing treatment, there is still a daunting amount of untreated disease. Of a representative sample of 12,250 children aged 5–15[1], two thirds had active caries requiring treatment; and when gum disease, malocclusions and other conditions such as fractured incisors were taken into consideration, 9 out of 10 children over the age of 6 were found to be in need of dental attention. Caries represents the major dental problem in children and the report of the survey clearly points to the failure to contain it by conventional treatment, particularly amongst the younger age groups. It also shows a high prevalence of gum inflamation (gingivitis) in all age groups. Gingivitis in children is the precursor of chronic periodontitis in adults, the major cause of tooth loss in later life.

TABLE 1

Dental Disease in Children at different ages in England and Wales 1973

Children (per cent)	Age (years)		
	5	9	14
Untreated caries	63	76	62
Periodontal disease	47	78	74
Malocclusion	17	55	28
Needing some dental attention	79	96	90

TABLE 2

Dental Caries in Children at different ages in England and Wales 1973

Age (years)	Total Caries Experience df + DMF*	Treated by Conservation %	Active Caries %
5	3.4	21	76
9	5.0	48	50
14	7.4	65	26

* DMF Mean number of permanent teeth decayed, missing or filled.
  df   Mean number of primary teeth, decayed or filled.

[1] Todd, J E (1975). Children's Dental Health in England and Wales, 1973. HMSO, London.

197

Whilst these tables illustrate the broad picture the full extent of the problem is shown in the Statistical Appendix, Tables D6 and D7.

13.3 To find remedies we must first consider how dental disease affects particular groups of children, how it can be prevented and how far needs are being met.

Dental Disease at Different Ages and in Particular Children

Babies and Young Children

13.4 There is less known about dental health in the first five years than in later childhood. In the survey referred to above, 71% of 5 year olds had decay experience yet only 60% of mothers, interviewed when their children were entering school, considered that children should be taken to the dentist early in life. This means that for many the opportunity to achieve a natural, atraumatic relationship with a dentist was missed and the familiar rejecting attitude to dental care was established.

13.5 There is a rampant form of dental caries affecting infants and young children and causing early and rapid decay of the primary incisor teeth. It is associated with the protracted use of a "dummy" or hollow feeder, used as a comforter and containing a sweetened liquid, often a fruit syrup. The persistent use of a bottle, containing sweetened milk or orange juice, after weaning, has a similar effect, and excessive caries may also follow the frequent administration of "medicines" in a syrup vehicle. Harm results not only from the effects on the primary dentition but from starting a craving for sweet things that may eventually cause the destruction of the permanent teeth as well.

13.6 The School and Priority Service devotes 5% of all sessions to the treatment of pre-school children and in 1973 78,000 were treated. In the General Dental Service in the same year over one million estimates for young children were approved and nearly 500,000 of these related to treatment. Dentists are certainly giving time to this group but the need for treatment shows that present preventive measures are not yet effective. However the 5-yearly surveys carried out since 1948, the last in 1973, show a considerable improvement in the dental health of 5-year olds.[2] The reason for this is not clear. It may reflect the success of persistent dental health education or it may be associated with a change in the pattern of confectionery consumption rather than a change in the quantity consumed.

13.7 If the dental care of the pre-school child presents problems it can also be said to provide opportunities, as dental decay in the very young is particularly responsive to prevention. Many of the dietary faults accepted as inevitable at a later date occur because they have been mistakenly adopted when the child was very young. At a time when spare capacity amongst dentists is at a premium it is unfortunate that so much time is involved in the treatment of disease that could have been prevented. If a clearly-defined system of priorities were to be drawn up the permanent dentition of the older child would warrant more attention, but it does not seem reasonable to deprive any child of necessary care

[2] Department of Education and Science (1975). *The School Health Service 1908–1974.* HMSO, London.

198

and there is good reason to believe that an early relationship between child and dentist is more likely to be fruitful than one developed at a later age.

Schoolchildren

13.8 *Caries* Of the 12,250 children aged 5 to 15 examined in the children's Dental Health Survey, two out of three had active caries. This suggests that in a school population of nine million, six million were in need of treatment. Of children aged 5, 29% were caries free and 31% had five or more decaying teeth and by 8, 15% were caries free and 29% had five or more decaying teeth; this high level of disease continued and at 14 only 4% were caries free and in 72% five or more permanent teeth were affected.

Periodontal Disease Children in the school years were more likely than young children to develop disease of the gums, and from the age of 7 onwards, at least half the children were affected. There is a strong relationship between debris on the teeth and inflammation of the gums. Gingivitis in childhood leads to chronic periodontitis in adults which is a further major cause of tooth loss.

Malocclusion Between 7 and 15 years of age at least half the children were found to have some degree of crowding, and in addition many other variations in occlusal development may occur.

Accidental Injury In the later years of school life, between the ages of 12 and 14 years, 20% of boys and 10% of girls had damaged their front teeth through accident.

If all the disorders reviewed in the survey were taken together, then 9 out of 10 children needed dental treatment; and because dental disease recurs this means continuing surveillance and treatment. Early decay of the first permanent molars and permanent incisor teeth indicates a higher incidence of caries; and as this will be maintained such children are a group at special risk.[3]

Adolescents

13.9 By fifteen years of age, 33% of the children had already lost one or more teeth, and 8% five or more teeth by extraction for caries. Neglect in childhood and adolescence diminishes the prospect of good dental health in the adult. A survey in 1968[4] showed that whilst few young adults had lost all their teeth, the proportion of those between the ages of 15 and 34 in the North who had suffered total tooth loss was over 15%. Whilst this was higher than the national average, the fact that 37% of the adult population was found to be edentulous remains a sad statistic which could be related to dental ill-health in childhood and adolescence. The problem in adolescence is dental neglect as part of a natural rejection of authority at this age with an unwillingness to arrange continuing dental care.

[3] Sutcliffe, P (1974). Longitudinal Study of Caries Experience and Extraction of First Permanent Molars in Children. *Comm. Dent. and Oral Epid.* 2, 182–186.

[4] Department of Health and Social Security (1970). *Adult Dental Health Survey 1968*. HMSO, London.

The Handicapped

13.10 The range of handicap and the number of affected children are described in Chapter 2. Here we have in mind the 164,000 children in England and Wales in 1973 who were receiving special education in a variety of institutions or at home. Many of these children present special problems for dental treatment and much of their disease remains untreated at the present time. A study of severely mentally handicapped children between 6 and 9 years in three London Boroughs showed that 77% of carious lesions in permanent teeth were untreated, suggesting that the level of restorative treatment in severely handicapped children falls well below that for normal children in the country as a whole.[5] Another study over 3 years of physically and mentally handicapped children of all ages found a similar level of dental decay and an excessive level of periodontal disease, but demonstrated that preventive dentistry was possible.[6] It stressed the advantage of mobile dental clinics going to the institutions where the children were living or to their schools, but in view of the greater need for general anaesthesia for routine procedures in such children, this approach should be linked with centres where skilled anaesthesia is available. In view of the dental needs of the handicapped and their inability to seek treatment for themselves, society has a special responsibility for providing them with dental care. Many health authorities are making special provision for the treatment of handicapped children and we are encouraged by this. Yet although there are centres of excellence, in many parts of the country the necessary experience and facilities are not available, and for the country as a whole none of the services are providing adequately for this group.

Prevention of Dental Disease

13.11 Although genetic constitution will influence the development of the individual's mouth and teeth, historical and epidemiological evidence points to powerful environmental factors as the major causes of dental caries. In this country, the epidemic increase in dental disease began in the second half of the last century and has been repeated in other industrially developed and affluent societies. The common factor was an increase in the consumption of refined carbohydrate foods and, for children, greater consumption of foods with a high content of refined sugar, especially the many varieties of biscuits and sweets.

13.12 The cause of both dental decay and periodontal disease is the occurrence of bacterial plaque on the teeth. In the presence of frequent exposure to sugar, acids derived from it attack the tooth enamel beneath the plaque initiating the process of tooth decay. Bacterial action within that part of the plaque in contact with the gums causes them to become inflamed, and this gingivitis can lead to advanced destruction of periodontal tissues later in life. Current feeding habits such as the use of reservoir feeders, continuing to drink from a bottle after the age of two, eating in the school break and free access to the biscuit tin at home, increase the incidence of caries.[7] Some decay and most gingivitis can be prevented or controlled by removal of plaque by tooth brushing. The prevailing

(5) Murray, J J, and McLeod, J P (1973). The dental condition of severely sub-normal children in the three London Boroughs. *Brit. Dent. J.* 134, 380.

(6) Pool, D (1975). *The dental needs of handicapped children.* RSH Vol 95.

(7) Todd, J E (1975). *Children's Dental Health in England and Wales, 1973.* HMSO, London. Tables 21.11, 21.12, 21.13, 21.15, 21.16, 21.17

indifference to cleaning teeth at home and at school is therefore of great importance. The low priority of dental hygiene in the scale of family discipline is also reflected in the tendency to avoid the dentist unless in trouble; a third of all children attend a dentist for the first time because of toothache and the need for an extraction. There is moreover a social class gradient in attitudes towards dental health, with the result that those in the higher social classes tend to take more care of their teeth, to have less active decay, and to make more extensive use of the existing services. It is important to redress this situation with better directed and more understanding dental health education.

Dental Health Education

13.13 Dental health education is part of general health education. Seeking to change behaviour by explanation and persuasion is a slow process, and present methods have not so far proved very successful. Yet establishing sound habits of dental hygiene in childhood remains an important aspect of dental health. There are three areas where the education of the public is particularly important: the practice of personal oral hygiene, regular seeking of dental care, and restraint in the consumption of sugar. With regard to the latter, the frequency and nature of sugar intake are more significant than the quantity consumed.

13.14 It is the responsibility of the individual dentist to inform his patients on these matters. However at present his educational opportunities are limited by the fact that only a minority of children are regular attenders, and all too often by the time of the first attendance, resistance to dental hygiene and faulty dietary habits are already established. *Education for dental health should therefore be part of the routine care of expectant and nursing mothers and regularly provided for mothers of pre-school children.* As the direct involvement of the dentist may be limited the aid of those who have a natural contact with mothers and children in those early important days should be enlisted. There should be increased emphasis on dental health education in the training curricula of midwives, child health visitors, GPPs, paediatricians and paediatric nurses and they should be encouraged to include it in their health education in the home, practice or hospital. A dental hygienist visiting an ante-natal clinic or a children's ward could possibly achieve more by educating the other professionals than by direct contact with mother and child.

13.15 Parents will read leaflets, magazines and see TV programmes and it is the duty of the educator to see that they do not face conflicting advice; this would be achieved if there were better communication between professionals. *We believe that the Health Education Council should continuously transmit to the media up to date information on the subject of dental health.* The influence of television is considerable and can be favourable or unfavourable. On the credit side it is probable that more people learn of the dangers of plaque from this source than any other. The advertising of confectionery represents the debit side and therefore the responsibility of those who devise and monitor the content of advertisements is great. It was noted that in the Netherlands there are restrictions on the content and timing of sweet advertisements. While we do not advocate the complete adoption of the Dutch system in this country we do consider that care should be taken not to encourage the frequent eating of confectionery between meals.

13.16 At the community level dental health education should be the responsibility of the Health Education Officer in consultation with expert dental opinion and in particular, the Area Dental Officer. *The Area Dental Officer should, if there is no Dental Health Education Officer, appoint a suitably motivated and trained person who is enthusiastic and acceptable to children, parents, and professionals.* We hope that the Area Dental Officer will regard funding and supporting this person as one of his most important duties. The Dental Health Education Officer would of course need to cooperate closely with the Health Education Officer.

13.17 Dental health education should continue during school life; a cooperative effort between dentists, teachers, school nurses and parents. *Dental health should be taught as part of general health education in teachers' training colleges, and schools should promote dental health projects and from time to time hold a dental health week.* Area Dental Officers should be active in promoting dental health education in schools, remembering particularly the end of school life, as this is a common period for self-neglect. *Experiment should be encouraged in the evaluation of different methods of dental health education.* As effective methods are found they should become part of the education of children, and the special education of expectant mothers and the parents of young children, and of all professionals concerned. It is useless preaching control in sugar consumption and improvement in oral hygiene if there is a practical indifference to these precepts. Discretion should be exercised in the items sold in school tuckshops, for the sale of sweets, biscuits and other foods containing sugar on the school premises must imply that the schools approve of their consumption. In the future facilities should always be available in school cloakrooms for the practice of oral hygiene. Children should be encouraged to clean their teeth after school lunch.

Fluoridation

13.18 The control of sugar consumption and the self-removal of dental plaque require the cooperation of the public. There is one measure that would prevent a great deal of dental caries without individual effort: water fluoridation. *The presence of fluoride, to a level of 1 part per million in all public water supplies, would substantially reduce dental caries in children and restrain it in adults, and the procedure is safe, effective and cheap.* "The solid justification of the safety of 1 part per million of fluoride in water rests on the health experience of generations residing in the temperate areas of the United States who have consumed naturally fluoridated water. No illness of infants or adults has been unequivocally attributed to fluorides from these sources. Fluoride is accepted as a safe and effective prophylactic agent in the prevention of dental caries whose benefits, strikingly apparent in childhood, continue, with continued use, into adult life".[8]

13.19 Comprehensive surveys[9] in this country as well as in the USA have confirmed the facts and rigorous scientific and professional examination the

---

[8] Hodges, C H (1974). Fluorides in Paediatrics. *Amer. J. Dis. Child.* 128, 291–293.

[9] *Department of Health and Social Security Report No 122* (1965). The fluoridation studies in the United Kingdom and results achieved after eleven years. HMSO, London.

validity of the conclusions. The recent report of the Royal College of Physicians "Fluoride, Teeth and Health" (1976) concludes that:

> "There is no evidence that the consumption of water containing approximately 1 mg/litre of fluoride (1 ppm) in a temperate climate is associated with any harmful effects, irrespective of the hardness of water."

A resolution of the 28th World Health Assembly (1975)[10] on fluoridation and dental health considered that:

> "Sufficient evidence on the safety and effectiveness of the use of fluorides as a method to prevent dental caries has already been obtained" and recommended: "approved methods for the prevention of dental caries especially by optimisation of the fluoride content of water supplies".

No public health procedure has been subjected to such long and stringent testing. In terms of protection for the whole community, including those most in need, fluoridation is beyond doubt the most effective public health measure for the prevention of dental disease. The effect on dental services has been impressively demonstrated in New Zealand where children are largely treated by "dental nurses" who correspond to our dental auxiliaries. Prior to fluoridation one nurse was capable of caring for 450 patients; ten years after its introduction, each nurse was able to care for between 700 and 1,000 children, and the average number of fillings inserted annually had fallen from 5 to 3 per child.[11]

13.20 If decay is preventible, why is it not being prevented? At present 8% of the people of Britain enjoy the benefits of fluoridation; why then are 92% being deprived? If caries killed, fluoridation would have been mandatory for twenty years. The real obstacles are public apathy, minority prejudice and governmental reluctance to impose a political solution. The cost in unnecessary disease, personal pain and discomfort, misuse of professional resources and national expenditure has been immense. *We recommend that immediate steps should be taken to introduce fluoridation on a national scale, if necessary with new legislation.*

Other Preventive Procedures

13.21 The Report on Preventive Dentistry of the Working Party on the Dental Services[12] considered a variety of systemic and topical methods of administering fluoride. It recognised that each raised problems in their application to pre-school and school children, and affirmed that the best means was the fluoridation of public water supplies. Nevertheless, we are satisfied that properly formulated fluoride applications applied by dentists or their licensed representatives effect a reduction in incremental caries over a two to three year period, which is the usual span of clinical trials so far. Their use is recommended for individual children at special risk from dental caries and its sequelae, especially the severely handicapped child. Evidence is lacking at present on the longer term effect and the cost benefit of such applications, and until this is available, we suspend

---

(10) WHO Assembly Resolution (1975). *Comm. Dent. Oral. Epid.* 3, 149.

(11) Kennedy, D P (1970). School dental nurses in New Zealand. *New Z. Med. J.* 72, 301–303.

(12) Department of Health and Social Security (1973). Report of the working Party on the Dental Services: Preventive Dentistry. HMSO, London.

judgement on the question of their routine use in the total child population. *We consider that serial studies should evaluate the long-term effect of fluoride applications and that they should include feasible forms of self-application, such as mouth rinses.*

13.22 We noted the Swedish study by Axelsson and Lindhe[13] which showed that children who had their teeth cleaned frequently and fluoride topically applied by hygienists were virtually free from dental caries and gingivitis. There are a number of difficulties in the way of implementing such a programme in England and Wales, one of which is the lack of a sufficient number of hygienists or dental auxiliaries to carry it out. However the results were sufficiently impressive to justify a serial study in this country to evaluate the method, and its cost effectiveness.

13.23 Studies of the efficacy of fissure sealing have shown conflicting results and again there is a need for longer term evaluation. At present, therefore, we can recommend their use only for children at special risk from dental caries and its sequelae e.g. children suffering from heart disease or from bleeding or clotting disorders and for caries prone children. *In general, we recommend that the value and cost effectiveness of different preventive procedures aimed at individuals and groups should be evaluated.*

Are the needs being met?

13.24 During the past two decades there has been a steadily increasing amount of dental treatment provided for children and a better pattern of care. More teeth are conserved and fewer extracted, so that the problem of gross sepsis in young mouths is less common.[14] At the same time the prevalence of dental disease in school children has remained as high as ever during this period, with the result that care is still needed by large numbers of children. The present system of records, which registers courses of treatment, makes estimation of their number difficult. We know that in 1974 the School and Priority Dental Service treated 1.5 million children and it is unlikely that the General Dental Service treated more than 3.5 million. This means that 5 million received some treatment for dental decay, and of the remaining 4 million approximately 3 million who needed treatment did not receive it. As far as the management of irregular teeth (orthodontics), is concerned, crowding of the permanent teeth should have been treated by the age of 14. However in a sample of children of this age, 50% were suffering from this condition which, in many cases, could have been dealt with simply by limited and selective extraction.

13.25 Another serious aspect of the problem is the regional variation both in disease and services. This is shown in Tables 3 and 4.

---

(13) Axelsson, P, and Lindhe, J (1974). Effects of preventive programme on dental plaque. *Journal of Clinical Periodontology.* 1. 126–138.

(14) Evidence from British Association for the Study of Community Dentistry.

TABLE 3

Caries in Schoolchildren in Wales and in the SE Region of England

Region	Age (Yrs)	Caries DMF	Experience df	Children with one or more extractions for caries (per cent)	Children with active caries (per cent)
SE England	5	—	3.1	—	57
	15	8.1	—	19	50
Wales	5	—	4.0	—	71
	15	10.1	—	50	72

TABLE 4

Dental Manpower in two Health Areas in England 1974

Area	Maintained School Population	Number of General Dental Practitioners	Community Dental Services	
			In post Number	wte
Avon	162,070	287	37	32
Humberside	172,139	118	30	21

Through more and better treatment, and with immense effort, dental disease in children is partially contained. The most astonishing fact of all is that we are describing a preventible disease.

13.26 Dental disease is universal and recurrent; dental decay is in part preventible; present services are only meeting half the need. We received evidence to the effect that dental care in Britain had in the past, been largely directed towards adult treatment, and while this work had been necessary, nonetheless many dental situations had only become inevitable because of neglect in childhood. We believe from the evidence that if we could get the first 12 years right, the picture would look very different. *The emphasis should move away from adult dentistry and repair, to children's dentistry and prevention.*

13.27 The straight way to this objective is plain; reduce the amount of disease and so make it possible for the service to meet the need. Fluoridation could reduce dental decay in children to half its present level and the effects would be evident within ten years. This is the first priority; without it a comprehensive service for children cannot be achieved at a reasonable cost. In the meantime the service goes on, under strain, unequally distributed, administratively divided, only partly containing the problem.

13.28 Dental services for children are provided by: the General Dental Service, the School and Priority Dental Service, and the Hospital Dental Service. The staffing of these services is shown in Table 5.

TABLE 5

Professional Staff in the Dental Services in England and Wales (1974)

Professional category	GDS	SPDS	HDS
general dental practitioners	11,408 (No)	—	—
general dental practitioner orthodontists	120 (No)	—	—
school dental officers	—	1,585 (wte)	—
consultant dental surgeons	—	—	339 (241 wte)
consultant orthodontists	—	12 (wte)	98 (81 wte)
other hospital dental staff	—'	—	637 (510 wte)
dental auxiliaries	—	205 (wte)	
dental hygienists	*	12 (wte)	59 (wte)

* There were approximately 400 hygienists working in the general dental service in 1974 (United Kingdom Statistics = 418).

The General Dental Service

13.29 There are 11,528 practitioners in this branch of the service. Since 1948, an increasing proportion of "courses for treatment" for children has been carried out by them; in 1949, 7% were for children under 15 years and by 1974 this had risen to 31%.[15] The national survey found that 75% of the children in the sample had used the General Dental Service at some time, and half the 14 year olds had always done so.[16] Treatment is free for all under 16 and for those over 16 who are full time at school. For those between 16 and 21 who have left school, it is free apart from the charges for dentures. The general categories of treatment are known, in a collective sense, but its consistency and effectiveness in the individual is difficult to elicit. Payment is based on "items of service"; it does not include specific fees for preventive procedures, although the fee for the first attendance covers "clinical examination, advice and report", and for periodontal conditions "any necessary instruction in oral hygiene". This service provides orthodontic treatment for 130,000 children annually; and 120 practitioners confine their practice to the treatment of malocclusion which is mainly a problem of growth and development.

The School and Priority Service

13.30 This branch of the service has a statutory duty to provide dental inspection and treatment for all children in maintained schools without charge. In 1974, there were in terms of whole-time equivalents about 1,500 dental officers in this service assisted by about 200 dental auxiliaries and 20 dental hygienists. In 1974 they inspected almost 5 million school children—56% of the school population under 16—and the total number given treatment was 1.4 million, 16% of the school population. Their work included

(15) Dental Estimates Board reports (1948–1974).
(16) Todd, J E (1975). *Children's Dental Health in England and Wales, 1973.* HMSO, London.

15,000 sessions for dental health education, and 5% of their time was given to children under 5. 3% of school dentists specialise in the management of malocclusion and approximately 20,000 children are treated each year by the use of appliances; the full extent of their contribution to orthodontic care is unknown. The service operates by school dental officers visiting schools, inspecting children, notifying parents of any treatment required, offering to provide it at a named clinic or suggesting that it can be obtained from a general dental practitioner. There is reliable evidence that almost half the school children in the country do not receive an annual inspection and with it the possibility of treatment within the school dental service. This is primarily due to the difficulty of recruiting the necessary number of dentists and ancillaries for the work; Wales and the North of England are particularly handicapped in this respect. The General Dental Service and the School and Priority Service tend to care for different sections of the community, with the latter mainly providing services in rural areas and for children from the lower social classes and disadvantaged families. In areas where there is a low dentist population ratio, it may be the only practicable source of treatment.

The Hospital Service

13.31 This provides specialist surgical and orthodontic advice and treatment. In 1974 the total staff for patients of all ages was 1,074 (wte 832) of whom 437 (wte 322) were consultants and 637 (wte 510) other grades. Of the consultants, 339 were "consultants in dental surgery" and 98 "consultant orthodontists"; the proportion of time the first group give to children is unknown but the consultant orthodontists are mainly concerned with children. In the Departments of Children's Dentistry in the University Dental Schools, there are 21 members of academic staff with honorary contracts in the National Health Service. As the category of consultant in children's dentistry does not yet exist in the National Health Service (it has recently been approved in principle) the members of academic departments carry the main specialist responsibility in a general paedodontic sense. This in no way underestimates the contribution of consultant orthodontists with their primary concern for children and their developmental approach to the subject. Each year, they see 70,000 children sent by the other two services, accept half of these for personal care, and return the others to the referring school dental officer or general dental practitioner.[17] The Hospital Service also provides treatment for long-stay children in hospital.

The Uneven Distribution of Services

13.32 The inadequacy of services is exacerbated by regional variations in staffing and facilities. In an improving service, the proportion of teeth filled to those extracted increases. Figures from the Dental Estimates Board for 1973 show this ratio to be 1 tooth extracted to 4.2 filled in Wales, increasing to 1 to 5.9 in the North, 1 to 7.2 in the Midlands and 1 to 13.4 in London and the South East. The disparity in services which they reflect is not acceptable.

---

[17] Consultant Orthodontist Group Report on Treatment Statistics, 1973.

Developing the Services—where should we go from here?

13.33 The underlying facts and the professional context within which this question must be answered are clear: widespread disease, official reluctance to prevent, insufficient and unevenly distributed manpower, a divided service. It was put to us that the three parts of the dental health service in the past had often worked with an independence which had done little to ensure that the convenience and clinical needs of children were met: services had sometimes been duplicated, sometimes neglected, and there had been no consideration of the overall cost to the community either socially or economically.

13.34 We are well aware that in children's medicine the divided care provided by general practitioners, child and school health doctors, paediatricians and allied specialists has been incomplete, confusing to parents, professionally divisive, and wasteful in its duplication of manpower and facilities. The pattern of general dental services for children has a broad similarity to the present child health services but there are important differences. Unlike the General Medical Services, there is no "list of patients" whom a practitioner accepts for continuous care, and a patient must seek acceptance from a dentist for each course of treatment. The School Dental Service differs from its medical counterparts in that, in addition to surveillance and individual preventive care, it provides a considerable amount of treatment. Treatment is available not only for children but for expectant mothers and for women who have had a child in the previous year.

The Present Situation

13.35 Before 1948, the School Dental Service was the only source of free dental treatment for children. After that date free treatment was also available from general dental practitioners in the National Health Service. The question therefore arises as to whether the two branches of the Service are in competition with each other or whether they are complementary. There are important factors which should be considered in relation to this question.

13.36 Many areas exist and are likely to exist within the foreseeable future where the proportion of general dental practitioners to the population is so unfavourable that it precludes the possibility of their alone extending a comprehensive preventive and therapeutic service to the child population. The situation is exacerbated by the fact that 97% of children need dental treatment during their school years and that the treatment required is of a continuing nature. Moreover, general practitioners have a pressing and continuing commitment to the adult population.

13.37 The School and Priority Dental Service on the other hand is specifically responsible for children, and, in providing surveillance and preventive care, is similar to the School Health Service. In addition it provides a considerable amount of treatment. We noted earlier that it provides a service for those sections of the community who are less likely to seek it, and where dentists are in short supply, it may be the only practicable source of treatment. We therefore see the two services having

208

complementary rôles, which will vary with the needs, demands and resources in different areas. The School and Priority Dental Services provide care for priority groups and we envisage a strengthening of these services to provide supporting services which for one reason or another cannot be provided by the General Dental Service.

13.38 We have also considered the future rôle of the General Dental Service and anticipate that with greater numerical recruitment to general practice the present trend for more children to be treated by this service will continue. Yet the advantages of one practitioner, with a special interest in children, providing total therapeutic and preventive dental care as a member of a group practice for all children in a particular area are readily apparent. Whilst from manpower shortage and other difficulties such a service is not practicable in many parts of the country at the present time, we consider it essential that this type of service should be investigated. Only when the advantages and disadvantages for children and for dentists are clearly seen can the profession fairly consider a major change of this kind, involving, as it might, a change in the method of remuneration for one branch which has been in use for 25 years.

13.39 *We are of the opinion therefore that a model should be set up to investigate and evaluate a primary care service for children based on the General Dental Service with a system of remuneration provided by a capitation fee.* Our proposal is that in one or more districts with a high ratio of dentists to population, good professional relationships, a sympathetic Area Dental Officer and a community-minded dental school, a model service along these lines should be introduced. The viability of such a scheme would depend upon the establishment of suitable training programmes; the provision of more dental accommodation in health centres; and the acceptance by the profession and government of payment for children by capitation or annual fee. Such a change in remuneration either to a capitation fee as in medicine, or to an annual fee for maintaining a child dentally fit, should encourage the practice of preventive as well as reparative dentistry for children. We accept that a primary care service of this sort might be a desirable pattern, especially where dental group practices have been developed but until it has been tested there are no grounds for wider recommendation. To mount effective experiments will take time and must not weaken existing services. *Recruitment to the School and Priority Dental Service must be maintained and the service strengthened.* In-service or continuing opportunities for special training in children's dentistry should be available equally to members of the General Dental Service and the School and Priority Dental Service.

Ways Forward
13.40 Currently the most serious problem is the unacceptable difference in the provision of services in different parts of the country: 57% of the school population and 53% of the total population live north of a line drawn from the Severn to the Wash, but only 40% of general dental practitioners and 45% of school dental officers work there. *A sustained effort to attract dentists to areas deprived of adequate dental care must*

be made and effective incentives sought. Among these, a system of preferential remuneration acceptable to the profession and the DHSS, and good accommodation, should be high on the list. This latter could be provided most satisfactorily in health centres, with the advantage of bringing dentists into everyday contact with other members of the primary health care team. This also strengthens our view that the continuing development of health centres should have high priority. Even greater regional differences exist in the school service while many areas have a serious shortage of both.

13.41 From the beginning of the Health Service, the General Dental Service has provided a steadily increasing part of children's dental care. The increase in its work with children can hardly continue at the same rate without an increase in manpower. In 1956, the McNair Committee recommended that the strength of the profession should be raised to 20,000 and with an annual intake of 942 students this should be reached by 1980. Yet in such a situation, a general increase in dental manpower as recommended by the McNair Committee is not the complete answer nor necessarily the right one. *For this reason we believe that it is time to review the manpower needed for the provision of a satisfactory dental service which accords priority to children, taking into account the implications for undergraduate and postgraduate education.*

Cooperation in Primary Care

13.42 A new type of service lies in the future and redressing regional inequalities will not be easy, so what steps can be taken now? The General and the School services could work more closely together, with both services providing a greater contribution to the dental care of certain groups of children, particularly the handicapped. This will mean some increase in dental manpower in the school service with special training in children's and community dentistry, an acceptable career structure, and rewards more closely in line with the general dental service. Another important area where collaboration would help concerns school children receiving regular attention from the School Dental Service when they leave school. Continuity of dental treatment is left to individual initiative and at this age a break readily occurs. We believe the transfer of school children to general dental practitioners should occur during the last year at school; helped at this stage they are more likely to continue regular dental care in adult life.

Ancillary Personnel

13.43 Two classes of ancillary dental workers provide care in the mouth, the hygienist and the "New Cross" auxiliary. The hygienist's duties include health education, scaling and polishing teeth and undertaking preventive measures. They are capable of making a considerable contribution to child dental health and it is likely that their skills would be particularly valuable in preserving the dental health of handicapped children. However, most hygienists are employed in general dental practice and whilst they do carry out treatment for children we believe most of their work is devoted to treating the adult population. There is at present no way of persuading a larger proportion to work wholly with children.

13.44 The dental auxiliary on the other hand works almost exclusively with children and for this reason we gave careful consideration to her rôle. A survey of children in the last year of school life suggested that 80% of their treatment could have been provided by dental auxiliaries, had sufficient numbers been available.[18] The dental auxiliary (New Cross type) in this country, working in association with a dental surgeon in hospital or in the School Service, carries out simple fillings, extracts primary teeth under local infiltration anaesthesia, carries out certain preventive procedures and takes part in dental health education. She is well qualified to undertake much of the preventive and treatment care needed by children. "So far, research in the UK has been limited to the use of auxiliaries with established training backgrounds. It is desirable that this research should progress into the relation between training and the pattern of practice and should include the interaction between different members of the dental team."[19] The problem is their limited numbers. Since 1962, 691 have qualified, and 300 are at present in post in England and Wales, mostly in the south. This is not surprising when there is only one training school, in London, admitting 60 students a year for a two-year training. *Convinced that this type of professional ancillary can make an important contribution to child dental health, we recommend the establishment in the provinces of two new training schools, similar in size and approach to the School for Dental Auxiliaries, New Cross.* This has, so far, been a woman's profession and consideration should be given to ways of recruiting men. The gradual increase in the number of dental auxiliaries which we consider necessary would be absorbed by the School and Priority Dental Service who have available accommodation and manpower for supervision. In the long term, however, legislation would be needed to permit dental auxiliaries to work in general practice.

A Strengthened School Service

13.45 Moving from general principles to daily practice, we see the School Dental Officer as a general paedodontist, working closely with a dental auxiliary, and in collaboration with the General Dental Service, contributing more widely to the dental care of children. This extended rôle would include the following:

the identification, by annual dental inspections, of the needs of all school children

the provision of a treatment service for children complementary to that provided by the General Dental Service

the provision of a comparable service for the pre-school child

the provision of preventive procedures at an appropriate level for children in special need, eg the handicapped, the caries prone child, and the particularly nervous child

the deployment of ancillary staff in providing treatment and preventive procedures

---

[18] Bowden, D, Davies, R, Holloway, P, Lennon, M, Rugg-Gunn, A (1973). Treatment needs of 15-year old children. *Brit. Dent. J.* 134, 375.

[19] Allred, H, and Hobdell, M H (1975). Research in Dental Care. *Brit. Med. Bull.* 31, 149–151.

the organisation of dental health education in the community

the provision of a specialist service, within the new clinical structure, to provide for emergencies; for children requiring difficult or lengthy courses of treatment; for orthodontic surveillance assessment and treatment; and other such cases which might prove particularly time-consuming for the general dental practitioner

the collection of necessary epidemiological data.

13.46 We have seen on our visits the strain and disenchantment of men and women working in the School Service and their need for personal relief, an acceptable career structure, wider post-graduate training and better facilities and rewards. Personal relief means increased manpower, but this can no longer be estimated in terms of national dental manpower alone. The expected increase in the contribution of dental auxiliaries, the effects of redeployment, and the diminished work load in those areas where fluoridation has been introduced, must be taken into account. This is a good example of the need for area planning based on local epidemiological data which the new partnership between Area Dental Officers, Specialists in Community Medicine (Child Health) and District Planning Teams for children can produce. *We recommend that the School and Priority Service should be increased to a level which would allow it to undertake the functions outlined above.*

Consultants and Specialists

13.47 In dentistry as in medicine, primary and specialist care should be complementary aspects of a single service. In view of the key position occupied by children in the strategy for dental health we were surprised to receive evidence to the effect that the absence of a consultant service in paedodontics was a serious deficiency in the present system, not covered by either of the existing dental consultancies, and of the need for consultant advice to be available on the full range of children's dental care and preferably from one source. There have been consultant oral surgeons and consultant orthodontists since 1948; it has recently been accepted that a third specialty in restorative dentistry for adults should be added; the fourth need, for a similar consultant for children, has now been accepted by the Joint Committee for Higher Training in Dentistry of the Royal College.[20] The order reflects past professional development and the higher prevalence of malocclusions compared with unusual oral and dental pathology.

13.48 We have no wish to overlook the pioneer rôle of orthodontists in the development of specialist dental care for children. However the time has come for coordination of the orthodontic services at present available in the General Dental Service, the public dental service and the hospitals, to make the most effective use of existing resources and to ensure that skills are deployed to maximum advantage. These requirements can be met by an orthodontic team approach, involving school dental officers, general dental practitioners and hospital orthodontists. One group of hospital specialists believes this should lead to an integrated community and hospital service.[21]

---

[20] Report of Joint Committee for Higher Training in Dentistry (1972). Royal College of Surgeons, London.

[21] Parker, C D, and Bettles, R H (1975). Hospital and Community Orthodontic Services in Leicestershire: a report on cooperation between services. *Brit. Dent. Jour.* 139, 331–335.

13.49 If this is desirable for one aspect of specialist dentistry it is surely necessary for the remaining area of unmet need at specialist level. *For the present and the future, the consultant in paediatric dentistry is an essential not an after-thought.* The justification for such a consultant is not his expertise in carrying out advanced technical procedures, but his ability to apply knowledge of normal and abnormal growth and development, and of local and general pathology to all aspects of dental care—conservative, preventive, surgical and orthodontic. He would have a special responsibility for children with physical or mental handicap or psychiatric disorder, would be a member of the Regional Child Development Centre, and would visit special hospitals and residential schools to give advice or carry out treatment. (See Chapter 14 paragraphs 39 and 45.) *This new type of specialist would first develop in University Departments of Children's Dentistry, and in the starting phase there should be at least one in each region, especially in regions without a dental teaching hospital.* His training would have much in common with that of the consultant orthodontist.

Academic Departments concerned with the Dental Care of Children

13.50 There are thirteen undergraduate departments and one post-graduate Institute concerned with children's dentistry. Their design does not follow a single pattern, but the essence is a combination of orthodontics and other children's services. In some instances, mainly for historical reasons, the departments of children's dentistry and orthodontics are separate both physically and administratively; in others they are physically contiguous and administratively parallel; and in a few, conservative, orthodontic, and preventive care for children is undertaken in the one department and the aim is the study and teaching of comprehensive dental care for children. Academic integration is the basis of service integration and an ideal worth striving for. The historical priority of specialist orthodontics arose from the demand by practitioners for consultant help in orthodontics rather than in children's dentistry; and the academic departments of orthodontics (or the orthodontic component) have been responsible for the development of the orthodontic services at consultant level in university departments and in the National Health Service. Similar development has not occurred in the other aspects of children's dentistry. *There is therefore a basic need to strengthen the child dentistry component of academic dental departments for children.*

13.51 The conditions met most often in children with which they are involved at present are these: injury, heart disease, uncommon or complex dental pathology, handicap and psychiatric disorder, blood disorders, miscellaneous paediatric problems, cleft lip and palate and the normal child who is caries prone or particularly nervous. This distribution of illness emphasises the need for a strong professional partnership between paedodontists and paediatricians and allied specialists in service, teaching and research.

13.52 Yet if children's dentistry is to advance as a subject and a service,

213

undergraduate and graduate needs must be understood and attractively met. A good academic department would ensure the following:

Undergraduate paedodontic training to provide the potential dentist with the interest, basic competence and confidence in the dental treatment of children

Postgraduate training especially to improve the standards of primary care in the general and school services

In-service training of full-time rotating junior staff as the potential consultants of the future.

To fulfil these responsibilities the department would need to be involved in the following:

Full preventive and therapeutic dental surveillance of enough children to allow the student to develop the necessary techniques and confidence to treat and handle children in the dental chair

Preventive and therapeutic services for handicapped children to introduce students to the developmental understanding and dental techniques which their management requires

A close working and teaching relationship with other academic departments, especially paediatrics, child psychiatry, paediatric cardiology, paediatric surgery, haematology and with the Regional Child Development Centre

Epidemiological studies in collaboration with the Department of Social Medicine and the Area Dental Officer.

13.53 *The implication therefore is that if the primary and specialist dental care of children is to be improved to the degree which our recommendations require, academic departments of children's dentistry must be strengthened.* All departments are fully occupied with their present treatment, prevention, teaching and research responsibilities; and the 21 honorary consultants in such departments provide almost the whole of the consultant service in paediatric dentistry. *Further commitments could not be undertaken without an increase in teaching staff: at least one additional teacher to each undergraduate department and more than one to the one postgraduate department of children's dentistry in the country.* There is one other teaching experiment which deserves comment. *From the limited experience so far we suggest that schemes allowing final year dental students to operate under supervision in the School and Priority service should be extended and their educational and service value assessed.*

13.54 We are convinced that the emphasis in dental as in medical care for children should move to the community. The hospital is then one instrument in a network of community services. Its continuing importance is guaranteed by contemporary needs for specialist skills in the management of more complex disorders as well as its traditional rôle in research and teaching. Hospitals should examine their changing responsibilities and be willing to extend their practice, research and teaching into the community. In this sense the term "Hospital Service" for the third branch of the present service has an old-fashioned ring and might well be replaced by Supporting Consultant and Specialist Service.

214

13.55 We now consider the contributions of consultants and specialists to different aspects of the hospital service.

Outpatients

13.56 Outpatient dental care for children is provided by two types of hospital: large dental teaching hospitals and smaller specialist dental units forming part of many district general hospitals. All children are referred by a dentist or doctor with the exception that dental teaching hospitals will accept patients without referral for the relief of pain. There are four main reasons why they come: for the relief of pain, perhaps because general anaesthesia is necessary; for advice and treatment of malocclusion; because the child is physically or mentally handicapped; for the management of uncommon or complex disorders.

13.57 The use of outpatients by the first group is an extension of facilities available in the General or the School services, and whilst unavoidable with the present levels of manpower, should be generally discouraged as expensive hospital facilities are used. The exception is the more open door of the University Dental Hospitals. If referral cannot provide a sufficient quantity of common conditions the degree of open access should be agreed with the Area Health Authority. This would be comparable to the extended hospital provision in the Accident and Emergency Departments we have recommended for the inner city communities.

13.58 The largest group of children, estimated at 70,000 annually for all hospitals is the responsibility of Consultant Orthodontists; since a third of the children needing help do not receive it, this service should be developed. Half the children referred for a malocclusion return to the dental practitioner or school dentist for treatment. Yet each Regional Consultant sees on average over 1,000 patients in a year, without fully meeting the need. We share the view given in evidence to us that "orthodontics is an essential part of any child dental health programme and an essential background to the intelligent planning of general dental treatment in the child and in this way makes an important contribution to general dental health".[17]

13.59 *The best way to fill this gap in orthodontic care might be for every child to be examined in the tenth year by a dentist with special training in orthodontics.* This would identify children with a developing malocclusion and ensure that further investigation and treatment were carried out. The validity of orthodontic screening at this stage using a treatment index has been reported.[22] *However before this is widely implemented, preliminary trials should be carried out in areas where dental manpower is sufficient and the quality of dental services good.*

13.60 The Consultant's responsibility would be shared with the Area

[22] Scivier, G A, Menezees, D M, and Parker, C D (1974). A pilot study to assess the validity of the Orthodontic Treatment Priority Index in English Children. *Community Dent. Oral. Epid.* 2, 246–252.

Dental Officer, and include training programmes for the examining panel to ensure that criteria were clear and standardised. His services may be required in planning treatment for some children, but with specialised orthodontic training many malocclusions would be treatable by the School Dental Officer or General Dental Practitioner. *We advise a population norm for each orthodontic consultant and supporting staff of 100,000 children in the geographic area for which he is responsible.* Defining children for this purpose as birth to 15 years the minimum number of orthodontic consultants would be 120. The teaching and research commitment of academics holding honorary consultant contracts should be excluded from the calculation of this norm.

13.61 Whilst the Orthodontic Consultant is hospital based and should remain so, with an increase in manpower he could improve the service by taking it in certain circumstances to the community. The Regional Orthodontic Consultant, who has a defined geographic responsibility, should examine the distribution and size of his sources of patients. When large enough, he should consider travelling to the clinics, health centres, and one day to the general dental practices which refer most patients. On these visits he should examine selected new patients with prepared records or patients presenting problems in treatment. We noted previously[21] a successful example of this type of cooperation between specialist orthodontics and the school services; it involved 16 school clinics which were visited by the hospital consultant for joint clinics every two or three months.

13.62 The severely handicapped have special and largely unmet dental needs. *We recommend that in general their dental care should be brought up to and maintained at the level of that provided for other children and that in particular in certain types of physical handicap—for instance children suffering from heart or blood disease—the highest level of dental health must be maintained continuously.* Suitable preventive measures should be made available for handicapped children. Encouragement should be given to graduates to undertake this work and the dental education of consultants and specialists should include training in the treatment of handicapped children. *Although hospitals have a part to play, what is urgently needed in most areas is a unitary service which enables specialists, general dental practitioners and school dental officers to cooperate in providing dental care for all handicapped children at district level.* Working as a team they would regularly visit children at home or in special schools and decide what treatment was necessary and where it should be carried out. This would avoid excessive travel for children and parents. Dental hygienists would be particularly valuable in ensuring that these children are properly instructed, but at present they do not work in appreciable numbers in a field where they could be most valuable. *We are of the opinion that in day and residential institutions for handicapped children a dental hygienist should be employed whole or part-time according to the numbers of children in care.* Unusual and complex disorders in the handicapped would be dealt with by large regional or university hospitals with the necessary staff and facilities. The proposed consultant in paediatric dentistry could be a key

216

person in the design and development of this service. The training of such men and women, based in hospitals but with precise commitments in the community, is in our view a high priority and we would ask the Dental Schools to proceed as quickly as possible to train them.

In-patients

13.63 Children will be admitted for three main reasons: because they have a chronic illness, for a specific surgical procedure in the mouth and jaws, and where even a simple dental procedure carries a special hazard as with haemophilia. The chronic sick have much in common in their dental needs with the handicapped whom we have considered in the preceding paragraph. Children admitted for special surgical procedures or where there is a major risk of haemorrhage or other serious hazard, will always be under consultant care. In some centres, orthodontic consultants carry out their own surgery; in others the patient is admitted under the care of the consultant oral surgeon. When a medical condition is present, the relevant paediatric consultant is also involved. In future the consultant in paediatric dentistry will undertake an increasing part of the surgical aspect of child dental care, but the responsibilty for major oral surgery and the care of trauma in the face and jaws should remain with the consultant oral surgeon. *However, many dental surgical procedures needed by healthy children are particularly suitable for treatment on a day care basis, and the provision of facilities and their maximum use should be encouraged.* This would allow a more precise estimate of the number of beds needed for in-patient care. Ideally the in-patient beds should be in the children's ward.

13.64 This re-appraisal of the contribution of the hospital to the total services confirms the need for an increasing partnership with primary care. This will be seen in the collaboration of the new consultant in paediatric dentistry with general dental practitioners and school dental officers in seeking both a more comprehensive and a more local service for the handicapped, and in the collaboration of the consultant orthodontist in the joint orthodontic screening of all children in their tenth year which is to be evaluated. With hospital specialists moving into the community in this way the primary care services will become more discriminating in their referrals to hospital.

Procedures

13.65 Although we have not taken evidence on the use of general anaesthesia or the use of radiological equipment and we believe that great care is taken by the profession in both procedures, we feel it important to emphasise again that both procedures should be carried out according to the guidance or the codes of behaviour laid down.

Records

13.66 Detailed statistics of treatment in the general dental services and school dental services are available but they do not provide comprehensive information on dental treatment provided for school children because of their different basis of collection. Records in the general dental services are designed as an instrument of payment for the dentist, on an item-of-service basis, and relate to individual courses of treatment. They are collated by the Dental Estimates Board and could be produced on a national, regional or area basis but cannot by their nature identify the numbers of children treated. School dental service records are designed to provide a continuing record of each child's dental care. An omission which should be remedied is the lack of information about children who have orthodontic treatment by extraction only. Records are transferred to the appropriate health authority when the child moves from one area to another. The records are collated to provide annual statistics on a national, Regional and Area basis related to the numbers of children treated. Records for the two services should be comparable. We understand that only limited additional information could be obtained by modification of the present system of collation at the Dental Estimates Board.[24] It seems likely that comprehensive treatment statistics, showing the dental treatment given to children in whatever service they were treated, could only be achieved by bringing the school dental service records into line with general dental service recording methods. The improved system should permit the identification of patients which is not the case at present. *Since one of the difficulties in assessing needs at the moment is the lack of uniformity of dental statistics, the opportunity should be taken to improve the system so that needs can be measured and services more effectively monitored than at present.*

Dental Research

13.67 We decided here to limit our comments to the factors controlling the broad issues, though the need for specific areas of research are noted in different parts of this chapter. Considerable information is available on many aspects of child dental health: some is of a serial nature (eg some growth and development studies and the clinical trials of caries-preventing agents); most is based on cross-sectional prevalence studies, and though this is appropriate in some cases, in others more meaningful results would be obtained by the collection of serial data. Examples of areas where long-term serial research would be valuable include the evaluation of different methods of delivering dental treatment to children; the critical study of dental health education; and extended studies of preventive measures to allow long-term evaluation and assessment of cost benefit. Research funding bodies are in general reluctant to fund long-term projects which may extend over a period of 10 years. Research designed to improve dental services should therefore be based on the Central Departments and the Children's Research Liaison Group (see Chapter 21) would be the appropriate body.

---

(24) Anderson, J. Department of Dental Health, University of Birmingham—personal communication.

CHAPTER 14

HANDICAP

14.1 Throughout our report handicapped children have been identified as children with special service needs. No separate service has ever existed exclusively for their benefit; instead, their needs have been met through the normal services provided by general practitioners and hospital specialists in the NHS, by the local authority child health services, and by the facilities for special educational treatment that local education authorities provide for children from the age of two. We do not ourselves propose that there should be a special, largely separate service in the future. It is therefore important that we look at the way the integrated child health service that we propose will meet the special needs of handicapped children, and those of their parents and teachers.

Prevalence and Prevention

14.2 We have accepted the definitions of defect, disability and handicap given in the report([1]) of the National Children's Bureau working party on children with special needs, not only to further the use of a standard terminology but also because they make the essential distinctions:

> A DEFECT is some imperfection, impairment or disorder of the body, intellect or personality;

> A DISABILITY is a defect which does result in some malfunctioning but which does not necessarily affect the individual's normal life;

> A HANDICAP is a disability which for a substantial period, or permanently, retards, distorts or otherwise adversely affects normal growth, development or adjustment to life.

14.3 Neither incidence nor prevalence rates of disorders provide the requisite data for the planning of health, social and educational services, because not all children with a defect or disorder are significantly handicapped by it and because more than one disorder may occur in the same child. Authorities with responsibilities for services require to know the actual number of *children* with handicaps for whom they have to provide services. Since the incidence and prevalence of some conditions are known to vary between different geographical areas, between inner city and rural communities, and between social classes, *AHAs should conduct their own surveys of handicapped children to obtain appropriate data on which to base services to meet local need.* Local authorities are largely dependent upon information from staff of health services in order that they can comply with the Chronically Sick and Disabled Persons Act, 1970.

([1]) Younghusband, E, Birchall, D, Davie, R, and Kelmer Pringle, M L (1970). *Living with Handicap.* National Bureau for Cooperation in Child Care, London.

14.4 We can give only an indication of what this need is likely to be. Our estimates are derived from the published reports of a few reliable surveys[2-8] and they are applied here to an average health district having approximately 60,000 children under the age of 16 years (3,750 in each yearly age group). The estimates suggest that about 1,125 children aged 0–4 years will be moderately or severely handicapped by either physical (somatic), motor, visual, hearing and communication, or learning disorders which require special health care; 140 of them might need to attend a special school, full-time or part-time according to their age. About 4,125 children of compulsory school age will be similarly handicapped. Of these 700 might need to attend special schools. We must emphasise, however, that these are only approximate numbers; and they do not include children who are handicapped by psychiatric disorder (see Chapter 15). Furthermore, family circumstances and environment may act as external obstacles to normal function; they may predispose or contribute to dysfunction and sometimes cause it, especially in learning and behaviour. But they are not in themselves an intrinsic functional handicap and for this reason social handicap is not mentioned above either. Suffice it to say that adverse social factors occur more frequently in the many children slightly or moderately handicapped, particularly by learning disorders, than in the smaller number with severe handicaps of all kinds.

14.5 A reduction in the birth frequency of children with genetically determined handicaps may be expected as a result of the expansion in genetic counselling facilities we have recommended in Chapter 18, a declining birth rate among women over the age of 35 (who currently give birth to over one third of all children with Down's Syndrome), and more frequent use of methods of prenatal diagnosis followed by termination of pregnancy when fetal abnormality is present. Whilst every effort must obviously be made to improve obstetric and neonatal care where standards fall behind the best, the effect of such improvements as we have recommended (Chapter 8) on the incidence of congenital disorders is less certain. Better care is likely to reduce perinatal mortality but some of those babies who might not otherwise have survived may well be handicapped. We hope that the major impact of better obstetric and neonatal care would be in reducing brain damage that may contribute to or cause mental retardation and severe learning difficulties in those who survive.

(2) Miller, F J W, Court, S D M, Knox, E G, and Brandon, S (1974). *The School Years in Newcastle upon Tyne*. Oxford University Press, London.

(3) Rutter, M, Tizard, J, and Whitmore, K (1970). *Education, Health and Behaviour*. Longman, London.

(4) Rutter, M, Cox, A, Tupling, C, Berger, M, and Yule, W (1975). Attainment and adjustment in two geographical areas. *Brit. J. Psychiat.* 126, 493–519.

(5) Birch, H G, Richardson, S A, Baird, D, Horobin, G, and Illsley, R (1970). *Mental Subnormality in the Community*. Williams and Wilkie, Baltimore.

(6) Bain, D G H (1973). Health Centre Practice in Livingstone New Town. *Health Bulletin, Scottish Home and Health Department, Edinburgh*.

(7) Sheridan, M D, and Peckham, C S (1973). Hearing and speech at seven. *Special Education*, Vol 62, No 2.

(8) Dubissow, J (1975). An investigation into the incidence of congenital malformations and their call upon the resources of the community. Unpublished progress report.

14.6 *We believe the most important and most practicable contribution to the prevention of handicap lies in the effective treatment of potentially handicapping physical disorders and in the early recognition and prompt management of functional disorders (especially neuro-psychiatric disorders) of relatively moderate degree.* These are more accessible to modification and their numbers are very much greater than genetically determined severe handicaps that can be prevented by contraception and termination of pregnancy. Their prevention requires a higher standard of primary paediatric care (eg of convulsions in young children) through patient and consistent application of up-to-date techniques; a rational and determined concentration of services on children who may be regarded as "vulnerable" (eg the children of mothers who fail to make the best use of services that are available); and health education—or more precisely, health and development education. The whole tenor of our report is towards this end, for when dealing with chronic handicap, prevention (sometimes primary but invariably secondary) is inseparable from treatment.

Arrangements for the discovery of handicap

14.7 Severe, overt congenital abnormalities are usually recognised at birth, but slighter defects may be missed unless carefully looked for.[9] It may be some time before non-visible congenital disorders (eg deafness, congenital heart disease) reveal their presence by subsequent dysfunction unless they too are sought, and time must inevitably lapse before handicaps can be detected in skills only acquired as the child matures, as in the case of speech, and later, reading. Health services have been least successful in identifying the less severe disorders; and delay in helping handicapped children occurs most frequently in the case of school children with only slight or moderate neuro-developmental disorders that nevertheless cause quite serious handicap both to learning and behavioural or emotional adjustment.

14.8 The purpose of health surveillance, as we have stressed, is more than the detection of defects: but general developmental assessment is, nevertheless, an essential feature of arrangements that are required for the *early* recognition of handicap. Such recognition is clearly desirable—provided facilities and skills exist for intervention to be effective. The GPP and CHV pattern of staffing, and the recommendations we have made in Chapters 9 and 10 for adoption of a standard programme of health surveillance, should ensure that serial developmental assessment, carried out by doctors and nurses trained for the job, more nearly reaches all children. Given that, there should be an improvement in the early identification of handicaps especially those due to sensory and neurological disorders.

14.9 We attach particular importance to the medical examination of children prior to their entry to school, and to the regular visits of doctors and nurses to schools, because these are likely to reduce the delay in

---

[9] Pethybridge, R J, Vowles, M, and Brimblecombe, F S W (1975). Congenital malformations in Devon: their incidence, age and primary source of detection. In *Bridging in Health*. Oxford University Press, London.

helping pupils with learning and behaviour disorders. Today such delay is in part due to the late referral of children for investigation in spite of obvious difficulties in school; but in addition many school doctors do not always recognise handicapping conditions because they fail to notice less obvious defects that often underlie a child's difficulties. The entrant examination must therefore be undertaken in part as an exercise in the discovery of learning and behaviour disorder no less than of physical and sensory disorder. As education is compulsory from the age of five, virtually all children can be medically examined then, irrespective of whether or not they have attended child health clinics when younger. We expect too that more frequent meetings and discussion between health staff, teachers, social workers and psychologists will encourage earlier and informal requests for a medical opinion of children about whom teachers feel concern. CHV and SN thus have a central part in the recognition of handicapped children.

Facilities for the investigation and care of handicapped children

14.10 Diagnosis of handicap is not an exclusively medical responsibility; it may require the help of psychological, educational, social work and nursing personnel. The assessment of handicap is a prescription for action —which may be medical, educational or social.

14.11 A minority of handicapped children may require temporary admission to hospital for assessment and/or treatment but usually these can be provided on an out-patient basis rather than in hospital. On rare occasions long-stay hospital admission may be necessary. For many handicapped children there will be no specific medical treatment. Some children may require day admission to a school for effective assessment to be made and others may first need admission to a children's home. However all handicapped children need continuing surveillance after initial diagnosis and assessment. And because most handicaps are long lasting the child health services (no less than the educational and social work services) must continue to provide for the child's changing needs through adolescence, and until health services for adults effectively replace them.

14.12 The standard of diagnosis, assessment, treatment and care for children suffering from physical, mental or multiple handicaps whether in the hospital or the community does not reach that largely achieved by the National Health Service for the treatment of acute illness.

14.13 At the primary care level general practitioners are not trained to deal adequately with chronic disorders of children, and many GPs are not interested or are too busy to do so. Moreover the number of handicapped children on the list of a single GP is too small to enable him to keep up-to-date with developments in care and in services, and in his own skills, unless he has a special interest in these matters.

14.14 Consultant paediatricians are too few in number to do more than look after children with acute medical conditions and carry out diagnostic, medical assessments on cases of chronic handicap referred to them. They cannot at present look after the majority of handicapped children, whose disabilities are of moderate degree and whom they do not see. Nor are most paediatricians adequately trained in the educational and social aspects of chronic medical disorders, or familiar with the facilities and known to the staff of local education and social service authorities.

14.15 There is a prevailing but unacceptable lack of urgency in providing adequate assessment in the community for children with chronic and inter-mittent problems of ill-health, educational backwardness and behaviour disorder. The former local authority health services have not had (and still do not have within the reorganised NHS) a treatment rôle. In the absence of responsibility for treatment and outcome, assessment and advice all too readily become depersonalised and perfunctory. Consequently there is in these services a dearth of well-qualified people. The virtual absence of any career structure for doctors undertaking clinical work in the local authority services has also contributed to the present situation.

14.16 It can be said that the services for handicapped children are characterised by overlap and by poor coverage. The deployment of the scarce resources of staff and facilities leaves much to be desired: highly qualified staff spend much of their time doing work which could be done by others with less training. There is still a serious lack of communication between the various professional staff who actually provide help to handi-capped children and their parents. Nor is it always clear as to where or with whom the responsibility lies for the continuing surveillance of handicapped children.

14.17 We considered very carefully whether the needs of handicapped children called for a special service, staffed by personnel trained, ex-perienced and fully engaged in providing them with specialised primary and hospital care when necessary. If all handicaps were complex, severe or multiple we might have favoured this arrangement. However, only a minority of children have disorders that present difficulty in diagnosis and assessment and require intensive investigation; most disorders are of only moderate severity and complexity. That they too require proper diagnosis and assessment is not in question—but intensive comprehensive assessment is usually not warranted, and in any case the sheer number of children handicapped in their learning and development excludes any possibility of multi-professional examination in depth of each and every child. This we have surely learnt from the pioneering experience of multi-disciplinary child guidance teams.

The RÔLE of the PRIMARY HEALTH CARE TEAM

14.18 The need of parents of handicapped children for constant and ready access to experienced professional staff can only be satisfied by a local rather than a district based service, linked with educational medicine. Hence we believe that it would be a mistake to separate the special health services for handicapped children from those which all children receive as pupils at school. Accordingly, *the primary health care team should provide the main health service contribution in quantitative terms to the diagnosis, assessment and treatment of handicapped children.*

223

14.19 We think the GPP and CHV pattern of staffing, with allied services, would provide a more adequate and well-rounded health service for handicapped children than is at present available. It is the health visitor in the primary care team, and the social worker, who are the mainstay of these services. The health visitor is first and foremost a trained nurse with a background knowledge and experience of dealing with medical disorders. This knowledge is essential for a person to whom parents will look for an interpretation in day to day terms of medical information and instructions given them by a doctor, and for help in applying these in the daily care of the child. If health visitors at present often lack the skills and confidence to do this effectively this is because their knowledge is inadequate, and their case loads generally too large to allow them to spend as much time with handicapped children and their parents as they should. Nor is it possible for them to visit schools as frequently as is necessary. We anticipate that the training and rôle of a CHV will largely repair these shortcomings and that stronger links with the social work services will make for a more effective family service.

14.20 The social worker will not be involved with every family and will rely upon the needs of the family being made known to her either directly or by referral from other involved professionals. Her initial concern must be with the effective functioning of the family as a whole. Having a handicapped child may give rise to strains upon the marital as well as the parental relationships and may endanger the stability of the marriage. Other children may suffer and each member of the family may have to accept a changed rôle. While some families can adapt to this situation others may need considerable help and support. The social worker must ensure that every family with a handicapped child is properly informed, not only about rights, benefits and services, but about social life in the community that may facilitate and support their care of the child. She should enlist if need be the services of the occupational therapist to advise on aids and adaptations. Because of her experience of the ways in which children with intrinsic handicapping disorders can become socially handicapped, she will want to keep a watching brief to ensure that additional difficulties do not arise as a result of inadequate resource provision on the one hand and isolation of the family from the community on the other.

14.21 Our recommended pattern of staffing also allows for the fact that the handicaps of school children are frequently first apparent to teachers rather than parents. It is right and proper that teachers should exercise their own judgement in seeking opinions of colleagues in other professions: and a necessary corollary is that they should be able to consult freely with these colleagues. Instead of hierarchical arrangements therefore, whereby all requests for advice from specialists in other services are made through a single, administrative channel, flexible arrangements are required which permit those in different disciplines to work on a "mini-team" basis, making a direct approach to colleagues as and when they see the need and taking independent action as they see fit. If this is to happen, all professional staff must assume responsibility for their actions and be accountable for them. They must also see that relevant information is passed to their colleagues in other disciplines. What we are proposing is in accord with the spirit of Circular 2/75, issued in 1975 by the DES.[10] We welcome this as much as we support the practical advice on the assessment of handicapped pupils contained in the circular.

The RÔLE of the DISTRICT HANDICAP TEAM

14.22 A central feature of district health services is the district general hospital (DGH). This hospital, with its specialised facilities and consultant medical, nursing and allied staff, can provide the supporting knowledge and care needed to supplement the local, primary care service. It should provide this for the handicapped as it does for the ill child and in order that it may more effectively do so in the future *we recommend that a special handicap team be established in each health district, based in the DGH.* The concept of a handicap team is not new; already there are in existence a number of specialised hospital-based, usually multi-professional comprehensive assessment units serving the needs of the hospital catchment population. What is new in our proposal is that each district should formally organise such a team, which we see as central to our proposals for the comprehensive care of handicapped children.

Function of a District Handicap Team

14.23 The team would have two distinct functions, one clinical and the other operational. The clinical function would be:

i to provide investigation and assessment of certain individual children with complex disorders and to arrange and co-ordinate their treatment;

ii to provide their parents, teachers, child care staff, and others who may be directly concerned in their care, with the professional advice and support that can guide them in their management of the children;

iii to encourage and assist professional field-work staff in their management and surveillance of these and other handicapped children locally, by being available for consultation either in the district child development centre (paragraph 14.42) or in local premises;

iv to provide primary and supporting specialist services to special schools in the district.

14.24 The operational functions would be:

i to be involved with others at district and area level in epidemiological surveys of need; to monitor the effectiveness of the district service for handicapped children; to present data and suggestions for the development of the service; and to maintain the quality of its institutions;

---

(10) *The Discovery of Children Requiring Special Education and the Assessment of Their Needs* (1975). Joint Circular from Department of Education and Science (No 2/75) and Welsh Office (No 21/75). HMSO, London.

ii   to act as source of information in the district about handicap in children and the services available;

iii   to organise seminars and courses of training for professional staff working in the district.

14.25 We have avoided describing these latter functions as *administrative* because we do not mean to imply that the district handicap team should in any way assume the responsibilities of the SCM (CH) and AN (CH) for ensuring that satisfactory medical and nursing services for handicapped children exist in each area. The clinical team would of course be well placed to feed back to district and area management staff, directly or through district planning teams for children, the views of those working in the field about the organisation of the service and the measures required to maintain and improve its quality. But its rôle in doing this would be advisory rather than executive.

Staff of a District Handicap Team

14.26 *The basic staff of this team should comprise a consultant community paediatrician, a nursing officer for handicapped children, a specialist social worker, a principal psychologist and a teacher, together with supporting administrative staff. The medical specialist would be a consultant community paediatrician with special training and experience in handicapped children and in development and educational medicine.* A small proportion of his time would be spent in general or special paediatric work in the DGH, but he would concentrate mainly on the problems of handicapped children, and spend much of his time outside a hospital setting. He would not necessarily be the only consultant to whom handicapped children were referred; some GPs will no doubt continue to refer their patients to one of the general paediatricians and to other consultants. However, we see the consultant community paediatrician in the district handicap team as being in charge of the multi-professional assessment and treatment facilities in the child development centre; responsible for seeing that other consultants are aware of the district facilities for handicapped children and their parents; and responsible for the medical tasks that are part of the operational function we have defined for the team.

14.27 It is often suggested that the paediatrician should be responsible for coordinating the investigation, treatment, educational and social management, and subsequent follow-up of all children referred to the handicap team. This is a matter for each centre to decide. We do not think that all these tasks are best carried out by one person, nor that any one professional group is uniquely qualified always to take this leading rôle. It may be appropriate for the paediatrician as director of the centre to ensure that each child referred is fully investigated and to arrange case conferences, but thereafter we favour case-assignment arrangements whereby it is agreed which particular member of the handicap team should be responsible for supervision and follow-up of particular children. The choice will depend on the nature of each child's handicap, and hence the kind of help most needed, as well as on the rapport achieved between the parents and individual members of the team and the parents' preference. In the course of time responsibility for the supervision of a child's well-being might pass to another member of the team; but always it would be clearly understood by the centre, by the school, and by the parents who it was that carried this responsibility.

14.28 *A nursing officer for handicapped children (NO/CHV) should be a full member of the district handicap team.* She should be trained in the nursing and child health visiting aspects of the care and treatment of all kinds of handicap in children. Health visitors suggested in their evidence to the committee that such specialisation was necessary and this is also our view. We would not favour any narrower specialisation, for example a NO/CHV for mentally handicapped children; many of the more severely handicapped children who would be referred to the centre will be handicapped in more than one way and the NO/CHV like the paediatrician must have the knowledge to give advice on a range of problems.

14.29 The NO/CHV would be the nursing link for handicapped children between the DGH's maternity unit, its children's department (including the child development centre) and the primary care team. With the CHV she would visit families at home when her special skills were required, handing over to the field CHV full responsibility when the latter was ready to accept this. She would continue to be available in a consultant capacity. She would also herself provide CHV services to one or more special schools.

14.30 We visualise the NO/CHV as undertaking the CHV tasks that are part of the operational function of the team.

14.31 *A district handicap team should include a specialist social worker* with knowledge and skills additional to those currently obtainable within the framework of a generic training. This social worker should be involved either directly or in a supervisory capacity in the care of all families with a severely handicapped child living in the district. In the case of those with congenital abnormalities she should be informed of the birth by the paediatrician or the social worker attached to the hospital so that she may be available soon after the baby's arrival to help the family with the complex and painful feelings that evidence to this committee suggests are too often ignored by professionals. With her assistance parents may be helped to understand the implications of what they have been told and begin to plan for future management and care.

14.32 The rôle of the specialist social worker and the NO/CHV would have many areas of overlap in the early years of the child's life and they would need to work in close cooperation, both for the sake of the family and as a model for other non-specialist workers in the field of handicap. The specialist social worker would extend her concern for individual families, and the monitoring of adequate resource provision and community links to the district as a whole. She would be responsible for developing and mobilising the resources of the social service department on behalf of families with handicapped children and would carry a teaching responsibility in conjunction with the other members of the team. At planning level she would have a responsibility to see that the needs of handicapped children were taken into account by housing and environmental planners.

14.33 *The district handicap team will need the full-time services of a principal psychologist.* At present, psychologists who work with children are of two disciplines: educational psychologists are chiefly employed by LEAs, while clinical psychologists are usually employed by health authorities and work in hospitals. Both clinical and educational skills are needed in the investigation and treatment of handicapped children, especially those with psychiatric disorder (see Chapter 15), and further expansion of educational and clinical psychology is required. However if the needs of children are to be adequately met, it seems to us that a greater measure of unity in the profession has somehow to be achieved. Today great importance is rightly attached to the contribution of the clinical psychologist in the assessment of young handicapped children but this must take account of their educational as well as their developmental needs and the training of clinical psychologists does not extend sufficiently into the field of special education. Educational psychologists are skilled in the diagnosis and assessment of pupils who have developmental cognitive and educational problems but psychiatric problems commonly develop in association with these, and educational psychologists often lack training and experience in the considerable range of methods of psychological treatment applicable to children with psychiatric disorder. Furthermore, while all child psychologists dealing with the handicapped need skills to enable them to work with families, these have been developed mainly by clinical rather than educational psychologists.

14.34 The work of educational (but not clinical) psychologists was fully discussed in the Report of the Summerfield Committee[11] and their recommendations dealt adequately with the question of prior teaching experience in relation to their training. Clinical (but not educational) psychology has recently been the subject of a report by the Trethowan Committee.[12] This committee did recognise the overlap between the functions of clinical and educational psychologists and acknowledged the need for much closer liaison between their services so that "a comprehensive psychology service" was available for children. However they saw this being achieved through cooperation between individual psychologists and liaison at the administrative level. The need or otherwise for an integrated child psychology service was regarded as an academic matter for the profession.

14.35 We do not share this view. We think there is a limit to what personal endeavour can achieve in overcoming structural inadequacy in the organisation of a service, and regard some form of integrated child psychology

---

[11] Report of Committee on Psychologists in Education Services (Chairman: A Summerfield) (1968). Department of Education and Science. HMSO, London.

[12] Consultation Document from the Sub-committee reporting on the Rôle of Psychologists in the Health Services (Chairman: W H Trethowan) (1974). Department of Health and Social Security.

service, within which there should be some specialisation, as essential. The question of whether such a service should be organised independently or as part of health, education or social services requires further consideration. In the meantime, moves within psychology to bring the two disciplines together through common elements in training should be encouraged. (See also Chapter 15.)

14.36 In services for handicapped children, as also in those for children with psychiatric disorder (see Chapter 15), it is essential for psychologists to be actively involved in cooperation with other community services. Hence clinical psychologists must continue to develop their consultative and liaison work with schools. Until there is an integrated child psychology service it will be necessary for them to consult their colleagues in educational psychology with respect to any contact with schools, and to cooperate with them in ways that reflect the differing expertise in these two branches of psychology. In this we share the concerns of the Trethowan Committee. However, we disagree with their recommendation (paragraph 5.13.2) that educational psychologists should have the power to prohibit clinical psychologists from access to schools. Obviously this would only rarely occur, and when it did would reflect poor working relationships, but this power of veto runs counter to the principle we uphold that professionals of any discipline should not be able to erect barriers to referral or consultation. Head teachers should have the right to seek advice and help from whom they wish and it is not acceptable that their power to do this should be limited by educational psychologists. For this reason we regard the matter as part of a general approach to the organisation of services and not an issue specific to psychology.

14.37 *There is need for a teacher with wide experience of handicapped children of nursery and infant school age to be a member of the district handicap team.* She would have charge of the observation group in the child development centre and also participate in the assessment of individual children and the formulation of their management programme, enlisting as necessary the help of other teachers who may have highly specialised knowledge, eg a teacher of the deaf. She will need to be aware of the special education facilities available in the district, and to keep in touch with pre-school play groups and opportunity groups to which young handicapped children may go. If however the team is to be fully informed of the placements available in ordinary and special schools for young children both within and beyond the health district, an officer of the LEA concerned will need to be involved. There are at present about 85 advisers or local inspectors in special education employed by 57 LEAs. In others, advisory functions are carried out by assistant education officers or educational psychologists. Close liaison between the appropriate LEA officer and the teacher will not only ensure effective educational assessment and placement of individual children but also help to keep the LEA informed about the educational needs of handicapped children in general.

14.38 At any time, other consultants and professionals may need to examine and treat a handicapped child referred to the district handicap

229

team, and for varying periods theirs may be the most important part in the management of the case. On these occasions they must act as additional members of the handicap team. It is also essential that the staff of child psychiatric clinics and district handicap teams work very closely together, because of the greater tendency for behaviour and emotional disorders to occur in children with other handicaps, especially severe mental retardation: joint clinical sessions by various members of each team are needed. In paragraphs 14.66 et seq. we examine more fully the respective rôles of child psychiatric and district handicap teams in the health care of mentally handicapped children, and in Chapter 15 we discuss in detail the services required for children with psychiatric disorders. In paragraphs 14.55–14.58 we discuss the special contribution of speech therapists, audiologists and teachers of the deaf.

14.39 *The consultant community paediatrician will need to liaise with the consultant in paediatric dentistry* regarding dental treatment required by handicapped children. Much of this treatment will be of a routine nature but may need special facilities (eg general anaesthesia) so that it can be carried out by members of either the general or the community dental services by arangement with the Area Dental Officer.

14.40 *Finally, the district handicap team will need secretarial assistance* and help in maintaining its information and record systems.

Location of a District Handicap Team
14.41 The care of handicapped children entails the diagnosis and, where possible, correction of disorders. Diagnosis and treatment may begin at birth or in infancy. This initial paediatric and nursing care of very young handicapped children requires to be undertaken where there is a wide range of diagnostic facilities and where other specialists to whom young children may first be referred can readily consult the handicap team, and be consulted. For these reasons we think it best that the team be based on the DGH. However, this does not mean that it should only function within the hospital. Individual members and where practicable the whole team should seek every opportunity to work in local settings—health centres, play groups, and perhaps certain local authority children's homes, and especially in respect of older children in remedial education centres and schools. Health services for handicapped children cannot function effectively in isolation. Premises are static but staff are mobile, and it is the inter-mingling of different professional staff that maintains the join in a joint service.

14.42 The district handicap team will provide initial assessment and treatment of children referred by the primary health care teams. We also anticipate that education and social service departments will use the handicap team for much of the comprehensive assessment of children who first present to their staff with educational and social problems. *The handicap team is thus to be regarded as part of a common service.* They will of course concentrate their resources on the educational, remedial and caring

230

rôles for which they have a particular responsibility, the community providing various settings within which medical and nursing care, and periodic re-assessment, jointly with the primary health care team, take place. Since it will be the rule rather than the exception for assessment and treatment to be combined, and since assessment will take place in various premises and never as an isolated procedure divorced from treatment, it would seem inappropriate for any of these premises to be singled out as an "assessment centre". *We favour the term " child development centre" (for which there are already precedents) as a description of the unit in the DGH on which the district handicap team is based.*

14.43 We have been impressed by the contribution to the facilities for handicapped children that a special day and short-term residential unit can make that offers both treatment and care.[13] For instance, it can look after a newborn infant with a severe congenital deformity whilst the mother is given time to adjust to her situation, with expert help in learning to manage her child. And it can provide for parents a respite from the burden of unceasing care of physically handicapped children, or of those with profoundly disturbing behaviour, and in so doing often obviate the need for permanent residential care. This kind of unit needs to be provided at district level in order to be accessible to parents, but its size will vary according to the ascertained need of the district. In the opinion of those who have had experience of working in such units, they are best provided by health authorities—and this, so we have been informed, is also the parents' preference. However, there would seem to be room for arrangements for their establishment by health and social service authorities together; this would be a matter to which joint consultative committees should give some thought. It may be that day services could be incorporated in such a residential unit. We have considered the possibility that there should be a single focal point, a centre for handicapped children, in each district, acting as a common base for health, education and social work services for all handicapped children. The idea is certainly attractive. It might be the most effective means of achieving the degree of collaboration between professionals that we regard as essential; parents might also welcome a common point of information about services and of contact with professional staff. It would need to be sited close to the district general hospital to avoid duplicating some medical diagnostic facilities, and it would need to include child psychiatric services. A few small units of this kind exist but they have not been evaluated. However the cost of building an all-purpose centre would be prohibitive at present and we hesitate to recommend such a unit for each district. We would however like to see one established as a model for critical study.

14.44 In the meantime, we believe the development of the district services for the more severely handicapped children in the network pattern we have described would be feasible, economical and perhaps no less effective.

---

(13) Brimblecombe, F S W (1974). An Exeter project for handicapped children. *Brit. Med. Jour.* 4, 706–709.

Among its merits would be a measure of unit flexibility that does not exist at present.

The Regional Handicap Team

14.45 For children with disorders which need highly specialised personnel and investigation, *regional multi-professional centres for handicapped children should be established, in university hospitals*. They would inevitably but rightly be used to some extent as child development centres for the districts in which they are situated: it is important that regional staff should not lose touch with district experience. However, the main function of regional centres would be to offer short-term investigation, diagnosis and assessment of children for whom district handicap teams lacked the necessary facilities. We have in mind children with complex or dual sensory disorders, or who require extensive neurological examination or metabolic and genetic investigation. The new type of consultant in paediatric dentistry would also play a part in supporting diagnostic services for handicapped children at this level.

14.46 We emphasise the consultant rôle of regional centres. There should seldom be need for their staff to provide continuing treatment except for children in the catchment area for which they act as a district centre. They should aim, rather, so to advise staff at district child development centres that the latter retain overall responsibility for the treatment and management of the child. *The doctor in charge of the regional centre should be a consultant paediatrician with special experience of handicapped children. He should also be appointed on a sessional basis to the regional audiology centre*. The second relationship is easier when the regional audiology centre is situated in the regional child development centre. (See paragraph 14.57.) It is at regional level also that we see an important rôle for psychiatrists with special interest in mental retardation in children.

14.47 In serving these functions, regional centres should aim to be centres of excellence for teaching purposes, and undertake research into the handicapping disorders in children.

Parents, Professionals and Handicapped Children

14.48 Parents have much to gain, like their handicapped children, from the pattern of services we have proposed; but they also have their own special service needs, for they face problems in bringing up handicapped children which are additional to and to some extent different from the problems facing all parents. It is evident for instance, that families of handicapped children often get little relief from the economic and social difficulties that arise because they care for the handicapped child. These often mount as the child gets older and circumstances change. They are commonly worse off than families with children suffering from acute disease, though their burdens are usually more severe and last much longer. We foresee the advice, counselling, and practical help from NOs/CHV and social workers, the improved domiciliary service, and the increased day and residential facilities which we have advised, as substantially meeting many of these problems.

14.49 However, parents of handicapped children have two other service needs of a different kind. First is the need to be treated as participants and not by-standers in the process of assessment and decision-making. When the child lives at home it is the parents who have to report on his function and behaviour, and monitor his progress. And because it is usually best for the child to continue to live in his own home, it is they who will be largely looking after the child from day to day. It is therefore as necessary for parents as for professionals to understand the child's level of abilities, his strengths and weaknesses, and the association between his handicap and behaviour problems that may exist or threaten. And to care for the child successfully at home they need support in their wish to keep him at home, for most of these parents are affectionate, and interested to make the most of their child's ability however limited this may be and despite the cost to themselves. Frequently they need to be reassured that just because he is handicapped, even severely so, this does not mean that he would be better off in hospital or cared for by professional people. And when residential care or schooling is thought to be necessary for either the child or, as more often, the parents or their family, they need time to consider the complex issues, to overcome their reluctance to part with the child, or to resolve to keep him at home against advice if they wish. To make a decision they need such information and advice as is available about the likely consequences for the child and for themselves and their family, of different courses of action: and they need to be allowed to change their minds without loss of face.

14.50 We are concerned that parents of handicapped children are not sufficiently involved or even consulted when decisions about treatment and management are made; they are simply told of them. Thus they frequently feel excluded from the treatment régime, caretakers of the child rather than partakers in his treatment. They are not given to understand how their day to day management of the child is an essential feature of therapy nor are they sufficiently often instructed in specific therapeutic procedures (eg physiotherapy, speech therapy, or behaviour therapy) to continue these at home. Consequently, they tend to see services as being offered too much as a substitute for, rather than a supplement to their own efforts. Successful care within the family would be much easier if the potential contribution of parents to assessment and therapy were more widely recognised and welcomed.

14.51 Arising from this partnership no less than because as front-line therapists they need access to health, educational and social service staff, *we think parents should have the right of direct access to the district handicap team and others concerned in the treatment of their child.* It is usually thought that to open professional doors to parents might lead to problems of overlapping responsibilities and uncoordinated care. But the possibility of such administrative difficulties should not be an excuse for denying parents access to the help they feel they need. It should serve only to underline the importance of each professional, when approached, accepting a personal responsibility for coordinating any action he may advise or take with that programmed by the team. We are aware that some parents may "shop" their handicapped child around, seeking for what professionals might regard as an unattainable cure but this is a manifestation of unmet need that should not be suppressed but recognised, and supported with the best advice and guidance.

14.52 We have referred in Chapter 8 to the sensitivity that needs to be shown in telling parents that their newborn child has a congenital defect. Similar understanding is required in discussing handicaps that may subsequently arise. At these times parents also need to feel that there is a network of people and services ready to help them. Such a network must include not only the statutory services but also self-help groups and voluntary bodies. These latter can be of particular importance in ameliorating any feeling of isolation and in providing continuing practical assistance when professional resources are limited. For parents to derive benefit from such groups, they must first be made aware of them. Hence professional health staff must see the dissemination of information as an important function of their job. Regrettably, in the evidence we received, lack of information was an often-mentioned criticism. The committee received one telling piece of evidence from the mother of a mentally handicapped child:—

> "On reflection we feel that, medically, everything possible had been done for Rachel. Now we were left to cope with the problem alone, a problem which we and our families had never before experienced; for the first time in our lives we needed help, and none was offered. The doctors could only suggest we treat Rachel as a normal baby (! !) and the health visitor, though a good listener, could suggest nothing.
> After the very, very unhappy months, literally torn between suicide or murder, as the only solutions to an otherwise insoluble problem, I happened to notice in the local paper a small advertisement for a Christmas charity dance—proceeds to the local playgroup for mentally handicapped children. I was staggered! Were there really enough of these children to support a playgroup? Why hadn't the health visitor known of such a group? This playgroup turned out to be my salvation . . . I met other young mothers of handicapped children, and through them I began to adjust to my problem and slowly to cope with it."

14.53 During the last two decades, voluntary associations of parents of handicapped children—not only the mentally handicapped but those with cerebral palsy, epilepsy, spina bifida, autism and sensory, motor and behavioural handicaps—have, in bringing parents together, given them both strength and knowledge to cope. In addition, much of the credit for the increasing public awareness of the needs of children and especially of children suffering from specific disabilities must go to voluntary and independent organisations. There are many rôles which they can and do fulfil to the benefit of parents, children and professionals. They can disseminate information about the quality and type of service available and, where

234

necessary, highlight deficiencies; they can raise funds to enable independent research to be undertaken (see Chapter 21), and they can give time and constructive help to specific projects, such as the organisation of self-help groups and the arrangement by Book Groups of story telling sessions at the homes of housebound or handicapped children. Many special schools and other services have been established and administered by independent organisations. We feel strongly that such cooperation between parents and professionals can only be for their mutual benefit and that of the children and should be encouraged. We have no reservations about this, notwithstanding that we think the resulting services should be adequately integrated with the statutory services.

14.54 Another special need of parents is assistance in reaching various day facilities such as clinics, health centres and educational groups. Some LASSDs provide free transport for children attending these services. If the child has been ascertained as a handicapped pupil having reached the age of 2, special transport is readily provided by the LEA for him to attend a school. The hospital car service is available to enable him to attend hospital for out-patient treatment when an ambulance is not for any reason available. But these forms of transport may only be available to a few children attending special clinics for assessment and treatment, or pre-school groups organised in health, social service or private premises. Not all parents of handicapped children have their own cars, and often those who do not have cars are most in need of the services. We do not think that ambulances are an appropriate form of transport for most of these children. To avoid the disputes that arise about which authority is responsible for providing transport for any reason, *we think each health, education and social service authority should assume responsibility for ensuring that transport, if necessary, is provided for handicapped children and their parents when attending their services.*

Services for CERTAIN GROUPS of Handicapped Children

Children with Hearing, Speech and Language Disorders

14.55 The interrelationship between difficulty in hearing and some disorders of speech is very close and for this reason we consider their service implications under a single heading.

14.56 We have not closely examined the *speech therapy services* because it is only a few years since they were the subject of enquiry and report by the Quirk Committee.[14] However, the evidence we received often expressed considerable concern at the delay in the implementation of some of the recommendations of that committee. We share this concern as fully as *we endorse the recommendations for a large expansion in the number of speech therapists and a substantial force of aides.* In 1974 there were some 1,186 whole-time equivalent speech therapists employed in the NHS in Great Britain (about 1,060 in England and Wales). The numbers

(14) Report of a Committee on the Speech Therapy Services (Chairman: R Quirk) (1972). Department of Health and Social Security. HMSO, London.

are increasing steadily but there is still a long way to go before the 20-year target of 2,500 for Great Britain, set in 1972 by the Quirk Committee, is reached. (No separate figure was given for England and Wales.) Close links between the speech therapy and paediatric services are essential. Better coordination may follow as a result of the integration within the NHS in 1974 of speech therapy services formerly organised separately by local health and education authorities, and of the appointment of Area Speech Therapists. However, we wish to draw attention to the need to guard against two likely consequences of this transfer. First, there might well be a redeployment of speech therapists that would be to the detriment of pupils, notwithstanding the importance the Quirk Committee attached to speech and language disorder in young children. Second, insufficient emphasis may be given to the wide range of communication disorders in children when planning the additional training of speech therapists the Quirk Committee recommended. For example, it is essential that such training include an understanding of the development and disorders of hearing in children.

14.57 In the past a number of local authorities have organised *audiology clinics,* sometimes jointly with staff seconded from regional hospital authorities. We understand the need for special skills and facilities to be available for the investigation of children with hearing loss but we are not happy that these are so often separated from more general, diagnostic and assessment facilities. There is real danger that the holistic assessment of the deaf child may be overlooked in a unit which is geared to focus attention on a specific defect. On the other hand, whilst a single centre for all handicapped children might avoid this we very much doubt whether the prevalence of disorders of hearing in children in a district is sufficient to warrant the full-time appointment of the specialist staff required for full audiological investigation. *We reluctantly conclude that an area-based audiology service would be more realistic; but we strongly urge that it have at least a functional link with the child development centre in the district in which it is situated.* This could best be procured by the *teacher of the deaf and the paediatrician having joint appointments to both audiology and child development centres.* Both services would gain from adjacent siting of their premises or better still accommodation within the same building.

14.58 There remains the question of the relationship between speech therapy services and child development and audiology centres. We regard delay and disorder in the acquisition of speech and language as having specific but not exclusively medical implications. Therefore we see the need for the speech therapist to be an integral member of the team investigating a child with a disorder of hearing, speech or language. We realise that speech and language disorders occur sufficiently often for speech therapy services to be organised on a district rather than area level. *We think that an area audiology service will need the equivalent of a full-time speech therapist* but doubt whether each district child development centre should sustain this. *We suggest that an experienced and senior*

236

therapist should be attached to each development centre but the number of sessions worked there, and her relationship to other speech therapists and the extent to which she might contribute sessions to the audiology service (and hence maintain liaison between development and audiology services) should be a matter for local decision.

Children with Disorders of Vision

14.59 The needs of children of all ages with visual handicap were considered by the Vernon Committee[15] in 1972. We have not thought it necessary to retrace that Committee's steps, and with one exception (see next paragraph) we endorse its recommendations in relation to health services for these children.

14.60 The strictures we have made about the separation of audiology clinics from general assessment facilities apply equally to ophthalmology clinics. We therefore welcome the understanding shown by the Vernon Committee and the Faculty of Ophthalmologists of the need for investigation and assessment of children with visual handicap to be carried out in association with a child development centre. *We would hope that the ophthalmological and educational expertise required could be organised at area level as well as at regional level* along the lines we have mapped for audiological services. We recognise that some children with exceptional visual problems will need to be referred either initially or subsequently to a consultant ophthalmology team at regional level, liaising closely with a regional handicap team. But *we think it should be possible for the majority of severely visually handicapped children to be seen initially in one ophthalmological clinic in each area, appropriately staffed and linked to its district child development centre.* Subsequently, medical supervision should then be undertaken in the districts with support as necessary from the area ophthalmology service. We see no reason why the re-assessment of the child attending a special school should not normally be carried out by the teaching and medical staff of the school.

Children with Physical (Somatic) and Motor Handicaps

14.61 These children will benefit as much as any from the development of the local and district facilities we have recommended. However, three features of the services they require call for comment. The first concerns therapy. The term "therapist" is used to describe a number of workers, some of whom are highly trained and intimately involved in treatment, others of whom are marginally if at all involved in direct therapy with individual patients. Among the former are staff of the three remedial professions: physiotherapy, occupational therapy and remedial gymnasts. In 1973, their rôles were studied[16] by a working party which recommended their gradual amalgamation to form a single remedial profession within which there should be scope for specialisation. No particular reference was made to remedial services for children—but there is the world of difference between rehabilita-

[15] Report of a Committee on Education for the Visually Handicapped (Chairman: R Vernon) (1972). Department of Education and Science. HMSO, London.

[16] Report of a Working Party on the Remedial Professions (Chairman: E L McMillan) (1973). Department of Health and Social Security. HMSO, London.

tion of adults and the primary habilitation of growing children. Whether or not amalgamation takes place we think that therapists working with children should be specially trained to do so. This is already occurring in physiotherapy and should be extended to occupational therapy and remedial gymnastics. We also think there should be no delay in bringing the pattern of training for these professions into line with that recommended for other professions: there should be a basic training to equip a therapist to treat patients of all ages with advanced specialised training for those wishing to work with children.

14.62 In principle we support the concept of a unified remedial profession but for children we wonder whether the concept needs broadening to include nursing and teaching expertise. We feel sure there is a limit to specialisation within the health and education services, and that ways must be found of reducing demands made upon fully qualified specialists. The use of speech therapy "aides" is one such way, and we have noted with interest the assistance given by "helpers" to qualified teachers in their care of young children with maladaptive behaviour disorders in schools.[17] Our terms of reference have been too wide to allow us to pursue this possibility in depth but it would be a profitable area for closer study and research.

14.63 The second feature of services for physically and motor-handicapped children concerns aids and appliances on which some may be wholly dependent. We are disturbed at the evidence we have received pointing to short-comings in the supply and quality of these, and in the administrative machinery for ordering and paying for them. The number of children needing them is small, and the cost to health and education authorities of an adequate service cannot be said to be prohibitive. An efficient service can be justified on the simple ground of humanity. To this can be added a pragmatic argument: it is a short-sighted policy, after money and effort has been spent on treatment and social education, to fail to equip a handicapped child so that he may fully exploit his limited opportunities. We are not in a position to make specific recommendations that might rectify the deficiencies in the present services, *but we recommend that DHSS and DES should look into the complaints we have received as a matter of urgency. We also recommend that in future it should be a responsibility of each district handicap team to keep a constant watch on the supply of all aids and appliances to children in their district.*

Children with Epilepsy

14.64 The emergence of the GPP and district handicap team, with support from a regional handicap team, offers a solution to the long-standing problem of providing better facilities for the investigation and management of children with epilepsy. The establishment of special epilepsy clinics, recommended by the Cohen[18] Committee, met with opposition for a variety

---

(17) Boxall, M (1973). *Multiple deprivation: An experiment in nurture.* British Psychological Society Occasional Papers, No 3.

(18) Central Health Services Council: Report of a Sub-committee on the Medical Care of Epileptics (Chairman: Sir Henry Cohen) (1956). HMSO, London.

of reasons. The Reid Committee[19] conceded that if epilepsy clinics were set up in isolation they might provide a second-rate service because they would fail to attract staff of the requisite calibre; it advised that special sessions for patients with epilepsy should form part of any appropriate hospital department, such as neurology, psychiatry or paediatrics. We think neither committee emphasised enough that a better understanding of epilepsy in childhood and greater expertise in its management was required of doctors and nurses working in the primary health care services, because the long-term care of children with epilepsy cannot be satisfactorily carried out by intermittent and infrequent attendance at hospital.

14.65 The opportunities for the joint investigation by district handicap and child psychiatric teams should prove especially beneficial for epileptic children with associated behavioural disorders. Some of these children are to be found in mental subnormality hospitals although they may not be seriously mentally retarded. Others are to be found at home, often having been discharged because of their behaviour from one of the six special residential schools for pupils with epilepsy. Paediatricians and neurologists have not always paid sufficient attention to the behavioural and emotional problems of these children; child guidance clinics have until recently been equally reluctant to become involved in treating children with behaviour problems when they also suffer from epilepsy. The special schools have been slow to engage the services of child psychiatrists. We are glad that among the three special epilepsy centres taking part in an operational research project, recommended by the Reid Committee, there is one that is for children only.

Services for Mentally Handicapped Children

14.66 Mentally handicapped persons of all ages present great problems not only to their families but to the health and personal social services. Their numbers are not large, but the expense of providing services is very considerable: 4.9% of the total capital and current expenditure of DHSS is today allocated to services for mentally handicapped adults and children[20] and the proportion is expected to increase to over 5% by 1980.

Mildly Mentally Handicapped

14.67 In considering services for children, it is useful to make a distinction between the mildly retarded and the more severely mentally handicapped. Mildly retarded children constitute approximately $2\frac{1}{2}$% of the child population. Their common characteristic is intellectual retardation. At school they are "slow learners"—so slow indeed that a proportion (one-third to one-half) are to be found in special schools or classes for the educationally subnormal. Compared with normal children, a disproportionate number have associated physical or behavioural problems. Mildly retarded children are born to parents in all social classes but the prevalence rate among children of unskilled manual workers (Social Class V) is many times that found among

[19] Department of Health and Social Security and Welsh Office (1969). Report of Joint Advisory Committee on People with Epilepsy (Chairman: J J A Reid). HMSO, London.

[20] Department of Health and Social Security (1976). *Priorities for Health and Personal Social Services in England:* Consultative document. HMSO, London.

children from other social groups. Furthermore, while about one third of all mildly retarded children show on clinical examination signs indicative of central nervous system pathology, two-thirds do not. This latter group is composed almost exclusively of children from manual working class households and in particular, those in Social Class V. The reasons for their backwardness are usually obscure, but it is well established that families that are socially disadvantaged (poor, overcrowded, unskilled, ignorant, in ill-heath) or socially incompetent are at special risk of having children who are mildly mentally retarded.

14.68 To assist families to identify, and to assess, treat, educate and generally cope with retarded children, are major tasks for the child health and personal social services—and for the education service: the strategy of intervention is the same for all handicaps. The first responsibility is that of the primary health care team and the local social work services. They have the duty to bring to notice all families and children at risk, and to ensure that the services they require are made available to them. The CHV has a central part to play here. But she can only do this if she has a responsibility for the oversight of *all* families with children in a geographically defined area. The same applies also to the social worker.

14.69 Thereafter, *the health and social services that mildly mentally retarded children need should be met by the general services provided for the child population as a whole.* They include the initial discovery, assessment and remedial measures for mental handicap presenting in school children, undertaken by GPPs, CHVs and SNs together with teachers and psychologists. The GPP and CHV should provide the primary medical and nursing care that the children need in relation to sickness, their health and their handicap. We have emphasised (Chapter 9) the great importance of regular and systematic surveillance of all young children. For vulnerable children, at risk of mental handicap caused by or exacerbated by the circumstances of their upbringing, the need for such surveillance is particularly great. Responsibility for the oversight of individual mildly retarded children should be assigned specifically to one of the above professionals. Where further advice or additional measures are required, the child should be referred to the district handicap team or to the child psychiatric service. The psychiatric problems of mildly retarded children are broadly similar to those of children of normal intelligence and can for the most part be dealt with by the general child psychiatric services.

14.70 Whether or not they are mentally retarded, the need of young disadvantaged children for nursery and day care facilities is a pressing one. Social service departments and LEAs have a responsibility to provide these but in all health areas (which are geographically coterminous with local authorities), joint planning teams should be set up to coordinate and expand these facilities.

14.71 A proportion of mildly retarded children require residential care for social reasons. This may be in children's homes or in foster homes, or in the case of children of school age in residential schools in term-time. The arrangements that normally require to be made for the health care of children living in local authority children's homes or with foster parents should apply to those of them who are mildly retarded. Likewise the arrangements for mildly retarded school leavers and young adults need be no different administratively from those for other young people, though as with many other children leaving special schools mildly retarded adolescents are likely to need more help and closer supervision than ordinary adolescents.

Severely Mentally Handicapped

14.72 The health and personal social services required by mildly retarded children thus fit easily, and naturally, into the framework of services for the general population of children. However severely retarded children present problems of such complexity that they require special consideration. Their intellectual retardation (IQ <50) is so great that their development is extremely limited and appears qualitatively different not only from that of ordinary children but even from the mildly retarded.

14.73 About 4 children in every 1,000 who survive to adolescence are severely retarded. There is little social class gradient (ie a severely retarded child is as likely to be born into a professional household as into an unskilled manual working class household). Nearly all severely retarded children (at least in this country) have some form of severe brain damage, and the mortality of those who are most profoundly handicapped is high; many have additional handicaps. In one notable survey,[21] it was found that among those aged 15–19 years 28% suffered from Down's Syndrome (mongolism), 10% had cerebral palsy (and three-fifths of these were unable to walk), and 12.5% suffered from epilepsy. Among the younger children (aged 0–5), 16% were nonambulant, 17% had a severe behaviour disorder and 10% were incontinent. The remainder (two-thirds of the total number) were continent, ambulant and had no severe behaviour problem.

14.74 The small number of children for whom services are required should be kept in mind. Assuming an incidence at birth of 4 per 1,000 severely retarded children, in the course of a year 15 such children would be born in an average health district with a total population of 240,000 (60,000 children aged 0–15 and 3,750 births a year). A service planning unit for primary care having 3,000 children aged 0–15 will have only 12 severely retarded children under the age of 16; and in a whole district only 240 children aged 0–15 will suffer from severe mental handicap. These are manageable numbers for a developed health service in an industrial country. Moreover, these estimates are based on the situation which exists today. The number of retarded children may decline with advances in prevention and treatment and if fewer children are born to older women (see paragraph 14.5).

---

[21] Kushlick, A, and Blunden, R (1974). The Epidemiology of Mental Subnormality. In *Mental Deficiency: The Changing Outlook* (Ed Clark, A M, and Clarke, A D B). 3rd Edition. Methuen, London.

Services in General

14.75 In the past, responsibility for the administration of special services for severely mentally handicapped children has lain (as for adults) with regional hospital boards and local health authorities. Changes in this pattern of organisation of services—which have reflected a need for fundamental changes in the pattern of care of the children—have been foreshadowed and to some extent achieved, during the last 20 years. Throughout, the trend has been to transfer the major responsibility for providing particular aspects of care to the authority whose duty it is to provide such services for the general child population and for other handicapped children. The Education (Handicapped Children) Act 1970 placed upon local education authorities the responsibility for organising special education for severely retarded children where previously arrangements for their training had rested with local health authorities after the children had been ascertained as ineducable. Following the lead given in the Report of the Royal Commission on the Law Relating to Mental Illness and Mental Deficiency in 1959, the Seebohm Committee[22] in 1968 affirmed and the DHSS in 1971[23] strongly urged that local authority social service departments should provide residential care in the community for severely retarded children not needing either the special medical or nursing care that it is the function of hospitals to provide. We welcome these trends in the care of seriously mentally handicapped children because we endorse the underlying concepts from which they stem.

14.76 For the same reason *we recommend that the paediatric and child psychiatric services should assume responsibility for providing supporting health services for severely retarded children,* thus completing the cycle of changes initiated more than 20 years ago. In our view, severely mentally handicapped children have more in common with other children because of their childhood than they have with severely mentally handicapped adults because of their common disability. Services for these children need to offer a full paediatric and nursing service, alongside child psychological, social and educational expertise. As among all children some severely retarded children require additional help from the child psychiatric services and some will need in-patient hospital care for varying periods because of physical and/or psychiatric disorders. But neither the acute nor the chronic problems of severely mentally handicapped children are exclusively or mainly psychiatric. Supporting services for them should therefore no longer be so sharply differentiated from those for more intelligent children, nor should they remain so predominantly the professional responsibility of specialists in mental subnormality. These specialists are psychiatrists and they need to be freed of their other responsibilities to enable them to provide the *psychiatric* services which are in such short supply.

14.77 The pattern of services we have proposed for other handicapped children can offer a more rational and more adequate service than exists

---

[22] Report of Committee on Local Authority and Allied Personal Social Services (Chairman: Baron Seebohm) (1968). Cmnd 3703. HMSO, London.

[23] Department of Health and Social Security and Welsh Office (1971). *Better Services for the Mentally Handicapped.* Cmnd 4683. HMSO, London.

today for the severely mentally retarded and their families. All severely retarded children (but only the minority of mildly retarded who present special problems) would normally be referred for diagnosis, assessment and treatment as necessary to the district handicap team, exceptions being children referred direct to a general consultant paediatrician or the child psychiatric services (see Chapter 15). The primary health care team would retain responsibility for the medical and nursing aspects of the day to day management and care of the child while the district supporting paediatric services would in the first instance provide consultant out-patient and in-patient care, more particularly for problems of a non-psychiatric nature. The regional handicap team would be available if needed.

14.78 Many severely mentally handicapped children have psychiatric problems, and because these differ in important ways from the psychiatric problems of normal and mildly retarded children, their treatment requires a special expertise. For this reason, *when specialist psychiatric advice and treatment are required they should be provided by child psychiatrists with a special interest in mental handicap.* Similarly, the in-patient care of severely retarded children with psychiatric problems requires a very different orientation from that of normally intelligent or mildly retarded children and different units have therefore to be provided although there should be no rigid demarcation. To a considerable, though lesser extent, the same applies to day units. At present the supporting facilities for these children are seriously deficient. Out-patient services are inadequate and sometimes totally lacking; in-patient units are badly staffed and lack key facilities; and day units are few. Detailed consideration and proposals for improving this state of affairs are given in Chapter 15.

Services for Children LIVING *at Home*
14.79 In addition to day hospital units there must be adequate provision of other forms of day services in the community. The parents and families of severely mentally handicapped children usually face great difficulties in their management. There are also not infrequently problems of acceptance by parents, sibs, other relations and friends or the general community. Today specific help in dealing with these problems is usually not available to families; nor do social service departments usually provide the practical assistance that many of these hard-pressed families need at home. *We see it as a function of district handicap teams to ensure that such help is provided. Parents and child should attend the child development centre and members of the handicap team, especially the social worker and NO/CHV, should regularly visit the family.* And the efforts of the district handicap team should be coordinated with those of the primary health care team and the field social worker. This necessitates a considerable expansion in community services for mentally handicapped children and their families .

14.80 Educationally, the greatest shortcoming lies in the lack of day places for severely retarded pre-school children. Experience suggests that at least half of these children would benefit from daily attendance at a nursery centre, not necessarily full-time. This would require about 35 places to be

243

available in a district of 240,000 persons (60,000 children aged 0–15.) A few children are so handicapped that it might be thought that they would gain no benefit from going to such a centre. However, recent research has shown that appropriate educational practice, based on behavioural principles, can be very effective in raising the level of competency in severely retarded children; and though further research is required, we already know that the outlook for such children is not as hopeless as is often assumed. There is the further point that these profoundly retarded children are likely to be the very ones whose parents might most need a break from the 24-hour care of their child.

14.81 It is by no means the case that severely retarded pre-school children invariably require to be educated in special nursery units taking only handicapped children. The majority might be better placed in ordinary nurseries provided these are adequately staffed to meet their special needs, and have ready access to the district handicap and child psychiatric teams. Research is needed to show how this can best be given, and how parents and the staff of nurseries can be effectively helped to manage and bring on these severely handicapped children.

14.82 Education is mandatory for all severely mentally handicapped children of school age, of whom there would be approximately 170 in a district containing 60,000 children. The district handicap team can actively collaborate in the development of curricula, and assist teaching staff as well as parents in the problems of management. Likewise they can advise planning authorities about the needs that arise in the transition from school to sheltered workshop and help ensure that the social and educational needs of severely mentally handicapped adolescents are suitably provided for. Research and development programmes to devise more effective, enjoyable and stimulating curricula are very much needed.

Residential Services

14.83 If each district is to have a full range of facilities for severely mentally handicapped children it will need both short-term and long-term residential accommodation, of different kinds. Short-term accommodation is needed for social crises at home and to afford parents a brief respite from the constant care of their child. In such cases children would best be placed in the residential unit described in paragraph 14.43. There also needs to be short-term psychiatric in-patient units to deal with acute psychiatric disturbance requiring hospital treatment and nursing. *We advise that about 10 beds for the use of short-stay children should be included in the in-patient accommodation planned in each district for severely retarded children with psychiatric disorder.* Where other short-term hospital accommodation is required (eg for investigation, treatment of surgical conditions, and for episodic illness), *it should normally be provided in paediatric wards in the DGH.*

14.84 The majority of severely retarded children live at home with their parents but long-term residential accommodation is required for the upbringing of those whose families cannot provide the necessary care at home (especially older children with associated physical handicaps) and those with chronic behaviour disorder requiring psychiatric treatment in hospital. In 1974, about 4,700 children were in long-stay mental handicap hospitals; over two-thirds had been there for 2 years or longer. About another 1,600 were in residential places available to local authorities. Approximately half the children in mental handicap hospitals suffer from severe physical or behavioural problems and these disabilities have in the main been the reason for their admission. Nonetheless, for every such child in hospital there is at least one similarly affected living at home. Furthermore, it has been presented to us that of the children in hospital who had medical problems warranting admission, one fifth could have been discharged following short-term treatment. It is generally agreed that there is no medical or nursing reason why half of the children at present in long-stay care in mental subnormality hospitals should have been admitted in the first place: their major need was for a home. Thus, it would seem that three-fifths of those at present in hospital would be appropriately placed in residential accommodation in the community—and would have been so placed had the recommendations made in the White Paper "Better Services for the Mentally Handicapped" in 1971 been more fully implemented. As there was in 1970 a waiting list for admission to hospital of 1,792 children, the shortage of local authority provision can be seen to be very great.

14.85 *We think there should altogether be long-stay accommodation for approximately one third of all severely mentally retarded children—that* is, for about 80 living in a district with a population of 240,000 persons (60,000 children aged 0–15). We have not been able to make a firm estimate of the distribution of these places that will eventually be required as between local authority and hospital premises. It would appear that at present *at least half (40 places) can and should be provided in local authority domestic accommodation.* Current need for long-stay psychiatric in-patient facilities is in the order of 20 beds per district, but we feel sure that fewer beds would be necessary for long-stay purposes if the services we have recommended above for severely retarded children were provided in full.

14.86 In "Better Services for the Mentally Handicapped" and in HM(71)22,([24]) a number of suggestions were made for the siting of long-term hospital in-patient accommodation for severely mentally handicapped children. *We hope that AHAs will generally opt for special units forming part of the children's department of district general hospitals.* These should be situated near the hospital rather than in the hospital grounds. This is a more appropriate setting and one that would improve the prospects for the integration of the children into the community and facilitate the involvement of people in the community in the lives of the children in hospital.

14.87 A recommendation was made by the Briggs Committee on Nurs-

---

([24]) Department of Health and Social Security and Welsh Office (1971). *Hospital Facilities for Children.*

ing([25]) that mental handicap nursing should be carried out by a new profession of "care staff" drawing on both residential social work as well as nursing. From the point of view of children who need hospital care there are some who require more or less continuous skilled attention from nurses. Whilst we would like to see a larger content of instruction in theoretical and practical child care in the training of these nurses, we think their predominantly nursing rôle is indispensable. However it does not follow that all hospital units should be staffed exclusively by nurses, *and experiments are needed that examine in practice the feasibility of providing "technical" nursing in units that are run as far as possible as residential homes.* The model of a residential school for severely handicapped children provides a precedent. The children who do not need this kind of nursing care should not be in hospital. If for the time being they have to because there is no suitable residential accommodation in the community, a radical social re-organisation of their wards as "homes", in the charge of existing child care staff and with support from "visiting" nurses and doctors, would in our view be of greater benefit than the introduction of a new caring profession. We understand that a committee chaired by Mrs P Jay is at present looking at the whole question of the nursing and care of mentally handicapped adults and children, both in hospital and local authority settings. As part of their remit they will be considering the training implications of any recommendations they make.

14.88 We realise that at a time of severe financial stringency our unqualified support of the principle that subnormality hospitals should only admit children who need special in-patient medical and nursing care may add to the demands upon social service departments that they cannot possibly meet out of local resources. There is already evidence, that, *faute de mieux,* they are placing a number of mentally handicapped children in voluntary and private homes; and whilst many of these are satisfactory, others are not. Nevertheless, we think this situation should continue to be countered by efforts to safeguard the care that is given in such homes.

14.89 The report of a study group,([26]) chaired by Miss D E Harvie and set up by the DHSS, is a timely reminder of the problems that may arise from these placements. We believe that many of the group's recommendations would be met if the pattern of services for handicapped children that we have advocated were to be adopted. The health care of these mentally handicapped children should be provided like that of other handicapped children by primary health care teams of GPPs and CHNs, supported as and when necessary by the district handicap team. Given this assurance of the quality of health care *we think the methods, including the frequency of medical examinations, should be a matter for professional discretion. It would seem to us reasonable, however, that an authority should require a report on each child in a voluntary or private home following the annual review that every handicapped child should have.*

([25]) Report of the Committee on Nursing (Chairman: Asa Briggs) (1972). Cmnd 5115. HMSO, London.

([26]) Report of a Study Group on Mentally Handicapped Children in Residential Care (Chairman: D E Harvie) (1974). Department of Health and Social Security. HMSO, London.

Transition to a New Pattern of Services

14.90 For a country which a century ago introduced compulsory education for children in a short space of time, and which at the same time greatly expanded the number of places in institutions whose very permanence is now a barrier to progress, the problems of providing a first class service for four children with special needs in every thousand are scarcely insuperable, and with good will and intelligent planning they are fully manageable. We trust that AHAs and LAs will jointly plan an ordered transition to the new type of service we have advocated.

14.91 We cannot stress too strongly however that if the transition is to occur without a serious deterioration in an already unsatisfactory situation several conditions must be met.

i *Ways must be found to retain the services, and utilise to the full the experience, of those at present professionally employed in the mental handicap service.* We have in mind in particular the nurses, and those consultants in mental handicap with a training in child psychiatry. They are the mainstay of the present service, and in the short run are simply irreplaceable. The future of nursing in a reformed service is, as has been noted, being considered by the Jay Committee and we believe that a satisfactory outcome, acceptable both to the nursing profession and to the client group, will emerge.

ii Our recommendations presuppose that there will be a steady build-up in the number of GPPs and consultant community paediatricians, and that these will assume paediatric responsibility for mentally handicapped as for other handicapped children. *Their training must be such as to ensure that they can do this adequately.* For the most severely handicapped, many aspects of primary care will need to be provided by the paediatrician (or psychiatrist) rather than the GP.

iii *There must be adequate mechanisms for the handing on of adolescents to the services that deal with the adult handicapped and disordered.* This is a matter which is of primary concern to the Warnock Committee at present considering special education; we discuss some of the issues in Chapter 11. As far as mentally and physically handicapped children are concerned we make just two points. The first is to draw attention to the serious deficiencies in the amount and quality of our services for young school leavers, and handicapped adolescents due to leave children's institutions and go into a more adult environment. This is tragic in itself, and leads to the retention of young adults in children's units because there is nowhere for them to move on to. Thus places become blocked, and waiting lists lengthen. The second point is a warning: as the quality and adequacy of provision improves, more cases will come to notice since, in a limited way, the supply of services which meet a need uncovers latent demand. Unless therefore the needs of young people and adults are provided for, an improvement in the services for children will accentuate some of our current problems and in time will prove self-defeating. However

247

if the improvement in services for children reduces the level of serious handicap in adults, as we believe it may, the load will be reduced. If the reduction in numbers going into long-stay hospitals frees some beds for adults, pressure on accommodation will be reduced. If there is a steady expansion in local authority homes and an extension of short-term placements and weekly boarding arrangements (more feasible in locally based units) money and resources will be saved. Finally, we have emphasised, better day care service will reduce the demand for residential services.

iv Our recommendation that the psychiatric care of mentally retarded children should be the responsibility of child psychiatrists with a special interest and experience in the field of mental handicap means that there must be a comparable group of psychiatrists to deal with the psychiatric problems of mentally retarded adults (paragraph 15.69). The current group of mental subnormality consultants, without special expertise with children, would obviously form the core of such a service. Precisely how such services for adults should be organised requires full and careful consideration. We believe that it should be possible to make arrangements, parallel to those we have suggested for children, which not only would retain the strengths of existing services for mentally handicapped adults but also would remedy the present weaknesses. However, consideration of these arrangements is outside our remit.

Children in Long-stay Hospitals

14.92 Severely mentally handicapped children in mental subnormality hospitals form the greater proportion of children in long-stay hospitals but a significant minority of long-stay children are not mentally handicapped. In a survey of 7,823 long-stay children in 1969,[27] there were 1,423 who were physically handicapped. Most of these were motor—or multipli— handicapped but some had physical diseases, such as asthma. Such children may require hospital admission only intermittently for medical or surgical treatment, but repeated spells in hospital may amount to a sizeable slice of their childhood. As these physically handicapped children are to be found in small groups in many hospitals, rather than in large numbers in a few hospitals as are the mentally handicapped, the problems they present in child care occur throughout the hospital service.

14.93 Evidence to the Committee suggests that although some progress has been made in identifying and solving the problems associated with the care of long-stay children in hospital, in many instances progress has been slow or non-existent, and the standard of child care is still low.[28] A paper issued by the DHSS in 1974[29] outlined the problems and made a number of excellent proposals whereby hospitals could provide "home care" for long-stay children. *We recommend that this DHSS paper should be given more publicity.* Continuity of care, therapy and education

---

[27] Department of Health and Social Security (1970). Report of a Survey of Long Stay Hospital Accommodation for Children, April 1969.

[28] Oswin, M (1971). *The Empty Hours.* Penguin Press.

[29] Department of Health and Social Security (1974). Paper circulated to Regional and Area Health Authorities following a conference on Long-Stay Children in Hospital.

should be the prime objective and the first step must be the creation of good relationships and understanding between health, teaching and care staff, otherwise the child's world becomes confused by opposing philosophies. Some of our observations on the long-term hospital care of severely mentally handicapped children apply with equal force to that of other handicapped children.

CHAPTER 15
PSYCHIATRIC DISORDER

15.1 In this chapter we consider the services needed for children and adolescents with psychiatric disorder. In this context, we have taken psychiatric disorder to comprehend conditions in which an abnormality of behaviour, emotions or relationships is sufficiently marked and sufficiently prolonged to impair social functioning and/or to lead to disturbance in the family or community. This definition excludes mere oddities of behaviour, variations in personality or life-style, and minor problems not leading to social impairment, but it covers a considerably wider range of disorders than would ordinarily be subsumed under the heading of "mental illness" or "mental disease".

Nature and Prevalence of Psychiatric Disorder

Nature of Psychiatric Disorder

15.2 For the most part, child psychiatric disorders do not constitute diseases or illnesses which are qualitatively different from normality. Rather they differ *quantitatively* in terms of both severity and social impairment, but minor variations of the same thing can be found in many essentially normal children. Hence psychiatric disorders must be viewed in the context of normal child development where isolated "symptoms" are extremely common and usually of little significance. Also, it is quite common in childhood for disorders to be partially, or even entirely, specific to certain situations[1] and for problems to lie in the interaction between a child and his environment, and not just within the child himself. Since treatment often needs to focus on this interaction, services should be available where the problems are manifest—in the home, school or community as well as in the clinic.

15.3 Nevertheless, different types of disorder have different causes and require different varieties of treatment. The two largest groups of common conditions consist of emotional disorders (in which the main problem involves an abnormality of emotion such as anxiety, fear, depression, obsessions or hypochondriasis) and conduct disorders (in which lying, fighting, bullying, destructive behaviour, stealing and poor relationships with other children are frequent features). Specific delays or disorders of development (including speech retardation, enuresis and encopresis) also constitute an important part of child psychiatric practice. Additionally psychoses (although infrequent in early childhood) need to be taken into account when planning in-patient services, especially for adolescents.

Educational Disabilities

15.4 The very considerable overlap between child psychiatric disorder and severe learning difficulties means that many children with psychiatric disorder will also show educational disabilities and may require special help with their schooling. The reasons for this association are multiple and by no means fully understood but some of the explanation may lie in a predisposition to psychiatric disorder caused by educational failure. In so far as this proves to be the case, there may be possibilities of preventive action.

---

[1] Rutter, M (1975). *Helping Troubled Children*. Penguin.

250

Psychiatric Disorder in the Handicapped

15.5 Psychiatric disorder is three to four times as frequent in mentally retarded children as in those of normal intelligence.([1]) Among mildly retarded children the types of disorder are roughly comparable to those found in individuals with an average level of intelligence but among the severely retarded, psychoses and other profound disorders are much more common. Children with a chronic physical disability have a slightly increased rate of psychiatric disorder and those with cerebral palsy, epilepsy and other conditions involving brain pathology have a much increased rate of disorder.

Social Influences

15.6 Research findings indicate that psychiatric disorder is particularly likely to develop in children from discordant or disrupted families, who have mentally ill parents, or who are from a socially disadvantaged background. Schools vary markedly in rates of delinquency, psychiatric disorder and reading difficulties. Although much of the variation is attributable to selective intake some is due to school influences on children's behaviour and development. In short, child psychiatric disorder may be attributed to a complex interplay of factors both in the child and in his social and psychological environments.

Prevalence

15.7 Well-based epidemiological studies demonstrate that, at a conservative estimate, over the course of one year between 5 and 10% of children have disorders of sufficient severity significantly to handicap them in their everyday life. In most cases the disorders will have been present for several years at the time of identification, and follow-up studies show that many disorders persist into adolescence and adult life. The prognosis for emotional disorders is considerably better than that for other child psychiatric conditions, but even so half persist for at least 4 years. At present only a tiny minority of children with psychiatric problems receive any type of professional help or treatment although at least a third to a half require some kind of therapeutic intervention. We recognise that a problem of this magnitude is far beyond the resources of existing child psychiatric services and indeed the type of help needed is in many cases more appropriately provided by other means which we shall later discuss. The same studies have shown that prevalence can vary considerably according to circumstances. It is, for instance, higher in metropolitan areas than in towns or the countryside, in adolescence than in middle childhood, in boys than girls. Accordingly we feel that the aim should be a rational and equitable rather than an equal distribution of resources.

Existing Services

Staffing

15.8 In Chapter 4 (paragraph 4.44) we noted the interdisciplinary basis of psychiatric services with psychiatrists, psychologists and social workers as the principal agents. In England and Wales, the number of consultant child psychiatrists (180.3 in whole-time equivalents at September 1974) remains substantially below the very conservative target for 1965 set by the Underwood

Committee in 1955[2] of 288 when adjusted for the increase in child population and the inclusion of pre-school children, and far below that set by the RMPA in 1960.[3] The number of social workers in child psychiatric clinics also remains well below both targets, even if those without specific training in psychiatric social work are included.[4] Although the number of educational psychologists (638) now exceeds the Underwood target it too remains below that of 850 set by Summerfield.[5] However, the number of clinical psychologists working with children (though not exactly known) is very much smaller. There are huge disparities in staffing (particularly of child psychiatrists and psychiatric social workers) between different parts of the country, with London and the South being the best provided.

In-patient Units

15.9 Since 1964, the number of psychiatric in-patient units for children has doubled. In 1972, there were 742 places for children and 502 places for adolescents in in-patient units for a child population (0–16 years inclusive) of 13 million. A survey of these units in December 1974 (see Appendix H) showed that most functioned at a high bed occupancy and that the average waiting time for admission was some six weeks. About half reported that in-patient facilities were adequate to meet the service needs of pre-adolescent children, but this was so for less than a third in the case of school age adolescents and only a sixth of adolescents above school age.

Other SERVICES *for Psychiatric Care*

15.10 Psychiatric services extend far beyond psychiatric clinics. Educational psychologists not only act as forerunners in referral for assessment and treatment but have a long tradition in the provision of direct help to schools as part of the separately run School Psychological Service. LEAs employed 742 of them in 1973 and in the same year there were 13,354 children in special schools for maladjusted pupils. This represents an almost three-fold increase since 1962, yet during the same 10 years the waiting list had doubled to 1,822.[4] Community homes also cater for children, many of whom have psychiatric problems. Unfortunately no figures are available on the extent and nature of many of the services provided. We know though that some nursery schools or playgroups cater for handicapped children and in certain areas tutorial classes of various kinds provide help for children whose educational difficulties co-exist with emotional or behavioural problems. The development during the last few years of counselling services in schools seems to be meeting a need[6, 7] though there has been little assessment of their rôle. In 1970 there were 236 school health service clinics for enuretic children, although the numbers dealt with are not known. School doctors also assess and advise both in child health clinics and in

[2] Report of the Committee on Maladjusted Children (Chairman: J E A Underwood) (1955). Ministry of Education. HMSO, London.

[3] Royal Medico-Psychological Association (1960). Memorandum on the Recruitment and Training of the Child Psychiatrist.

[4] Department of Education and Science (1974). *The Health of the School Child 1971-72.* HMSO, London.

[5] Report of Committee on Psychologists in Education Services (Chairman: A Summerfield) (1968). Department of Education and Science. HMSO, London.

[6] MIND/NAMH (1970). *School Counselling and School Social Work.* Wiley, London.

[7] Rose, G, and Marshall, T F (1974). *Counselling and School Social Work.* Wiley, London.

schools, and paediatricians help many children in need. Speech therapists provide services for mentally handicapped children and for children with speech delay or language impairment, some of whom will also have psychiatric problems. Voluntary organisations and social workers outside the clinic setting deal with families involving children with psychiatric disorder and health visitors assist with pre-school children.

Deficiencies in Services

Lack of Staff and Facilities

15.11 For historical reasons, psychiatric services have developed in a number of different ways with resulting fragmentation, duplication and lack of communication. Frequently, there has been a lack of both central and local co-ordinated planning. As examples, the Child Guidance Service has developed rather separately from Hospital Clinics; and in training, organisation, employment and career structure educational psychologists remain separate from clinical child psychologists, in spite of the fact that the two services meet rather similar needs. Despite a serious lack of information on the extent and value of existing services, it is apparent from available figures that there is an overall shortage of adequate facilities for treating children with psychiatric disorder. We are concerned to note that conservative estimates of staffing needs set two decades ago have still not been met. Such facilities as do exist are very unevenly distributed and are not necessarily the most appropriate. Facilities for children with chronic physical or mental handicaps and for helping adolescents and pre-school children are particularly underdeveloped, as is secure psychiatric provision for the small group of severely disturbed and anti-social adolescents who require it. Although the British system of special schools is one of the most extensive and advanced in the world, placement has too often been based on category of disability rather than individual needs.[8] Furthermore, there has been a serious lack of evaluated innovation in the special educational treatment of children with psychiatric disorder. The facilities for help in ordinary schools remain inadequate and unsatisfactory.

Training of Professionals

15.12 The training and experience of professionals treating children with psychiatric disorder has been very variable and sometimes inadequate. Although potentially able to help, many professionals working with children have not had sufficient training in normal and abnormal child development to recognise different types of psychiatric disorder or to treat them when appropriate. The relative professional isolation of many clinic personnel, together with heavy work loads, has made it difficult for them to keep up with advances in knowledge so that a choice of relevant treatment is often not available. At the moment, the majority of social workers are untrained and recognised training for nurses working in the field of child psychiatric disorder is only just beginning. Although the recently revised career structures in social work and in nursing have brought about worthwhile gains, clinical skills are still down-graded since promotion is largely available only to administrative posts. This has a deleterious effect on clinical practice because many people of high ability are obliged to leave clinical/fieldwork and because staff turnover tends to be high in areas of work

---

[8] Department of Education and Science (1973). Reports on Education No 77.

with children where continuity is important. Another disadvantage is that many teachers of professionals are no longer engaged in active practice of the work for which they are training people, and so run the risk of lacking day to day experience of the practical issues upon which they teach. However, much is already being done by the various disciplines to improve training and provide refresher courses and we feel that these efforts need to be supported and extended.

Prevention
15.13 Although there is ample potential for primary prevention and there are many good leads as to possible preventive action in the field of child psychiatry, there is—with a few notable exceptions—a grave shortage of proven measures. On the basis of what is already known, *a variety of preventive programmes should be instituted on an experimental basis with evaluation "built in".* We are especially concerned about measures for preparing young people for better parenthood, since it is evident that many of the problems in parenting stem from deficiencies and distortions in the parents' own childhood. This provides an important opportunity for preventive action although we do not know what would be effective. Clearly we recognise the inherent difficulties in learning through planned programmes what should primarily be spontaneous experience acquired through the years. It is possible that discussions at school with teenage boys and girls about the needs of young children, together with supervised practical experience in looking after children (such as by volunteer work in nursery schools or Children's Homes), may help in improving parenting skills, although such measures have yet to be evaluated. Any measures to improve the quality of family life are likely to have long term benefits and for those children brought up in institutions, improved residential care should foster more normal psychological development. As we have made clear in Chapter 12 improvement of the conditions associated with acute hospital admission can reduce the frequency of children's distress in this situation and should therefore be more widely undertaken. *We have concluded that both innovation and research are needed in the area of preventive services.*

Treatment
15.14 Again there is evidence of the efficacy of certain methods of treating children with psychiatric disorder and families with parent-child problems.[9,10] Nevertheless, many methods remain of unknown value. *Further research into treatment and systematic study and evaluation of therapeutic techniques are urgently required.*

Remedies: Staffing

15.15 The extent of child psychiatric disorder is great and psychiatrists treat only a small proportion of children in need of help. In many cases the nature of the disorder is such that children and families can appropriately be helped by other professionals. Although the rôles of professionals of different disciplines necessarily and properly overlap, the focus and emphasis will differ according to training and background. Thus, health visitors will have a special contribution

(9) Robins, L N (1973). Evaluation of psychiatric services for children in the United States. In *Wing*, J K and Hafner, H (Eds) *Roots of Evaluation: The Epidemiological Basis for Planning Psychiatric Services*. Oxford University Press, London.

(10) Graham, P (1976). Management in Child Psychiatry: recent trends. *British Journal of Psychiatry*. 129, 97–108.

to make with respect to pre-school children, particularly in cases where psychiatric problems arise in association with eating or sleeping difficulties or with problems in child care. Paediatricians, general practitioners and clinical medical officers will have most to contribute when emotional problems present in the form of somatic complaints or when psychiatric disabilities are associated with physical illness or handicap. Social workers have a special responsibility with respect to psychiatric problems arising in the setting of family difficulties or social disadvantages. Psychologists are particularly needed when emotional or behavioural problems are associated with educational difficulties or developmental delay and when disorders are most likely to benefit from the special treatment techniques developed by psychologists. Teachers are most concerned when difficulties present in the classroom situation or when special educational treatment is required. Nurses have most to offer in in-patient and day-patient settings but may also be useful in community services in providing practical help for parents with respect to child care. Counselling in schools is most important in the care of secondary school children with problems manifest at school. Child psychotherapists have special expertise in the treatment of children when the psychiatric difficulties stem primarily from emotional conflicts or turmoil within the child. Child psychiatrists have a consultative rôle in relation to a wide range of problems and of disciplines but are most needed for diagnosis and treatment of the individual child and family in the case of the more severe psychiatric conditions, or disorders associated with parental mental disorder.

Estimates of Staffing Requirements

15.16 If professionals from this range of disciplines are to be so utilised it is necessary that their numbers be increased, that they be appropriately trained and supervised, that the services be suitably coordinated and linked, and that there be an adequate career structure. In the paragraphs that follow, we have wherever possible given requirements. However the serious lack of data on the present numbers of staff and on the scope and quality of services renders precise numerical estimates of future needs meaningless, particularly since the requirements for any particular service necessarily depend on the extent and quality of other services. As a result, rather than arbitrarily fix staffing requirements for a decade hence, *we recommend that there should be regular monitoring on a much wider basis than hitherto to determine how far the development of new and possibly more effective services alters the need for longer established services.* Certainly, in some circumstances it would not be appropriate (even if it were possible) to provide detailed quantification. This applies particularly to the proportion of time which should be spent on child psychiatric work by professionals largely concerned with other issues. In many cases, the psychiatric aspect of their work is so closely intermeshed with other aspects that separation of the two would be misleading.

Psychologists

15.17 Both clinical and educational psychologists have a major rôle to play in the assessment and treatment of children with psychiatric disorder. Psychiatric problems commonly develop in association with developmental cognitive or educational problems and psychologists are particularly skilled in the assessment of these disabilities. In addition during the last two decades psychologists have developed a considerable range of methods of treatment applicable to children

255

with psychiatric disorder. The expansion of both educational and clinical child psychology needs to be continued, but if the needs of children are to be adequately met a number of developments are needed.

15.18 As we have made clear in Chapter 14 we feel that it is desirable that existing moves within psychology to bring the two branches of psychology closer together by considering common elements in training be encouraged. We recommend that there should be some form of integrated child psychology services, within which there would be the possibility of specialisation. Whether such a service should be organised independently or as part of health, education, or social services, requires further consideration. We appreciate that this recommendation goes beyond that of the (Trethowan) Report of the former SMHAC Sub-committee on the Rôle of Psychologists in the Health Services[11] which referred further consideration of the desirability of a new discipline of child psychology to the profession itself but we feel strongly that the split between the two branches is no longer appropriate. Furthermore we could not support the Trethowan view that clinical psychologists should not intervene in a school situation without the consent of the educational psychologist (see 14.36). The training of all psychologists working with children needs to include an understanding of normal development, of family dynamics and of group interaction, of pre-school problems, of learning disabilities, of counselling techniques, of school influences, and of parental psychiatric disorder, as well as the more traditional psychological methods of assessment and treatment. Emphasis needs to be placed on the acquisition of a range of therapeutic skills and of the particular skills involved in helping other professionals. Recruitment of psychologists into clinics and educational psychology raises the question of prior experience, especially as a teacher. The recommendations of the Summerfield Committee dealt adequately with this issue. Knowledge in child psychology is expanding and it is essential that psychological services as well as training schemes should have satisfactory academic links in order that staff should learn how to evaluate and apply research findings in their work. Refresher courses are also necessary.

15.19 Although their rôle in inter-disciplinary clinic teams will remain crucial, psychologists also have much to offer in helping children and advising other professionals (such as teachers) outside the clinic setting; we believe that this aspect of their work should be increased. More psychologists should be involved in the assessment and treatment of young children as well as those of school age. It is also necessary that there be a closer liaison between psychological (and indeed all other) services for children and those for school leavers and young adults. The services for older adolescents are particularly weak and need strengthening.

Social Workers
15.20 The central characteristic of psychiatric social work with children lies in its emphasis on the social context of behaviour. Social workers pay special

---

[11] Consultation Document from the Sub-Committee reporting on the Rôle of Psychologists in the Health Services (Chairman: W H Trethowan) (1974). Department of Health and Social Security.

256

attention to the way in which social attitudes influence behaviour and should be expert in knowing how social resources may be utilised to help families. Children's problems frequently arise in the setting of family difficulties or social disadvantage and the social work perspective is very relevant to child psychiatry. Providing help for families of children with pyschiatric disorder demands knowledge of normal and abnormal child development, of family pathology and interaction, and of methods of treatment beyond the scope of generic courses. Specialised courses after generic training for selected social workers are now being developed to fill this gap. Further impetus should stem from the conclusion in the recently published report of the Working Party on Manpower and Training for the Social Services[12] that extended further training (as opposed to short courses) is essential to the development of adequate specialist expertise. *If they are to contribute as they should, the number of social workers specifically trained to work in the field of child psychiatric disorders needs to be very substantially increased.* For the Underwood target of 1955 to be reached a three-fold increase would be needed. Given an increase in further specialised training something approaching this target might be possible if priority were given to this area of work.

15.21 However there are few advantages in providing extra training unless job opportunities are available. Accordingly, we welcome the growth of specialisation within social services departments and *recommend the further development of field work posts with teaching and consultative responsibility so that senior social workers of high calibre can remain in direct practice without loss of salary or status.* This is an essential requirement if social workers are to provide a good service, to expand clinical understanding, and to develop new and better ways of providing help. Furthermore social work theory and practice remain underdeveloped and if knowledge is to advance and be applied it is necessary that social work have an adequate academic basis with a considerable expansion of research. The present growth of University departments of social work is an important step in that direction.

Child Health Visitors

15.22 Traditionally, health visitors have been generalists but as we have said, it is unrealistic to expect them to deal adequately with all areas of community work. Specialisation as a child health visitor will allow them to concentrate on the pre-school period. Their present syllabus of training includes relevant aspects of psychology and sociology but in future more attention should be paid to psychiatric disorders in the pre-school period, to modern methods of psychological treatment, and to how to identify family stress. Because of their potential contact with all infants, child health visitors will be well placed to note parents under stress, to identify psychiatric problems in the pre-school period and to aid parents in their management of these problems. By virtue of their knowledge of families and of child development, they could provide an important counselling service for parents with respect to the more common emotional and behavioural problems in pre-school children.

---

[12] Department of Health and Social Security (1976). Report of the Working Party on Manpower Training for the Social Services. HMSO, London.

15.23 There have been considerable benefits from the attachment of health visitors to particular general practices. However, there have also been two main disadvantages. First, a disproportionate number of families with social problems do not register with a general practitioner and so do not come in contact with attached health visitors. Second, the closer the links that a health visitor has with general practice, the more tenuous the links are likely to be with other health services, because general practice has not been organised to serve particular geographical areas in the way that all other services are. *If child health visitors are to serve their coordinating function it is essential that ways be found to facilitate contact with community services (health, education and social services).* Clearly greater contact between child health visitors and social workers would be beneficial since both are concerned with the effects of social disadvantage on children's health. A further need is to develop ways of encouraging parents to bring older pre-school children to child health clinics for advice on emotional and behavioural problems. If such clinics are to provide such help for pre-school children *it is necessary that more consultative advice and supervision be available from psychiatrists, psychologists and social workers.*

General Practitioners

15.24 At present most general practitioners play a rather small part in the assessment and treatment of child psychiatric disorders. This is partly a function of the neglect of child psychiatry in undergraduate medical training in the past, partly a reflection of lack of interest and partly a result of lack of time. It is most important that child psychiatry have an important place in the medical curriculum in the future (as it already does in many medical schools) since child psychiatric problems will frequently be encountered by any doctor who cares for children. *Some teaching of child psychiatry should be a mandatory part of undergraduate training and greater experience in the form of elective periods should be available for those who wish for them.* We welcome the emphasis placed upon human behaviour by the Royal College of General Practitioners in the training of future general practitioners. Child psychiatry also needs to be a feature in the training of GPPs and CHPs. Given proper training, GPPs and CHPs should be able to provide help for more children with psychiatric disorder than at present but in view of time pressures it would still be unrealistic to suppose that many could themselves treat more than a minority of such children. Nevertheless, all should continue to play an essential coordinating rôle for services and to provide medical supervision of children primarily treated by non-medical professionals. *We believe that doctors with a particular interest and expertise in child psychiatry should have the opportunity to exercise those skills; postgraduate training in child psychiatric work should be made available by means of seminars, courses and on-going supervision.*

Child Psychotherapists

15.25 The number of child psychotherapists being trained is small. In general, their training is rooted exclusively in psycho-analytically based psychotherapeutic techniques. In some trainings this is grafted onto a prior degree in psychology but in others, this is not the case and the quality of professional experience prior to training is the selective factor. The field of psychotherapy as a whole includes work with groups, families and marriages and the relevance of brief focussed treatment methods; but we believe that the breadth of general

258

therapeutic practice is not adequately reflected back into the training of child psychotherapists. The relevance of other forms of psychologically-based interventions in families with psychiatric disturbance also needs to be understood.

15.26 Child psychotherapists have contributed in a particular way to professional understanding of disturbance in children and are often the only members of a clinic team able to offer the long-term, intensive treatment needed for some children. Because of their expertise they are used in a consultative capacity by many other medical and non-medical services and they contribute actively to some undergraduate and postgraduate training. *We believe that they could be even more effective as a professional group if an awareness of other psychiatric techniques complemented that of their own and if they could develop further skills in making their particular understanding of childhood disturbance relevant to the needs of other professional frameworks and settings.*

Counselling in Schools
15.27 Counselling in schools is a recent development with as yet no generally accepted coherent and systematic theory upon which to build practice.[13] There are at present several, sometimes competing, developments in counselling and as the subject progresses comparative evaluations will be required. It is universally agreed that those offering counsel must have an intimate knowledge of schooling but there is less unanimity on whether they necessarily have also to be practising teachers. Views also differ on how closely counselling should be linked with careers guidance, on whether it should cover families as well as children, and the extent to which its function is directly therapeutic as distinct from providing coordination with clinic staff and other professionals. Such differences in views can only be resolved by further experience. Nevertheless, while there is necessarily some uncertainty about the scope and direction of school counselling there is no doubt that it has an important and valuable rôle to play in helping children with emotional or behavioural problems, especially in secondary schools. Training in counselling should be extended and developed and schools should be encouraged to provide the necessary facilities for counselling to be carried out. Coverage on a much wider scale is needed and *we would hope that local education authorities will be prepared to support and encourage the growth of counselling and that the consultative services of psychologists and child psychiatrists will become more readily available to teachers.*

Teachers
15.28 It is evident from the epidemiological findings that teachers in ordinary schools are likely to have several children with psychiatric disorder in each class they teach. At present, teacher training often includes little on the practical aspects of what teachers can do to help such children and more needs to be done to give them knowledge in this area. In addition, in-service training in pastoral care, in teacher-child interaction and in the social structure of schools should continue to be fostered. Teachers need to have the opportunity to observe each other in the classroom and to be kept in touch with research findings relevant to teaching. *Some local authorities make use of specialist advisers to help with this aspect of school work and we feel that it would be of benefit to extend this*

(13) Schools Council (1967). *Counselling in Schools*. Working Paper No 15. HMSO, London.

practice. It is also essential that teachers have ready access to support and advice from clinical personnel. All clinicians need to be prepared to meet with teachers to discuss problems.

15.29 There are close links between certain forms of psychiatric disorder and difficulties in reading. Because in some cases the educational retardation may serve as a contributory cause in the development of emotional or behavioural problems, the early identification and remedy of scholastic difficulties might reduce the rate of psychiatric problems. *Services for children with reading difficulties are inadequate at present and we support the recommendations of the Advisory Committee on Handicapped Children*[14] *and of the Bullock Committee*[15] *to remedy the situation.*

School Doctors
15.30 The rôle of the doctor in school is rightly changing and training is being extended and modified to include more on normal and abnormal child development. At the moment, their main therapeutic rôle is in the child health clinics and in special investigation clinics. Little detailed information is available on the work carried out in special clinics, such as those for children with enuresis, but such as there is suggests that where they are run by someone with the proper experience they can perform a most valuable function. Unfortunately, this is often not the case and it is important that the doctors running such clinics should be appropriately trained to do so.

15.31 Increasingly the problems of children in school are behavioural rather than physical. *Being properly trained in developmental paediatrics and in the psychiatric aspects of this subject, the GPP or CHP as school doctor should become more involved in the treatment of children with psychiatric disorders.* Both they and consultant community paediatricians must be aware of the influence of the school as a social organisation and be prepared to play a much more active part in helping both children and teachers. Courses in child psychiatry for school doctors are run from time to time by the Inner London Education Authority and by Postgraduate Medical Centres. These are most useful when they involve a clinical attachment, as well as seminars or lectures, and where the course is followed by the opportunity for consultation with and support of clinical psychiatrists.

Paediatricians
15.32 Of necessity and quite appropriately, paediatricians already deal with many children with psychiatric disorder, particularly those in whom emotional problems take the form of somatic complaints (eating and sleeping difficulties, recurrent abdominal pain, etc) and those in whom the psychiatric disturbance develops in relation to a chronic handicap. However if they are to treat these children most effectively, *paediatric training must regularly include psychiatric experience.* Since children's disorders so often arise in the context of family difficulties, this experience should include knowledge of family and marital interaction and of parental psychiatric problems as well as of disorder in the child himself.

---

[14] Children with Specific Reading Difficulties: Report of the Advisory Committee on Handicapped Children (1972). Department of Education and Science. HMSO, London.

[15] A Language for Life: Report of the Committee of Inquiry under the Chairmanship of Sir Alan Bullock (1975). Department of Education and Science. HMSO, London.

Child Psychiatrists

15.33 As indicated above, we expect that the majority of children with psychiatric disorder could be treated by professionals other than psychiatrists. Nevertheless, *the rôle of and need for child psychiatrists should in future be greater than at present.* Certainly the shift to closer involvement of other professionals could not be accomplished without psychiatrists devoting more time to training others and providing a consultative service. Since child psychiatrists are currently in the best position to provide the necessary broad approach to children's disorders, they should continue to hold a key position in the co-ordination of inter-disciplinary clinic work. Psychiatric resources must be sufficient to provide time for research and to allow child psychiatrists to play their full part in the committees required to plan and coordinate the recognised health services. At the same time it is essential that they continue to be directly involved in the care of children with psychiatric disorders, particularly since many problems stem in part from psychiatric conditions in parents so that care needs to involve someone with knowledge of general psychiatry as well as of children's disorders. Furthermore, the more severe disorders necessitate assessment and treatment by persons specifically trained in psychiatry, and there are some conditions in which psychiatric problems are so closely inter-meshed with physical conditions that medical training is required. While some such disorders can appropriately be treated by paediatricians or school doctors, in many cases specialised psychiatric expertise will be required. Some of these disorders require treatment (such as medication) which cannot be prescribed by non-medical personnel. Additionally, child psychiatrists will in future be required to play a greater rôle than at present in the care of mentally handicapped children. (See Chapter 14 and paragraphs 15.65 and 15.68 below).

15.34 In view of this expanding rôle, *we recommend that over the next decade the aim should be to provide at least one child psychiatrist per 35,000 children as recommended by the RMPA in 1960.* If this is to include the psychiatric care of mentally retarded youngsters, of pre-school children and of adolescents under the age of 16 years, some 13 million children are involved. This would give a figure of 371 child and adolescent psychiatrists which, if it is to be realised, would require a major expansion in training. In view of the expanded rôle in work with mentally retarded children and in training research and consultation this should be regarded as an underestimate of the true need. It also takes no account of the needs of adolescents over the age of 16 years (see paragraphs 15.55–9 and Chapter 11). We judge that to meet these needs in full, the equivalent of two full-time child psychiatrists would be required in each model district of 60,000 children but we recognise that such a target is impracticable when we are still so far from achieving the more modest 1960 RMPA ratio. It should also be appreciated that in inner city areas where the rate of disorder is considerably greater, the ratio of child psychiatrists to child population needs to be higher than in other parts of the country. Nevertheless, even taking this into account, it is evident that more child psychiatrists are particularly needed in the less well-staffed northern parts of England.

15.35 For the number of consultant child psychiatrists to be increased as recommended, *there must be an expansion of senior registrar training posts in child and adolescent psychiatry. The scope of training programmes should also be increased and their quality improved.* We welcome the activities of the Joint Committee on Higher Psychiatric Training in providing both criteria for training programmes and also the means by which training programmes can be regularly reassessed in order to ensure a maintenance of high standards.

Paediatric-Psychiatric Liaison

15.36 Paediatricians care for many children with psychiatric problems which occur both with physical disease and also in isolation. Psychological factors often influence the course of physical conditions, and families need to be helped with the emotional strains which stem from chronic illness or which follow the death of a child. In addition, admission to hospital constitutes a stress for many children. Not only does paediatric training have to take account of these issues, but also psychiatric consultation should be readily available. Psychiatric clinic staff should be able to advise ward staff on the handling of difficulties as they arise in hospital. If psychiatrists are to provide such a consultative service to paediatric in-patient units, their training must make them familiar with these problems and it is desirable that they should have had some paediatric experience.

Child Psychiatric Nurses

15.37 Nurses already provide an important service by their work in psychiatric in-patient and day-patient units for children but *an increase in their numbers is needed if they are to play a rôle in the development of day hospital facilities, and to exploit their largely unused capacity for counselling parents.* In general, their work requires skills in child care, in the use of a hospital milieu as a therapeutic agent, in the use of individual treatment methods, and in helping parent-child relationships, as well as more traditional nursing skills. At the present time child psychiatric nursing does not constitute a distinct subspecialty, the nursing rôle lacks clear definition, and there is as yet no recognised training scheme in operation. The Joint Board of Clinical Nursing Studies' outline curriculum for training in this field of work should serve to raise training standards and to help the profession develop its own expertise once programmes become established. However, much has still to be done to get training schemes organised. Furthermore, if the training is to be widely taken up it is necessary that it aid career prospects. We therefore recommend two developments.

15.38 First, *there must be a proper career structure in child and adolescent psychiatric nursing, providing links with the field of mental retardation, in so far as it deals with children showing psychiatric disorder.* Only by bringing together different types of psychiatric nursing for children and adolescents can there be sufficient posts to warrant a recognised subspecialty. Secondly, *there is great need to modify the salary structure to enable the best nurses to remain in clinical work (if they wish to do so) without loss of pay or status.* The Briggs report[16] recognised that some ward sisters (often in specialised fields) already have consultancy functions, exercise advanced clinical teaching skills and participate in clinical research. It is recommended that these abilities and responsibilities should be accorded increased status and financial reward. The

(16) Report of the Committee on Nursing (Chairman: Asa Briggs) (1972). Cmnd 5115. HMSO, London.

Halsbury report([17]) went some way towards this end by suggesting the introduction of a higher level of ward sister. This constituted a very important step in its provisions for recognising higher clinical skills. If child psychiatric nursing is to develop its own expertise and advance its own subject it is necessary to attract academically able people into the work and to provide facilities and career structure for them to develop clinical research and teaching.

Training
15.39 All workers with children and psychiatric disorders will need some knowledge of normal and abnormal child development, of family pathology and interaction, of the effect of parental personal problems, and of a range of treatment techniques. They should be aware of the services provided by, and the expertise of, other staff dealing with children, and should know how to obtain the assistance of other disciplines and specialists who can contribute in helping a particular family. Training should include practical examples of how to deal with problems as well as providing a sound academic base and knowledge of relevant research. Because knowledge and practice are continually developing, all disciplines need further training throughout their career. Short courses and seminars are needed to keep staff in touch with developments both in their own, and in related disciplines. However, if the training involves therapeutic skills it is also necessary that the courses include supervised clinical work and be followed by some form of clinical attachment in which consultation, advice and supervision are available. Furthermore, if in-service training is to be widely taken up it is necessary that employing authorities have an obligation to enable people to undergo further training. How this should be organised must be left to the individual disciplines which are involved.

Parental Mental Disorder
15.40 Psychiatric problems in children are frequently associated with mental disorder in their parents.([18]) As a consequence, *those professionals who care for children must be familiar with the needs and problems of mentally ill adults as they impinge on the family.* This has implications for the training of paediatricians, child psychologists, social workers, health visitors and others. It also requires that there be close and effective links between child psychiatric and adult psychiatric services. This means, amongst other things, that within the Cogwheel system child psychiatry needs to be linked with both adult psychiatry and with paediatrics. The training of workers dealing with adult psychiatric patients and the organisation of services for this group must ensure that mental illness is viewed in the family and community context, with due attention to the effects on other members of the family.

University Departments or Sections of Child Psychiatry
15.41 If the training of child psychiatrists is to be strengthened and *if knowledge in child psychiatry is to advance, more resources must be put into teaching and research.* When staffing needs are being determined, teaching, training and educational responsibilities must be allowed for. In particular, there is urgent

---

([17]) Report of the Committee of Enquiry into the Pay and Related Conditions of Service of Nurses and Midwives (Chairman: Lord Halsbury) (1974). Department of Health and Social Security. HMSO, London.

([18]) Rutter, M (1975). *Helping Troubled Children*. Penguin.

need to develop within university medical faculties departments of child and adolescent psychiatry, including mental handicap in children. Such developments would provide a much needed expansion in teaching and training facilities; promote necessary research; stimulate interest and recruitment to the specialty; and contribute to the development of services and facilities within the child health service.

Staffing and Career Structure

15.42 It is important that staff working with children and adolescents should be those with whom young people can communicate easily and should be able to create a relaxed and friendly atmosphere in which a rapport can be established. Continuity is also important if confidence is to be maintained. In order both to provide a good service and to expand knowledge and develop new and better techniques, ways must be found to ensure that in terms of career structure and financial rewards there is sufficient encouragement for workers of high calibre in all the disciplines mentioned above to remain in active clinical/field work and to develop great knowledge and skills. It has already been noted that in several disciplines the present career structure serves as an active discouragement.

Interdisciplinary Collaboration

15.43 As we have made clear, child psychiatric services involve collaboration between many different disciplines, and it is necessary to consider how this may be facilitated. The reorganised health services already involve a complex committee structure at district, area and regional level. Child psychiatrists will have to play their part in this and it is necessary that they be involved in committees dealing with adult psychiatric services, paediatric services, social services and educational services where these may concern children with psychiatric problems. Nevertheless, in our view collaboration and communication are not best brought about by a primary reliance on committees. The complex nature of services is likely to require large committees (which are inefficient) and many committees (which are time-consuming). Already, there are too many, too large, committees without a clear remit. Rather, collaboration and communication should be facilitated by joint working arrangements and by joint elements in training (both basic and later in-service). This would in itself facilitate interdisciplinary thinking about the relevant and selective use of committees in planning and policy making.

Remedies: Facilities for Treatment

Child Psychiatric Services

15.44 *We recommend that the distinction between Child Guidance Clinics and Psychiatric Hospital Services should be dropped.* Both are, and should be recognised as, part of an integrated Child and Adolescent Psychiatry Service, which includes clinics in a variety of settings and with varying emphasis, all of which apply the same body of knowledge. All clinics, regardless of site, need to work closely with non-medical agencies (schools, social services, etc.), with hospital and community paediatric facilities, and with adult psychiatric services. We would envisage that, as in the past, parents should be free to approach the service directly (although, of course, clinics work closely with GPs and often they will be involved in the referral).

Child Psychiatric Clinics

15.45 *The out-patient services for children with psychiatric disorder should be developed on the basis of a well integrated interdisciplinary team providing a coordinated service.* As noted in the Joint Circular on Child Guidance[19] in order to achieve cohesion as a team, to provide continuity of treatment and to afford opportunities for interdisciplinary training, the same individuals will need to work together regularly. For the same reasons, and to ensure that children and their families should not have to go from place to place for multi-disciplinary assessment or treatment, the interdisciplinary teams should work from the same clinic premises. It is also essential that all psychologists and social workers who form part of the clinic team, but who are employed by Education Authorities or Social Services, should have a regular and lasting sessional commitment to the clinic. It is not acceptable that clinic professionals be employed on an occasional basis and, in the case of social workers, a full-time commitment should be the usual arrangement. We feel that on these points the Joint Circular recommendations are insufficiently strong. We would expect clinic professionals of all disciplines to spend a substantial proportion of time working with schools and other community agencies as part of a comprehensive clinic service.

Psychiatric In-Patient Units

15.46 The DHSS and Welsh Office draft discussion paper on child psychiatric services[20] recommends 20 beds per 250,000 child population. Clearly the need for in-patient facilities is heavily dependent on the quality of other services available, especially day services and residential special schools. This makes any estimate of need necessarily tentative and speculative, but given the planned expansion of other services the DHSS figure is probably about right in relation to short stay units for pre-adolescent children. This means that *for some parts of the country no expansion of in-patient services for pre-adolescent children will be required, although there are some areas still requiring such units. However, there is great need for a very considerable expansion of the facilities for adolescents including the provision of in-patient units. In addition it is also necessary to provide long-stay hospital units for severely disturbed children with chronic psychiatric conditions* such as occur with some psychoses and with some varieties of widespread brain damage. The number of such children is not large but they provide particularly severe problems for families. Because of the current lack of adequate in-patient provision, most of these children end up in long-stay units in mental handicap hospitals which are rarely equipped to meet their particular needs. The extent of this need should be assessed and we recommend that Health Authorities set up appropriate psychiatric units to meet it.

15.47 If in-patient units are to play their proper part in treatment it is essential that they all have effective links with community services and that they be properly integrated with out-patient facilities. Although all child psychiatrists should have access to in-patient services, one child psychiatrist should have administrative responsibility for the running of the unit as a cohesive whole.

---

[19] Departments of Education and Science and Health and Social Security and Welsh Office (1974). *Child Guidance*. Circular 3/73; HSC(IS)8.

[20] Department of Health and Social Security (1974). Draft Document on Child Psychiatric Services.

All permanent nursing staff working in such units should have had or should undertake specialist training in child and adolescent psychiatric nursing; the overall ratio should be at least one appropriately trained nurse per child patient.[20]

Day Hospital Services

15.48 Experience over recent years has suggested that many of the benefits of in-patient care, without the disadvantages of removal from home, can be provided for some children by means of day services which allow intensive treatment of a kind previously associated only with hospital admission. Day facilities should include attendance for children, for groups of parents and (especially young) children, and also work with families at home. The DHSS draft document suggested a total of 20 to 30 places per 250,000 total population, ie approximately 20 to 30 places per 60,000 child population. This figure may be accepted as a reasonable estimate but without further evaluated experience of the provision of day care it is not possible to determine whether this will meet the needs. If day hospital services are to fulfil expectations it will be necessary that sufficient adequately trained staff be provided. Apart from the saving on night staff, the level of provision should be comparable to that in in-patient units.

Work in Schools

15.49 The school is an important setting in which to provide help for children with psychiatric problems, both because that is where many problems are shown and because adolescents who would not attend clinics may accept help from someone they know at school. Several different needs arise. We have already pointed to the need for counselling of individual children with emotional or behavioural problems. Since personal problems may often stem from family difficulties, those offering counsel must be able to work with parents when this is appropriate and acceptable to the child. There is also need to help young children from a disadvantaged background so that they may better benefit from attendance at primary school. Although not yet systematically evaluated, special groups and classes at the pre-school and infants level, such as "nurture" groups[21] may be useful for this purpose and also to bring together parents and teachers to work towards a common goal. Recent research has shown the benefits of aiding optimal teacher-child interaction in the classroom and appropriately trained advisers can help their teaching colleagues to increase their skills in this aspect of teaching. THE recognition of school as a social organisation should continuously be borne in mind so that as an institution it is made capable of responding better to each child's needs. The evidence that schools differ markedly in their rates of behavioural disturbance indicates that efforts to improve school conditions should be of psychiatric benefit to the children. In all these areas psychiatrists, psychologists and social workers have valuable skills to offer and close liaison should be fostered between them and the school health staff. Their involvement should in no way detract from building on existing efforts to utilise teaching advisers with specialised knowledge in this field of work. All these types of service in schools need to be provided in such a way that there are good functional links with other services, and especially with child psychiatric clinics, the school psychological service and social services.

---

[21] Boxall, M (1973). *Multiple deprivation: An experiment in nurture.* British Psychological Society Occasional Papers No 3.

Special Schools

15.50 Both day and residential special schools are an important part of the provision for children with psychiatric disorder, and psychiatric clinical personnel are needed to perform a consultative service to these schools. Detailed consideration of the function of these schools is being undertaken by the Warnock Committee but certain needs should be mentioned. First, the system of schools is based on a category of disability rather than individual needs. This provides particular problems in the school placement of children with multiple disabilities. Second, because schools are scattered and are usually not linked to any particular catchment area the maintenance of links between schools and community services of all kinds presents considerable problems. Thus, it is unusual for children to return to ordinary schools having once been placed in a special school; we are uncertain whether this is sound practice. Third, there is little provision for weekly boarding which might make it easier to maintain family ties when this is desirable. Fourth, a high proportion of youngsters placed in schools for maladjusted children have reading or other scholastic difficulties but the provision for special remedial instruction is inadequate in many schools. Fifth, very little is known about the merits and demerits of particular educational methods in special schools and evaluative research is urgently required. Lastly, attention needs to be paid to the facilities required to enable handicapped youngsters to make a successful transition from school to work. This is a field where present services are particularly inadequate.

Community Homes and other Residential Facilities

15.51 Children needing care and treatment in special residential settings are likely to present with a range of problems, social, educational, and psychological, which will make demands on the residential staff. This applies particularly to hospital units, long-stay units for the physically and mentally handicapped, special schools and special community homes. In fact some of the most disturbed and disturbing children and young people will be cared for in these places. As a result, it will be necessary to ensure that residential child care staff have the requisite on-going training for this work (at the moment most are untrained); that there is sufficient consultative support from within social services and from psychiatric clinic personnel; and that the career structure and salaries for residential child care staff are sufficient to attract the right people for this important work. Psychiatric consultation is needed in Community Homes (previously Approved Schools and "Children's Homes") and in both independent and local authority special schools for help with individual children, for advising and supporting staff, and for planning. The time needed for these purposes should be taken into account when calculating the staff requirements for psychiatric clinics.

Pre-School Provision

15.52 In the past, child psychiatric services have been planned largely in relation to school age children so that pre-school children have received relatively little attention. This must now be corrected as epidemiological studies have shown the frequency of psychiatric problems in this age group and other investigations have indicated that problems of later childhood often have their origins in early life. *At the level of primary care, it is important that GPPs, child health visitors and consultant community paediatricians working in group practices,*

267

health centres and child health clinics should have the necessary training to recognise psychiatric disorders in this age group and the skills to provide therapeutic help and advice for some of the commoner problems. If these professionals are to provide such a service they must have clearly defined channels of access to further psychiatric consultation and referral when necessary. Psychiatric day services are particularly needed for this age group and it is important that there be facilities for parents to attend with their children.

15.53 The recent initiative to increase provision for pre-school education is greatly welcomed. It is encouraging to know that despite the difficulties imposed by the economic situation, the programme continues to progress quite widely and that LEAs have been given encouragement to provide places in priority areas. *Both innovation and evaluation should be provided from the outset to determine what sort of care is most beneficial for different sorts of children.* It is also necessary that pre-school education should develop in such a way as to increase parental involvement and to increase parental skills in dealing with their children. This means that particular attention should be paid to helping parents by practical assistance and counselling in the home and by their participation in playgroups and nursery schools. Their cooperation in nursery education can be of great help to teachers in extending their information about children.

15.54 The professional advice and consultation available to those involved in pre-school provision is in general inadequate. *Systems of regular support need to be devised at a local level to ensure that children showing difficulties can be identified and helped at an early stage.* Both professional and non-professional workers caring for children should be helped to understand the psychological needs of children and to have available clearly defined channels of access to further psychiatric consultation and referral when necessary.

Provision for Adolescents
15.55 The needs of adolescents have been discussed in Chapter 11 which raises several considerations in the planning of psychiatric services for them. First, the prevalence of psychiatric disorder probably rises in adolescence. Second, some adolescents are reluctant to accept the facilities available to children, and particularly among older adolescents there is a need for consultation outside the family confines. Third, there is a grave shortage of residential facilities—both school and hospital. Fourth, compared with younger children a higher proportion require a more secure setting. While data are lacking on the relative merits of different solutions, we consider that the following recommendations are most likely to meet the need.

15.56 In planning services, we must distinguish younger adolescents from those of about 16 and over. Disorders in the younger group are frequently continuations of problems first manifest in earlier childhood and psychiatric troubles are often associated with educational disabilities. Many problems are shown in the school setting, and in most cases the adolescent is financially and otherwise dependent on his family. For all these reasons, the particular training and expertise of the child psychiatrist is most appropriate to deal with younger adolescents. Of course, there are issues and concepts specially relevant to the adolescent period and there are particular issues which arise in the running of adolescent in-patient units. Nevertheless, these are matters of emphasis and *it is recommended that the psychiatric care of younger adolescents should be included as part of child and adolescent psychiatry.* The situation with older adolescents is rather different. As with many disorders in adult life, psychiatric problems may have their roots in earlier life but they are more rarely direct continuations of child disorders. Psychiatric problems in the late teens are less often associated with schools and with scholastic difficulties, and the older adolescent is usually much less dependent on his family. For these reasons *most services for older adolescents can be considered in relation to those available to young adults, provided that training in general psychiatry includes knowledge on developmental issues and provided that services for this age group are strengthened and expanded.* Nevertheless, psychiatric difficulties in the 16 to 19 year age period not infrequently arise from unresolved scholastic, vocational, and family relationship problems and child psychiatrists have expertise to offer with respect to this age group.

15.57 Within ordinary secondary schools, greater facilities than at present exist are required both to help individual children with personal difficulties and to give guidance to teachers faced with problems in the classroom. As we have made clear in paragraph 27, the provision of counselling in a growing number of secondary schools is an encouraging development of a supporting service to pupils. Nonetheless coverage on a much wider scale is needed to ensure that help becomes available to many more than the small minority of school children currently receiving it.

15.58 *Facilities such as "walk-in" clinics should be evaluated for their effectiveness in aiding adolescents to seek psychiatric help for themselves.* Advice on emotional difficulties may also be sought in the context of non-psychiatric services such as pregnancy testing or providing contraceptive advice. Staff running such clinics should be sensitive to the possibility that assistance may be required for more than the particular medical problems about which they are ostensibly being consulted. We support the suggestion that separate information sessions should be arranged for young people, so that counselling may be available on a wider range of health and social problems as well as on contraception and sexual matters. There may be a particular need for help with psychosexual problems during adolescence and if problems are not to persist into adult life, counselling should be freely available for this age group. Counsellors need to receive appropriate training for this work. Since such clinics may identify young people with psychiatric problems it is important that there should be liaison with the specialist services who should be prepared to provide support and to accept referrals as necessary.

15.59 *We recommend greatly increased provision of residential facilities in the form of hostels, schools, and hospital units.* Given adequate facilities and sufficient places, adolescent in-patient units should be able to provide sufficient security for the severely disturbed adolescent whose problems stem from an acute mental illness. However, greatest need arises with respect to adolescents who are not mentally ill but who show chronic socially disruptive behaviour. Most of these are not suitable for adolescent hospital units and much has still to be learned about the most suitable form of care. Systematic evaluation of alternative modes of treatment and alternative patterns of care is needed. In general, too many adolescents are unsuitably placed on adult psychiatric wards. However, some with adult-type mental disorders may best be treated there provided that adequate schooling is available and that a psychiatrist with special experience in adolescent disorders can advise when necessary.

15.60 The provision of services for children who transgress the law is largely outside our remit. Nevertheless, some such children have psychiatric problems and psychiatric services are relevant. The continuing development of psychiatric facilities will be needed for many of these youngsters. Psychiatric treatment as such is appropriate for only a small minority but psychiatric consultation should be available to Social Services both for the planning of specialised forms of care and for the aid of staff working in the community or in institutions. Psychiatrists will be needed for assessments and for Court reports and also to plan treatment in terms of the social organisation of the institution as well as in individual terms. Delinquency is often a consequence of social problems or of family difficulties and the Children and Young Person's Act, 1969, emphasised this by placing care within Social Services Departments rather than within a penal framework. Current difficulties centre on the lack of enforceable compulsion over placement in Community Homes and the need to create a viable system of care and control within a Social Services framework following the dissolution of the former Approved Schools System. In particular, a small minority of severely disturbed and antisocial adolescents present grave difficulties in special schools, community homes and adolescent units which cannot contain them. Youth Treatment Centres are being planned (on an estimate of 200 places for the country as a whole) to meet the needs of some within this group but for others different solutions may be needed. The same considerations apply to pre-adolescent children with problems leading to a need for more secure settings.

Transition from School to Work

15.61 The transition from school to work is a very difficult one for all adolescents but is particularly so for those with chronic psychiatric problems. Four steps would serve to ameliorate this process. First, local authorities should be encouraged to provide support for the continuing education beyond 16 years of those handicapped youngsters who would benefit from it (as many already do). Second, careers advice and counselling should be further developed so that greater knowledge is available on the needs and potential of handicapped adolescents and on appropriate job opportunities so that a better match can be made between the two. Third, an expansion is needed of hostel provision for handicapped teenagers who would be better away from home or for whom family support is lacking. Fourth, work training facilities for school-leavers with psychiatric handicaps should be developed. At present such a service can usually only be provided by Industrial Rehabilitation Units (which are designed for persons who have lost work skills rather than for those who have yet to gain them) or through services for mentally or physically handicapped persons (which are inappropriate in many cases).

Services for Mentally Handicapped Children

15.62 The needs of children with chronic handicap are considered as a whole in Chapter 14. However, services for mentally handicapped children are also discussed here because their psychiatric problems constitute one of the chief service demands.

15.63 In this country medical services for mentally handicapped people developed largely in terms of large long-stay hospitals and relatively little in the way of supporting community or outpatient care. This has had several undesirable consequences. First, hospital provision is used for many individuals who need residential care but who do not require in-patient medical or nursing services. Second, mental handicap specialists dealing with children have often had no training in either paediatrics or child psychiatry. Third, because consultants working in long-stay hospitals have had to cope with such a large in-patient population, there has not always been the opportunity to develop the specifically psychiatric treatments needed for the minority. Fourth, the lack of out-patient facilities in most areas and the lack of staff time for this work has led to under-developed services for families looking after mentally retarded children at home. Fifth, the organisation of services has often meant the professional isolation of mental handicap specialists with resulting ill-effects on morale and expertise. Recently there has been concern about the quality and quantity of recruits into the field.

15.64 In order to deal with these deficiencies it is recommended that a number of radical changes be made in the organisation of mental handicap services. These will take time to implement and the suggestions which follow refer to services as they might exist in a decade or so. Special arrangements are required to ensure a smooth transition in the lengthy interim period.

15.65 Special attention needs to be given to the provision of adequate community services for mentally handicapped children and their families. *Child psychiatrists should be an integral member of the team in district Child Development Centres.* Apart from psychiatric provision *it is also necessary that there be social workers and psychologists with the necessary knowledge and experience to provide counselling for all age groups and for children with all levels of handicap.*

15.66 *Local authority provision of hostels for mentally handicapped children and adults should be very greatly increased.* Experience in those areas where hostel provision already exists on a wide scale suggests that, with appropriate back-up services, the majority of mentally handicapped individuals requiring residential care can be looked after in that way.

15.67 *Consultant community paediatricians with a special interest in developmental problems should provide the paediatric care needed for mentally handicapped children.* For this to function satisfactorily, it is necessary that paediatricians undertaking this work should be appropriately trained, and that hospital units have the necessary facilities to admit severely handicapped children who may often have associated behavioural problems.

271

15.68 *Child psychiatrists should provide the psychiatric care needed for mentally handicapped children.* Mildly retarded children present much the same range of psychiatric problems as those shown by youngsters of normal intelligence and most can be adequately served by existing in-patient, day patient and outpatient psychiatric services. However, the psychiatric conditions in severely handicapped children differ in some important respects, and special provision will be required. Well staffed psychiatric in-patient units able to provide long-term as well as short-term care for severely retarded children with psychiatric disorders are essential. Very few exist at the moment and more will have to be provided. Altogether *there should be long-stay residential provision for just over a third of all severely mentally handicapped children.* The proportion of children needing residential provision is higher during adolescence and lower during the pre-school years. *Of those requiring long-term residential care, at least half could be adequately cared for in hostels if these were available.* A major increase in local authority hostel provision is required for this to be possible. Provided such hostels are available, provided there is adequate paediatric long-stay hospital provision for children with associated physical disabilities, and provided adequate schooling and psychiatric day services are available, fewer mentally handicapped children will need psychiatric in-patient care than is the case at present. However we lack adequate data to provide any accurate estimate of bed requirements. *At present it seems that there is a need for approximately 25–30 psychiatric in-patient beds per 60,000 children, of which about one-third should be for short-term admissions.* However, with the development of better community services and better hostel provision the number of beds needed might be substantially altered. For this pattern of services to be effective *it is necessary that training in psychiatric work with retarded children be routinely included in child psychiatry programmes.* This has already been recommended by the professional bodies concerned. It is also necessary that those child psychiatrists who run in-patient and day units for severely retarded children should have additional training in this aspect of their work. A few such child psychiatrists already exist and among mental handicap specialists there are already some with special experience and training in child psychiatric work with severely retarded children and their families. However, a marked increase is needed in psychiatrists with this expertise and interest.

15.69 In planning psychiatric services for mentally handicapped children, it is important also to consider the implications for adult services. It is suggested that the same division of responsibilities should be possible provided that those adult psychiatrists currently providing services for chronically handicapped psychiatric persons also take responsibility for the care of mentally handicapped adults with psychiatric disorder. Again, this has implications for training and for in-patient provision.

Organisation of Statistical Information

15.70 In our consideration, we have continually been faced with the lack of adequate statistical information. Hospital in-patient figures for psychiatric care are misleading in view of the failure to define what is meant by "children" and "adolescents", and bed occupancy figures are meaningless if the current practice to allow children home on leave for therapeutic purposes is not taken into account. Next to no data are available on psychiatric out-patient services for children and evaluative research of the efficacy of different forms of care and treatment is urgently required. Most children with psychiatric problems are treated by non-psychiatric professionals, often outside the Health Service, and no adequate data are available on this work. Thus, for example, data are lacking concerning children seen by Social Services, by school counsellors, and at special investigation clinics. Not only are figures lacking regarding work within any particular services but there are no means by which to integrate data across services. Furthermore, even when data are available, frequently the information provided is of little relevance in relation to modern methods of psychiatric practice. *It is strongly recommended that the organisation and collection of statistical information regarding services for children with psychiatric disorder be systematically examined by a group representing all the Government Departments involved.* On this basis, an improved system should be devised.

CHAPTER 16

A VOICE FOR CHILDREN

Introduction

16.1 In Chapter 5 we outlined the principles which informed our consideration of the child health services this country needs. High amongst these was a conviction that children have definable rights to health care and that, because they cannot articulate views of their own, society has a duty to ensure that their rights and special needs are fully recognised. In this chapter we set out those of our recommendations which stem from acceptance of this principle.

Rights to Health Care

16.2 Like William Morris, "we hold that children are persons not property and so have the right to claim all the advantages which the community provides for everyone" (1886). In this context, *we believe that children have a right to basic health care which comprehends not only treatment at times of illness or injury but also continuing surveillance to promote health and detect disability or handicap*. Currently the relationship between families and the child health service is informal; parents decide to what extent they wish to avail themselves of the services provided for their children. Fortunately most are caring parents but there are some who, through neglect or refusal to use services, fail to secure a minimal level of health care and surveillance for their children.

16.3 We have therefore considered at length whether the State should assume the ultimate responsibility for ensuring that the child's right to continuing and positive health care is upheld. This latter would not be without precedent. It is a duty enforceable under law[1] for parents to secure the education of their children at a standard considered suitable by the relevant education authority. This has long been accepted and does not appear to have damaged the relationship between children, parents and teachers. It could well be argued that a child's rights to health care are no less strong than to education. However, to extend the powers of statutory agencies further by a wholesale assumption by the State of responsibility for child health would have major social and political repercussions. We have therefore not sought general powers to over-ride parental decisions: we do not, for instance, propose any change in the present requirement that parental consent should normally be required before treating children under 16, save in emergencies or in cases of life and death. Rather we have isolated those situations where some additional confirmation of the child's rights seems to us essential. Most of our specific recommendations have appeared elsewhere in the text but we wish here to record the arguments which framed our decisions.

Health Surveillance

16.4 In Chapter 9 we have recommended a minimum programme of health surveillance examinations which should be made available to all children. However, in present circumstances, the child's participation in any such scheme

---

[1] Education Act 1944, s36-40.

would depend upon the voluntary co-operation of the parents. This has in recent months been the subject of some debate in the press and elsewhere and it has been suggested that the payment of family allowances should be made conditional upon participation. Comparisons have been drawn with the French system where proof of attendance for specified examinations is required for the payment in three lump sums of pre- and post-natal allowances. Since this country has no directly equivalent payments, any system of incentives would have to be based either on ordinary family allowances or on a new lump sum.

16.5 We feel that the former would be very difficult to defend in principle. The basic purpose of family allowances is to provide financial help for families with children. To reduce or withdraw this support for reasons unconnected with a family's bread and butter needs would be in direct conflict with this purpose and could cause great resentment among the recipients. Certainly the child concerned is unlikely to profit from the situation. Additionally the effectiveness of the scheme would be limited since on operational grounds the sanctions could apply to only a very few of the desirable number of examinations. Even so, it would be extremely expensive and difficult to administer in terms both of administrative procedures and manpower costs. Alternatively a system like the French one of additional lump sums given specifically as rewards for clinic attendance would of course involve very substantial extra expenditure. To be effective, instalments of the lump sum could hardly be less than £10 (and this is far below the French level) and a lump sum of £30 paid in three instalments would cost about £20 million a year. It seems to us very doubtful that, if £20 million were available for improvements in child health services, this would be the best way to spend it, both absolutely and also because the greater part of the money would probably go to families who would take their children for health checks anyway. Since the French system is a new one its effectiveness in reaching the others has yet to be demonstrated. It might prove to be the case that the attraction of lump sums would guarantee virtually total take-up, but in so far as it did not do so, and those not reached were the poorest and least capable families, it could be said that this was a regressive use of the money spent on the lump sums. And lump sums, while easier to relate to clinic attendance than weekly payments, would require additional administrative machinery.

16.6 This is a difficult area and there can be no totally satisfactory solution. Even so, we have accepted the arguments against financial sanctions or incentives as valid for this country at this time although we would not wish to close the door on future consideration of these policies. Instead we propose a limited increase in statutory powers. For the reasons set out in full in Chapter 10, *we have recommended the introduction of a statutory school entry medical examination:* we feel this to be of prime importance because of evidence of the value of a full medical and neuro-developmental examination at this stage. Beyond that we look to the child health visitor with her new geographical responsibility to lead the way in achieving whole population surveillance. Better record systems and more rigorous follow-up procedures should help her to identify families where health surveillance services are not being taken up. *In such cases, or where there is suspicion of serious ill-health for which medical help is not being sought, she should initially seek access to the child by persuasion but we recommend on a majority decision that in the event of failure, she should have the right to apply for a legally enforceable medical examination.* We do not feel that this proposal to strengthen the CHV's statutory position should jeopardise the relationship between the primary care team and its clients.

Suspected Ill-Treatment or Neglect
16.7 We have also been concerned to protect the interests of children in cases of suspected parental neglect or abuse. For children over 5, schools provide unparalleled opportunities for the identification and observation of those at risk. *We have therefore recommended that head teachers should have the right, on reasonable grounds for concern, to request the examination of a child under their charge, if necessary without the consent of the parents* (Chapter 10, paragraph 25). Children not at school, and not in the care or under the supervision of a local authority, present a more difficult problem. If our proposals in paragraph 6 above prove effective, the CHV should be better placed than hitherto to detect abuse.

16.8 At all times the Local Authority has a duty to investigate any case where it receives information that a child may be neglected or ill-treated or his health avoidably impaired. In addition it must bring care proceedings unless satisfied that this would not be in the child's interest or that some other authorised body—the NSPCC or the police—is about to do so. In the course of the investigation it may be desirable to carry out a medical examination of the child. At present this can be achieved without parental consent only by removing the child from home under a Place of Safety Order made by a Court. Removal from home in this way may not always be desirable and *we therefore recommend that the powers of a Local Authority under the Children and Young Persons Acts of 1933 and 1969 should be extended to enable a legally enforceable medical examination to be sought separately from a removal order.* We would hope that such a power would result in the early detection of cases of abuse which may now be missed because of the difficulties in getting an examination.

Professional Liaison
16.9 In this area, the boundaries between illness and neglect are often ill-defined and what matters is the effectiveness of the professional collaboration advocated here. We would expect that the child health visitor, when considering exercising the powers proposed in paragraph 16.6, would normally make contact with the Social Services Department to assess the overall needs of the family. If, despite the medical examination and subsequent discussion with health and social services staff, the parents still refused to have the child treated, then it would be for the Social Services Department to decide what action to take to protect the child under existing powers. Should the CHV's suspicions of abuse or other forms of neglect be roused, she should immediately contact the LASSD social worker who would normally take the lead in seeking a formal medical examination.

Ethical Issues
16.10 *While not proposing any change in the general requirements to obtain parental consent to the medical treatment of children, we should like to endorse the current exceptions which allow children under 16 to receive medical advice or treatment without parental knowledge in particularly delicate circumstances—*

276

usually concerning sexually transmitted diseases (s.t.d.) or contraception. So far as s.t.d. are concerned, the confidentiality of information obtained as a result of treating patients is specifically protected by statute. Practitioners are asked to make every effort to persuade patients under 16 to confide in one or both parents but not to the extent of running the risk of the patient's defaulting on treatment or of losing the patient's cooperation if his or her name is given as a sexual contact on a subsequent occasion. The basic philosophy is that if a patient is of such age and intelligence to be able to realise that examination is needed and to seek it without the benefit of parental prompting or advice, he/she is of sufficient age and intelligence to be able to give a sufficient assent to that examination. Likewise in the provision of contraceptive advice and treatment, doctors are advised that the parents of a child of mature age should not be contacted by any staff without his or her permission even though as a matter of clinical judgment the refusal of permission to involve the parents may effect the nature of the advice given to the child. It is for the doctor to decide whether or not to provide treatment, and if he does so for a girl under 16, he is not acting unlawfully provided he acts in good faith in protecting the girl against the potentially harmful effects of intercourse. He should of course always seek the patient's consent to tell the parents. *This is a particularly difficult matter and we must record that the Committee's decision to approve present practice was not unanimous.*

16.11 Equally sensitive issues arise in the cases of termination of pregnancy and sterilisation of minors. Both are complex subjects and have received considerable attention within the recent past. Indeed the DHSS is currently considering the need for a Code of Practice for the sterilisation of minors in the light of comments on a Departmental discussion paper from the various professional bodies concerned. We have therefore decided that there is nothing further that this Committee could usefully add.

16.12 Throughout the report reference is made to deficiencies in knowledge and to the need to develop new methods of treatment and improve paediatric skills. This cannot be done without active and vigorous research programmes but the Committee is aware that clinical investigations which involve children raise special ethical considerations. *We are of the opinion that no research investigations which involve children (including the fetus and newborn) should be undertaken without approval from the appropriate Ethical Committee.* Ethical Committees should scrutinise such proposals with special care and will normally require the advice of experts in obstetrics or paediatrics if these specialties are not represented on the committee.

Rights of Children in Long-stay Hospitals

16.13 There are currently around 6,000 children in hospitals for the mentally handicapped, many of whom have been there for considerable periods. There are also a further 2,000 or so children who have been in other hospitals for at least 3 months. Some of these 8,000 children are orphaned, some no longer have any contact with their families, and many more, though not abandoned formally, are seldom visited by their parents. This estrangement is a not uncommon occurrence in mental handicap hospitals and in the few other long-stay hospitals which are geographically isolated and which admit children from a very wide catchment area. Moreover, many parents—irrespective of their devotion and sustained support—are not in a position to assess their child's service needs and the frequency of reviews rests entirely with the consultant responsible for the care of the child.

16.14 We are concerned to ensure that the well-being and needs of such children are adequately reviewed at appropriate intervals and that within or alongside such reviews particular attention is given to the possibility of loss of parental contact or where, unfortunately, that has already occurred, to re-establishing it if that is in the best interest of child and parent. We have, however, been told that the National Development Group for the Mentally Handicapped are considering these matters with especial care. We therefore limit our remarks to a brief discussion of points which we believe the Development Group should carefully consider in relation to the recommendations that they may make. (These remarks also apply to children in other groups who may be in hospital for long periods.)

16.15 We believe that every child who is in hospital for more than 3 months should have a comprehensive review made of his service needs. This review should not be narrowly based but should extend to broader social and educational matters as well as to more strictly medical and/or psychiatric issues. It should, we believe, be carried out by a multi-disciplinary team drawn from an appropriately wide range of professional disciplines: it should particularly include those from the local authority who would be involved with the child at home or with his family. We think it will be found important to repeat these reviews at intervals, preferably every 6 months, and to consider where specific responsibility for the coordination of these reviews should rest bearing in mind that the involvement of local authority personnel is in our view essential.

16.16 So far as the specific problem of abandonment is concerned, we believe that there is a clear need for a much more positive approach than hitherto to its prevention in whatever residential setting. How this is to be accomplished will clearly require detailed study but we have been told that the Development Group are considering the possibility of pre-admission (or very early post-admission), multi-disciplinary consideration of the medical, social and educational needs of the child, including the likelihood of abandonment and of the action which should be taken. The particular problem as we see it is to ensure effective coordination between those health and local authority staff whose concern will be with the family at home and those professional staff whose responsibility is the care of the child while he is in hospital (or elsewhere) in order to ensure that abandonment may be avoided or where it has occurred, to re-establish links between parents or child. We hope the Development Group will consider carefully the possibility of assigning specific responsibility to initiate review action and to ensure adequate coordination of follow-up activities to a named individual.

16.17 It may be that in some cases where a helpful bond no longer exists, the desirability of promoting rehabilitation with the blood parents should not be overstressed. The Development Group should therefore consider what efforts could be made to develop meaningful, alternative ties with concerned long-term visitors from outside the hospital. Schemes of this sort could be organised by the LASSD in whose area the hospital is sited, following the precedent set for utilising such resources within the community for children in long-stay children's homes where the parents prove unreliable. The benefit to the child of regular stimulus and contact from outside the institution is self-evident. In addition, thought should be given to the arrangements needed to ensure the assumption of parental rights by the responsible local authority where, in spite of all efforts, abandonment does occur. While we see much scope for a more effective approach to prevent abandonment, there is a current problem with children who are already in this situation. We hope that the Development Group will make urgent recommendations for the speedy review of all of them.

16.18 A further matter which requires detailed consideration has been brought to our attention during the course of our work. It is that mentally handicapped children who attend residential schools have frequently to be admitted to hospitals during school holidays because there is nowhere else for them to go. We understand that our concern about this is shared by the National Development Group and no doubt by the Warnock Committee on Special Education. We hope they will be able to recommend effective steps to improve the situation.

The Advocacy of Children's Interests

16.19 Thus far we have been concerned with the need to protect the interest of the individual child in certain specific situations. We need now to go beyond this to consider the interests of children as a group. *It is our belief that children have special needs which they cannot articulate for themselves and that society has therefore a duty to ensure that these are identified and cogently represented.* Over 300 bodies, both professional and voluntary, exist to promote the interests of children yet despite some real achievements—(for example, at national level, the Children Act 1975 and central government initiatives on non-accidental injury)— there still remain unacceptable deficiencies in the present fragmented provision of services for them. Some deficiencies may, at least in part, be the consequence of financial restrictions, as with the urgent need for better care of mentally handicapped children. But this is by no means always so. Sometimes central recommendations which could be implemented without difficulty or great expenditure are overlooked or ignored by the peripheral authorities. For example, the DHSS accepted in 1959 the recommendations of the Platt Report on the Welfare of Children in Hospital[2] that children and adolescents should not be nursed in adult wards and that parents should be allowed to visit whenever they could, helping as much as possible with the care of the child. Nevertheless these practices are still not universally accepted by hospitals, despite repeated Departmental exhortation and the pressure exerted by NAWCH. A deficiency of an entirely different scale is demonstrated by the failure of the three main services concerned—health, social work and education—to act in concert to meet the needs of children in long-stay hospitals. In the light of these deficiencies we have given some thought to the practicability of strengthening the advocacy of children's interests.

---

[2] Central Health Services Council, Report of a Committee on the Welfare of Children in Hospital (Chairman: Sir Harry Platt) (1958). Ministry of Health. HMSO, London.

16.20 *We have identified the following fundamental needs:—*

   (i) to keep under critical review the needs of children and the adequacy of the services provided by both voluntary and statutory bodies to meet them;

  (ii) to coordinate the work of existing bodies to prevent unnecessary duplication and omissions;

 (iii) to respond to and to influence public opinion in the interests of children and to press for the fulfilment of their needs to be accorded due priority;

 (iv) to disseminate advice on good practice, the recommendations of official committees, and the results of research both in this country and abroad;

  (v) to ensure implementation by the responsible authorities of all such recommendations and advice.

16.21 The central question is whether these objectives can best be met by seeking individual solutions to individual problems and improvements in the way that existing agencies tackle their responsibilities, or whether there are structural obstacles to the effective and comprehensive representation of children's interests which require the simplification of already complex machinery by (paradoxically) a further addition to it. A similar decision faced the Working Party on Children with Special Needs set up by the National Bureau for Cooperation in Child Care in their consideration of the well-being of handicapped children. Their report, Living with Handicap,(3) outlined the lack of effective machinery at national level for comprehensive and coordinated appraisal and policy determination and argued the need for both an inter-departmental advisory council with a developmental, consultative rôle and an independent voluntary council to meet the objectives set out in 16.20 (i)–(iv) above. They considered whether this latter necessitated the creation of a new body but concluded that its functions could appropriately be discharged either by the National Children's Bureau (NCB) or a separate council under its auspices; as a consequence, the NCB set up the Voluntary Council for Handicapped Children.

A Children's Council?

16.22 Inevitably our discussions have covered similar ground and we have considered at length the desirability of creating a new comprehensive Children's Council. The main advantage of such a council would be its ability to take a comprehensive view of the child, transcending existing administrative boundaries between voluntary, statutory, health, educational, social and environmental services. Being newly created, it would be independent in its approach to existing agencies and policies and by publishing an Annual Report to be presented to Ministers, it could draw attention to its conclusions and recommendations. Clearly any such body would need to have strong communication links with Central Government Departments, and statutory bodies for the exchange of information, although formally it should be independent of Government and non-executive in function.

---

(3) Younghusband, E, Birchall, D, Davie, R, and Kellmer Pringle, M L (1970). *Living with Handicap*. National Bureau for Cooperation in Child Care (now the National Children's Bureau), London.

16.23 On the other hand, to carry out all the tasks described in paragraph 20 above would require a large multi-professional staff concerned not only with servicing the Council's meetings but also with the collection and analysis of much data covering all aspects of children's needs. Any proposal that the Council should monitor the local implementation of policy recommendations by expert committees and government, rather than confine itself to national issues, would be particularly demanding of staff. Furthermore, the effectiveness of such a Children's Council remains open to question. Certainly we doubt the feasibility of reconciling adequate representation of a wide range of interests with the need for a body of manageable size able to achieve a working measure of agreement. We are persuaded that a large committee with a broadly defined remit would achieve little; to be effective it should concentrate on no more than two or three issues per year or set up autonomous sub-committees concerned with particular issues.

16.24 It could be argued that the administrative effectiveness of a Children's Council in coordinating effort and focusing advocacy is of less value than its psychological significance to parents and professions caring for children. This argument supposes that parents and professionals would be encouraged and inspired by the belief that there was (as never before) a body speaking for children, whatever their needs. Valuable though this psychological function might be, it could hardly be the sole, or even foremost justification of a Children's Council. Inspiration and encouragement would be short-lived if the Council proved to be an ineffectual talking shop; practical results stemming from administrative effectiveness should be the touchstone. Using this as a criterion of judgment, *we have concluded that the arguments against a new comprehensive Children's Council are compelling. The functions outlined in paragraph 20 are too heterogeneous to be encompassed by any one body; rather they demand complementary action at both national and local level.*

Achieving Objectives at National Level

16.25 Different aspects of children's needs are already covered at national level by central Departments (eg DHSS, DES), professional organisations (eg the British Paediatric Association), and numerous voluntary organisations. Given the multiplicity of bodies, the creation of yet another might well be regarded as otiose and we have therefore considered the possibility of assigning responsibility for achieving the desired objectives to an existing body. None as at present constituted could meet all our requirements but we feel that with some modification, the Children and Family Life Group (CFLG) could achieve the main goals. This is a recently constituted sub-committee of the Personal Social Services Council, an independent body set up to advise the Secretary of State for Social Services on issues relating to local authority personal social services and to promote their development. The current terms of reference of the Children and Family Life Group are: to keep under continuous review all matters affecting the needs of children and their families; to be available for consultation by any interested organisation or group, statutory, voluntary or professional; to ensure that the views of such groups are taken into account by the Council; to encourage or promote enquiry or study; and to advise the Council and where possible and desirable to act on its behalf. The membership of the group represents a wide range of interests including Social Service

Departments, the British Association of Social Workers, Community Home Schools, the Association of British Adoption and Fostering Agencies, the DHSS Social Work Service and Children's Division.

16.26 Properly to fulfil an expanded rôle, its membership should be widened to include members with health service experience. To achieve this end and afford the Group greater autonomy, *we propose that the CFLG should be reconstituted as a joint sub-committee of both the PSSC and the Central Health Services Council (CHSC)*, a statutory body which advises the Secretaries of State for Social Services and for Wales on matters relating to health services. To retain effectiveness, this new joint committee for children must be a small expert body comprising no more than 12–14 members. Membership should be based on outstanding personal ability rather than representation of any particular profession or interest although its composition would ensure that knowledge of the personal social services, education and the health services was available. In addition, the joint committee might profitably invite DHSS, Welsh Office, Home Office and DES representatives as observers. Such a committee would have sufficient expertise to consider the broad issues of general care and upbringing. Any specific projects, either selected by the Council itself or referred by other bodies, would need to be dealt with by specially selected ad hoc groups.

16.27 The advantages of an extended Children and Family Life Group over other contenders are considerable. It would avoid the further proliferation of national bodies; its members would be able to draw on relevant past experience; it would have direct access to Ministers; it would enjoy strong links with local authorities as well as the professions; and, an important point, its recommendations would be channelled through parent Councils able to consider children not as an isolated group but in the wider context of the total distribution of resources on health and social services. Clearly this consideration of priorities would be of great importance in lending weight to the recommendations and in their gaining acceptance by Government, particularly at a time of financial and resource constraints. Such an overall view of priorities could not be encompassed by any group, including a Children's Council, which was narrowly focused on children. *We therefore recommend that the interests of children would best be served by the reconstitution of the CFLG as the Joint Committee for Children on the lines described above. We also recommend that the PSSC's manpower resources should be strengthened to enable it adequately to service the new committee with its considerably greater range of activities.*

16.28 We have also considered whether there is need for machinery supplementary to the joint committee for children which would be directly related to monitoring services at national level. In particular, we noted that several Acts concerning children (eg the Criminal Justice Act 1961, the Children and Young Persons Act 1969 and the Children Act 1975) have incorporated a duty for the Secretary of State for Social Services at given times to lay before Parliament a Report on the operation of the Act. Such reports are at present not synchronised and relate only to their own limited area of children's welfare. *We recommend that these duties should be brought together to lay upon the Secretary of State for Social Services in England and in Wales the Secretary of State for Wales a statutory duty to publish a single report on all aspects of their responsibilities for children, together with the relevant aspects of DES interests (special education and school health) and Home Office interests (children in trouble). It should be laid before Parliament every three years, beginning in 1979* when reports under the Children and Young Persons Act 1969 and the Children Act 1975 are in any case due. Such a report would necessarily review progress in implementing the recommendations of Committees such as our own, and preparation impose on the three Departments a more concerted view of their combined responsibilities. Its data would depend on close monitoring of services at local level and could incorporate material on the follow-up of recommendations from HMIs, the Health Advisory Service and so forth.

Achieving Objectives at Local Level

16.29 At local level, the two main needs are for co-ordinated planning for children and for close monitoring of the services provided. There is no dearth of bodies already in existence but while regretting the present complexity of administrative arrangements, we cannot recommend any further re-organisation in view of the substantial upheavals of the last few years. We have therefore tried to frame our recommendations within existing machinery.

16.30 A mechanism for planning co-ordination already exists in the Joint Consultative Committee (JCC) composed of members of the health and local authorities; its function is to examine jointly the plans of the authorities and to advise on the planning and operation of services in spheres of common concern. (A fuller discussion of its composition and function is given in Chapter 21, paragraphs 4–5). *We recommend that Joint Consultative Committees should be given responsibility for ensuring that the particular needs of children receive due priority and attention.* The method of discharging this responsibility should be for local decision. The JCC may wish to appoint a standing children's sub-committee to advise on the development of services for children, including children who are mentally or physically handicapped. Alternatively they may prefer to consider the matter themselves no less than once a year, inviting the participation of all services concerned with children including the probation, police and prison services.

16.31 A general and continuous responsibility for monitoring lies with the regional liaison group of Departmental professionals and administrators who liaise with the regional health authorities. They make general enquiries about the progress of regional planning and implementation of departmental policy as well as more specific investigations and individual problems (such as anæsthetic deaths, non-accidental injury to children, for example). Most of their activity is at regional level but they will be generally aware of what is going on at area or district level. Additionally members of the child health medical division maintain links, not only with the regional liaison group about what is happening to child health services in the regions, but also with the area Specialists in Community Medicine (Child Health).

16.32 Locally, the Community Health Councils (CHCs) have a part to play within their more general rôle of representing the views of the local community on their health services (see Chapter 21, paragraphs 33-36). Community

Health Councils should be given the fullest opportunity to consider and comment on the health services in their districts. Although they have no executive powers, they have right of access to NHS plans and to the AHA and its officers; they can visit hospitals and other health service premises and the AHA has a duty to consult them about any substantial development of the health services in their district and in particular about any important variations in services affecting the public such as the closure of hospitals or other services and the opening of new services. Their powers in the primary care field are rather more limited. We understand that in a number of areas there has been cooperation between Family Practitioner Committees and CHCs but equally we know that in others the contacts have been minimal; regrettably, in some the reaction to an approach by CHCs has been unfriendly or even hostile. It is accepted that CHCs have a legitimate interest in primary care services and have a right to information on the plans for and siting of new health centres in their districts but they have no statutory right of access to premises or parts of premises eg health centres, which, although controlled by the relevant AHA, are occupied by practitioners for the purposes of providing family practitioner services—although they may of course visit these premises with the agreement of the practitioner concerned. In view of the responsibilities for the health care of children that we have recommended should be placed with GPPs and CHVs, *we urge that CHCs should seek opportunities for discussion with members of the primary care team, if necessary in the practice premises. We believe that if the approach is made in the right spirit, they will meet with a constructive response. We recommend that the proposed Joint Committee for Children should in due course review the effectiveness of these arrangements.*

16.33 Some surveillance of general practitioners is already carried out by the Regional Medical Service, composed in England of 56 medical officers plus a headquarters division. It has two main functions: firstly to provide a second opinion on incapacity for work for sickness and invalidity benefit payments and secondly, to visit general practitioners in their practice premises every two years (if possible). A particular effort is made to pay an early visit to doctors newly settled in practice. These visits are intended to provide a two-way flow of information. The Regional Medical Officer takes the opportunity of a general professional discussion to put across directly or indirectly ideas about possible methods of improving the service provided by the general practitioner; prescribing and certification usually also receive attention. *We are inclined not to seek more formal monitoring machinery at this point when there is growing professional discussion of means of improving the delivery of health care.* In particular, we were interested to note the report of a Welsh BMA discussion document proposing a medical audit by peer review of practice. We welcome this as a positive step, albeit confined within a narrow span. There is also surveillance of services provided by General Dental Service practitioners. This is carried out in England by 29 Departmental Dental Officers who are regionally based. These officers examine patients who have been referred to them by the Dental Estimates Board either before or after treatment. They also carry out a small number of examinations at the request of dental practitioners or Family Practitioner Committees following complaints.

16.34 An NHS Hospital Advisory Service was set up in 1969 as a result of the Report on Ely Hospital.(4) Its functions are first by constructive criticism and by propagating good practice and new ideas to help to improve the management of patient care in individual hospitals, and in the hospital services as a whole; and second to advise the Secretary of State for Social Services about conditions in hospitals in England and the Secretary of State for Wales about conditions in hospitals in Wales. Recently the service has been renamed the "Health Advisory Service" to reflect a widening of remit to enable it to advise on the inter-relationships between hospital and community health care. A new multi-disciplinary team has been created to visit hospitals where children other than the mentally handicapped are receiving long-stay care; its specific objective would be to help the health service improve the quality of life for these children, looking at the whole nexus of health, local authority education and personal social services. Services for the mentally handicapped in England are to be reviewed separately by a new non-statutory National Development Team, who are to assist with policy implementation at local level. The Development Team intend to undertake a special and continuing commitment to mentally handicapped children's services, to enable it to provide an adequate review of specialist residential facilities for them.

16.35 We feel that together these bodies should adequately monitor services for children in long stay care given also our recommendations in paragraphs 16.13–16.18. We are however concerned to note that children in acute hospitals are excluded from the remit of the Health Advisory Service. The medical profession has in the past resisted any extension of the remit of the HAS to cover acute physical medicine but we feel that children are a special case given the evidence that even short stays in hospital are relevant to their total development. Since the HAS's concern is always with the services provided rather than matters of individual clinical judgement, they might profitably consider the life and welfare of children in hospital. *We therefore recommend that the new children's team of the HAS should be able to consider hospital and related services for all children other than the mentally handicapped.* Community Health Councils should request an HAS visit where they feel it to be necessary; this is particularly necessary since the workload consequences of extending the remit are likely to be great, rendering more difficult the problem of selecting hospitals to be visited.

16.36 Finally we might usefully repeat that many valuable ideas about improving the quality of health services for children are contained in the reports of official committees already published. Recommendations that do not demand immediate attention in the field tend to get overlooked, or shelved; in such cases inaction stems from lack of sustained publicity as much as lack of will or finance. We would hope that CHCs would strive to bring the recommendations of reports continually to the attention of health service management. To fulfil this function *CHCs should, as a matter of course, receive copies of all relevant circulars, reports and memoranda issued by the Department* and their own journal, CHC News, provides an excellent means of conveying information about important developments. Over and above this, *we believe that when the recommendations of official reports are endorsed by DHSS and passed on to*

(4) Report of the Committee of Inquiry into Allegations of Illtreatment at Ely Hospital, Cardiff. Cmnd 3687. HMSO, London.

health authorities, the Department has a responsibility to monitor the progress made on their implementation.

Conclusion

16.37 Much has been done to formulate policy on child health services to render them more suitable to children's needs but these efforts have all too often been ill-coordinated and insufficiently pursued. Our proposals have therefore been framed to tackle these major problems without elaborate new machinery. When implemented, they should act as a spur to all agencies concerned with the provision of services and provided a long-awaited voice for children.

286

PART III

THE WAY FORWARD: THE MACHINERY OF CHANGE

CHAPTER 17

ORGANISATION AND STAFFING OF PRIMARY CARE

17.1 Our central objective is to bring preventive and curative health services together within the framework of an integrated child health service and to ensure that the professional staff who provide this service to children and their parents are properly qualified for their rôles. For the reasons we gave in Chapter 7, we propose that this integrated service should be based upon the continuing development of a system of primary care supported by consultant services but with important modifications to each.

17.2 In this chapter we set out the organisation and staffing implications of the pattern of primary care services we described in general terms in Chapter 7. We do the same for supporting services in the Chapter which follows. In both chapters we are concerned with the picture as it would appear when the proposed patterns have been applied throughout the country. In Chapter 19 we discuss the arrangements that will be necessary during the important transitional period between now and then.

17.3 The chief modification we have proposed is that some GPs should be more widely trained in paediatrics as GPPs to ensure higher quality and more comprehensive medical care for children within and outside their practices. We have accepted the existing status that commonly applies to nurses working in the primary health care team, ie that they are employed by area health authorities but attached to general practices; and we have proposed that some should be trained to work exclusively as CHVs with children and their families providing comprehensive nursing care. Now we examine in more detail the arrangements that will be necessary for these new rôles to be successfully assumed, and we do this separately for the GPP and the CHV.

General Practitioner Paediatricians

Work Profile

17.4 We see the GPP as a primary care physician with special responsibilities for children in his practice and in the community of which it is a part. Although we are concerned here with the paediatric aspects of his work, we regard it as professionally essential as well as administratively necessary that he should provide general medical services to an appropriate number of adult patients, and share fully in other aspects of the life of the practice. To a great extent the nature of his work with children emerges from the chapters in Part II, where we discuss the effect of our proposed pattern of services on the principal functions of the child health services. It is drawn together here as a work profile of the GPP.

17.5 Within the practice we envisage the GPP assuming responsibility for the maintenance of high standards of child health care. He will be responsible for ensuring that the following health surveillance and preventive services are provided for all children registered with the practice; ie whether with him personally or with his partners:

(i) Health surveillance at 6 weeks, and $2\frac{1}{2}$–3 years jointly with the CHV.

(ii) Immunising procedures at the appropriate times.

(iii) Examination of preschool children referred by the CHV from her home visits and from child health clinics that she conducts herself.

(iv) Initial investigation, and when necessary referral, of handicapped children and their continuing care in collaboration with the district handicap team.

He will normally provide these services himself or share them with a GPP colleague when there are two in the practice. There will be times when this is not possible and other arrangements will need to be made (17.25). We also anticipate that his partners will consult him about their child patients because of his special training and interest in paediatrics in the same way that he would consult one of his partners with special knowledge of some aspect of adult medicine.

17.6 In the community he will act as school doctor to a number of primary and/or secondary schools in the neighbourhood. This will mean:

(i) in the case of primary schools carrying out the school entry examination;

(ii) regular sessions in these schools for health surveillance of pupils with the school nurse, advising teachers and monitoring environmental health;

(iii) in secondary schools, regular sessions for informal interviews with all school children in their 13th year, and for general advice on health matters;

(iv) examination of children referred by their teachers or school nurse, and their treatment when necessary in cooperation with the child's own general practitioner;

(v) examinations of children on behalf of LEAs regarding such matters as the continued issue of free milk in the junior schools, the employment of pupils out of school hours and the admission of students to teacher training colleges.†

17.7 He might also be involved in work for the local authority social services department. This would involve, for example, the examination of children for whom they have some responsibility although they are not "in care". One GPP would need to be nominated as medical adviser to the "area" social work department for such examinations and for medical advice of a general kind relating to children and families. GPPs would also be involved in giving advice to the staff of homes for children in care (see further paragraph 17.15).

---

† As part of the NHS, school health services are in principle available to all children although in practice the services that can be offered to private schools will be limited by resource constraints. However, since these schools normally use local general practitioners as school doctors, the establishment of GPPs will provide a further link between the NHS child health services and the medical services for independent schools.

17.8 We visualise a GPP as generically a general practitioner who has undergone the necessary vocational training and is under contract to the Family Practitioner Committee of the AHA to provide general medical services of the type usually provided by general medical practitioners to their registered patients. We anticipate that he would have more children and fewer adults on his personal list than the average general practitioner. There would be two other requirements to meet.

17.9 *First, the GPP will need to have successfully completed a more extensive training in child health than is at present included in most programmes of vocational training for general practice.* This should lead to a formal recognition which we shall refer to as accreditation. In addition to the management of acute illness, the training programme will need to concentrate on social and preventive paediatrics, educational medicine, and the primary medical care of children with chronic and handicapping disorders, including emotional and behavioural disorders. (See further Chapter 20.) *We recommend the RCGP and BPA should be asked to advise more specifically on the training and experience required, and to consider whether some form of assessment is desirable at the conclusion of training.* Criteria for a national system of accreditation could then be agreed with the profession.

17.10 *Second, the GPP would need a form of contract with the AHA, the final form of which must remain a matter for further discussion.* At present the GP's obligations under his terms of service do not include the medical examination of school children or of pupils for whom the LEAs may need to provide special education. The legal responsibility imposed on LEAs to make arrangements for the examination of school children has passed to AHAs under the NHS Reorganisation Act 1973, but LEAs retain their responsibility to ascertain handicapped pupils and the AHA has a duty to ensure that health staff are available to assist in the procedure. *It will therefore be necessary for GPPs to be under contract to the AHA to provide a service in educational medicine for the pupils and the teaching staff in specified schools* (see Chapter 10) and their contracts will need to specify a commitment to educational medicine of the equivalent of two or three sessions a week (see paragraph 7.18).

17.11 The position about the work we have described as health surveillance of children before they attend infant school is less clear. The rôle of the primary medical care services in the NHS has been defined to include the prevention of disease, the maintenance of health both physical and mental, and the detection of the earliest departure from normal in individuals and in families. We accept that this is the intention. But in the past, GPs have had neither the training nor the time to undertake this preventive work, and at present not more than a quarter (in the main urban areas probably not more than one in ten) do so. Furthermore, even when they provide this service for their child patients it is often covered by a separate arrangement with the AHA, or alternatively is carried out within their premises by AHA health visitors who are attached to their practices.

17.12 It is therefore arguable whether the health surveillance of pre-school children is practised by a sufficient number of general practitioners for it to be regarded as usual, and hence required by their contract with the FPC. If this were the case there would obviously be no need for the GPP's contract with the AHA to include a commitment to undertake the health surveillance of children under five either on his own list or on those of his partners.

17.13 On the grounds that health surveillance of pre-school children no less than that of school children requires the training and experience that we expect of a GPP and that both are elements in the preventive services which AHAs have a legal duty to provide, *we consider there is a case for the GPP having a single contract with the AHA for all his preventive work as a GPP, (ie both within the practice and in the school).* Depending on the number of children registered with the practice, the contract with the AHA would specify a commitment to developmental medicine of the equivalent of one or two sessions a week (see 17.18). We recognise however that there are arguments against such a course. In particular it could be argued that it would duplicate the GP's contract for work within the practice and would tend to perpetuate the division between prevention and treatment we wish to avoid. *We consider that the number and form of contracts should be left to negotiation between the profession and the Department of Health.*

17.14 Contractual arrangements will also need to cover the services which GPPs provide in relation to LASSDs. The latter have a statutory responsibility to make arrangements for the regular medical examination and health surveillance of children in care whether they are boarded out, or are in residential homes. At present all children in care are registered with GPs and it is customary for the local authority to enter into contracts with them for the additional services and examinations required. We envisage that in future LASSDs will wish to arrange for children in care to be registered with GPPs and we do not anticipate any difficulty in the provision of these services by GPPs.

17.15 However, in addition to these services in respect of individual children registered with GPPs, local authority social services departments have other needs for medical advice in respect of children. They may need advice for example, in respect of residential establishments, in particular community homes, reception centres, homes for adolescent girls or establishments for difficult children, and a GPP might appropriately be appointed as adviser to the staff of such a home. As indicated above the LASSD would normally call on a child's own registered practitioner for any medical examination that may be required. There will however remain a number of children, varying considerably between different LASSDs, for whom the authority has a responsibility but whose circumstances make it impossible for the doctor with whom they are registered to be called on, particularly in a crisis. For example, children who run away, or who move relatively rapidly between different forms of care. A LASSD will need to have ready access to medical advice in dealing with the problems of such children, and this situation could be met by the appointment of a GPP as medical adviser to each area social work office. He would also advise the office on paediatric matters of a general kind. Where such services were provided they would need to be covered in the GPP's contract with the AHA.

17.16 Accreditation would establish a doctor's eligibility to practise as a GPP. In order to practise as a GPP within the practice, however, we think he should also have a contract with an AHA for the medical services they require to meet the needs of local authority education and social services departments in respect of children. Although circumstances will vary between practices our estimate of the needs of LEAs and LASSDs (see below) suggest that this sessional commitment would in most cases largely be employed on work within the school health service. *We would therefore expect that, as a general rule, a GPP would be involved both in developmental medicine within the practice and in educational medicine in the community, and we consider this should be the aim in establishing GPP posts. We also consider that such contracts should normally be for not less than 2 sessions a week. However we recognise that it may be necessary to allow a flexible interpretation of these principles, particularly in the transitional period.*

Number of GPP Posts Required

17.17 Any attempt to estimate the number of GPP posts that would be required in a health district or an area inevitably runs the risk of over-simplification. Nevertheless, we felt bound to satisfy ourselves that the proposals we are making are practicable by estimating the number of GPPs needed to staff a national primary health care service for children.

17.18 Educational planning is sometimes based on a planning unit of 5 primary schools, with between them a population of 1,200 children aged 5 to 10 years, feeding one secondary school, with a population of 1,000 children aged 11 to 15 years inclusive (a total school population of 2,200 children aged 5–15 years). In the same neighbourhood there will be another 1,000 children aged 0–4 years. This gives a total child population of 3,200, about the average number registered with 5 general practitioners. *We have estimated that the health surveillance of the 1,000 young children would occupy 3 doctor sessions a week, the five primary schools during term-time would call for $2\frac{1}{2}$ sessions a week, the secondary school would need not less than 2 sessions a week and the LASSD commitment would be approximately $\frac{1}{2}$ a session a week—8 sessions in all during term-time.* The fact that the educational planning population and the population served by the 5 general practitioners would not comprise exactly the same children complicates the practical arrangements for primary child health services in a neighbourhood but does not invalidate the estimate of doctor-time they would require. We are confident that between them two GPPs could provide these 8 sessions, contributing 4 sessions each. This would allow each of them time for the equivalent of 3 sessions for therapeutic services to the children on their personal lists and for the equivalent of 4 sessions for general medical services to about 1,000 adults.

17.19 The concept of the GPP can be most logically applied within the framework of group practice and, as we have indicated above, most conveniently so within a group practice of 5 principals, 2 of whom are GPPs. And we note with interest that group practice has been strongly advocated by the Central Health Services Council and the forecast made that the optimum size of a group practice will be found to be 5 or 6 doctors, together with appropriate nursing and secretarial staff. However, group practice is not yet universal. Only 17% of principals in general practice in 1974 were in partnerships of 5 or more doctors while 20% still worked single-handed (Statistical Appendix, Table F1). The question therefore arises as to whether the GPP pattern is feasible in smaller groups than 5 or outside group practice altogether, bearing in mind that while seeking due priority for the health care of children our proposals for special interest in child health embodied in the GPP must not be inimical to the care of other patients by general practice as a whole.

17.20 We are satisfied that it is quite practicable for 2 GPPs to be accommodated in a 4-group practice and it is also possible for 1 doctor to be a GPP in a group of 3. It would be less satisfactory for a partnership of 2 to carry a GPP post unless it provided comprehensive (preventive and curative) care for more than half the children registered with the practice. It is theoretically possible for a doctor to be a single-handed GPP but this would not be a financially viable proposition without considerable adjustment to the capitation fee.

17.21 *We suggest that each AHA should establish a subcommittee including representatives of the FPC which would have the responsibility for approving GPP posts, so that they meet the criteria we have set out.* Although our proposed GPP system is rooted in general practice, we consider that the AHA should be formally involved in the approval of posts, first because the AHA has ultimate responsibility for the provision of all child health services, and second because whatever arrangements are made for contracts in respect of health surveillance for under-fives, GPP posts will normally involve a specific commitment to the AHA in respect of services for LEAs and LASSDs. We see the SCM(CH) playing a key rôle in advising this joint committee on the need for GPP posts, in consultation of course, with the LEA and the LASSD.

17.22 Where a GPP post could not be filled it would be the responsibility of the SCM(CH) to advise the AHA on making alternative arrangements for preventive health services for children registered with a practice. This would also be necessary if GPPs in post were unable to provide such services for all the children in their practices. In such cases there will be an obligation on the part of the practices to inform the SCM(CH). Whatever the reason may be, if alternative arrangements are required these will need to be discussed and agreed between the practice doctors and the SCM(CH).

Financial Arrangements
17.23 To those doctors attracted by the primary medical care of children, the proposed pattern of staffing offers increased professional satisfaction. At the same time financial recognition of the extra responsibilities will be necessary. Although confident that some satisfactory means of payment can be found, we have not thought it proper to suggest what these might be. *If our broad proposals are accepted, it will be for the Department and the representatives of general practitioners to negotiate how much should be paid and in what way.*

Implications for Medical Manpower
17.24 We have indicated above that we estimate that something of the order of 8 sessions per week of GPP time (ie excluding therapeutic services) would

292

be required during term-time (and about $3\frac{1}{2}$ sessions per week out of term-time) for every 3,200 children aged 0–15. On current population figures this would mean some 30,500 sessions per week nationally during term-time or a whole-time equivalent of about 2,800 more doctors. There are good reasons to believe that fewer than this number will be required. It is estimated that the whole-time equivalent of well over 1,000 doctors are still engaged in the clinical work of what were the local health and education authorities' services for children—some of these will be immediately eligible for accreditation as GPPs, others will undoubtedly seek the training and experience necessary for accreditation (paragraph 19.14). Moreover many general practitioners now find it possible to undertake extra work in addition to their practice responsibilities and a number are already providing some of the preventive and surveillance services for children. Taking all these factors into account we consider it likely that the number of extra doctors required will be considerably smaller than 2,800.

Child Health Visitors

Work Profile

17.25 The responsibilities of the child health visitor would be:

(i) to promote physical and mental health in all children in the practice to which she is attached, through health education and advice on the prevention of illness and accidents carried out on home visits, in practice and community health clinics, and when necessary in schools;

(ii) to ensure that such services reach all children in the neighbourhood for which she has a geographical responsibility;

(iii) to participate in close cooperation with others engaged in maternity and midwifery services, in antenatal programmes to prepare expectant mothers for child care;

(iv) to ensure that all children born within the general practice and the neighbourhood to which she is designated have an early postnatal visit;

(v) to provide health surveillance for all the children in her practice, with personal appraisal at the ages of 7–8 and 18 months and assessment with the GPP at 6 weeks, $2\frac{1}{2}$–3 and $4\frac{1}{2}$ years (this would involve responsibility for developmental records, making sure that growth is recorded on standardised charts and tests of vision and hearing are carried out). In the case of children from families with "social" needs it would involve working closely with the area social work office and, particularly, with the social worker linked with her own practice;

(vi) to maintain close contact with the NO/CHV working in the district handicap team as one part of the practice responsibility for the early detection and care of handicapped children;

(vii) to act as the senior member of the educational nursing team, providing advice and support to the school nurses in her primary health care team;

(viii) to provide health advice to the day nurseries, play groups, opportunity groups and for children in hostels for homeless families, in her neighbourhood;

(ix) to help children and parents to understand what a medical diagnosis means for them, and where this involves treatment of illness at home to guide and help the parents and endeavour to increase their capacity and confidence to carry it out;

(x) to provide, with the help of child health nurses, nursing care for children in their homes, or in group practice premises and health clinics and in this to work closely with the consultant paediatric nurse based on the district general hospital in the case of children discharged from hospital or for whom the latter's advice had been sought;

(xi) to accept management and teaching responsibilities for the school nurses and child health nurses who are members of her primary care team.

Numbers of CHVs

17.26 It is difficult to estimate with any precision the manpower necessary to carry out many of the above functions; some are so broad in concept and the need for others will vary so greatly between children, between families and between districts. We would emphasise that, particularly in a time of scarce resources, the specialist skills of the CHV should be concentrated on those areas of work which specifically require them. These we consider to be the health surveillance of the under-fives and their families, including antenatal teaching. In other areas of her work both within the practice, (eg the nursing of sick children at home), and in the neighbourhood, as in school nursing, she should be able to delegate a substantial amount of work to child health and school health nurses, confining her rôle to giving them guidance.

17.27 There is no information available nationally on the proportion of time which health visitors currently spend with under-fives although the DHSS have estimated, on the basis of 3 local studies, that it is about 60%. We have therefore begun by making an estimate of the number of visits or contacts that would be required to ensure health surveillance for 1,000 under-fives. This is set out below.

Age group	No. of children	Annual No. of visits/contacts per child	Total No. of visits/contacts per week
Under 1 year	200	12	48
1–	200	4	16
2–4	600	2	24
Total under 5 years	1,000	18	88

This is no more than a notional guide: not all children will need to be seen as frequently as this table suggests and a few will need to be seen more frequently. The duration of visits will vary; some will be short and others longer, especially if they include health surveillance as described in the programme set out in Chapter 9. Each expectant mother should also be visited twice during the pregnancy and each mother and child should have a visit within a few weeks of birth which would ensure that the CHV had established rapport with the mother and allow for an assessment of needs and risks within the family. This can only be done when the levels of staffing allow adequate time for it, and this we feel is rarely if ever the case at present. Against this background it is clear that the effective health surveillance of 1,000 children under 5, involving regular contact between the CHVs and their families at clinics and in the home, will take up most, if not all the time of two full-time CHVs. If as we propose the CHV is additionally responsible for oversight of nursing services to children in the community and school nursing services we believe it is essential that *there should be as a minimum 1 CHV per 1,600 children aged 0–15, and the ultimate objective should be 1 per 1,500*. On current population figures this would call for some 7,600 and 8,200 wte respectively.

17.28 In 1974 there were 9,137 wte health visitors in post of whom 2,236 were employed entirely in the school health service. As indicated elsewhere (17.26) we consider that much of the nursing work required within schools could appropriately be carried out by other nursing staff who do not require the special skills of a health visitor and in considering the potential supply of CHVs we have accordingly included health visitors currently working within the school health service. We cannot of course predict with any precision how many health visitors would in future wish to take the training required (see Chapter 20) in order to work full-time with children and their parents as a CHV. But we suspect from what we have been told by health visitors that it could well be of the order of 80%. Such a pattern of preference would obviously have major implications for the primary care services for other age groups, in particular for the elderly, and the needs of these other groups will still have to be met. To the extent that they are thought to require the skills of health visitors and that health visitors prefer to work with other age groups, then clearly, attainment of our staffing levels for CHVs will depend on an overall and considerable increase in the numbers of health visitors. It is important to bear in mind that nationally the health visiting strength is still 50% below the level recommended as long ago as 1956 by the Jameson Committee and restated by the Department of Health in Circular 13/72. And we note that the DHSS itself has estimated that the whole-time equivalent of 7,000 HVs would be needed to meet the health surveillance needs of the under-fives in England. It is against this background of an already seriously depleted service that our proposals for a substantial increase in the service given to children and their parents should be seen.

Child Health Nurses
17.29 The staffing level which we have proposed for CHVs assumes they would have the help of supporting staff. Within the primary care team there would be child health nurses and school nurses. Child health nurses would especially help the CHV in nursing children who are ill in their own homes but they would also carry out such other duties as the CHV felt able to delegate, including immunisations. The extent and nature of this delegation will vary from one CHV to another but it must not lead to a continued separation of therapeutic from preventive nursing. The CHV would be trained and expected to keep up to date in the nursing of sick children and it would be to her in the first instance that families should turn for advice and

295

doctors would direct their referrals. We think it likely however that generally the CHV would concern herself directly only with the more difficult nursing problems.

17.30 We envisage that the child health nurse will to a large extent be concerned with providing what is essentially a new service, both in as much as relatively little nursing support is currently available for families with sick children in their homes, and also because we see her as providing a valuable source of help and advice for families, for example spending time with parents in their homes to demonstrate how to prepare infant feeds, administer medication and apply child nursing techniques. To the extent therefore that child health nurses will be providing a new service it is particularly difficult to estimate the likely need for them. However, we have no doubt that the need for such a service exists already, and that it is largely unmet. And as with any new service, the provision of child health nurses will undoubtedly generate new demands.

17.31 In 1974 home nurses attended only 43 cases per 1,000 children under 5. No figures are available for visits to older children. It seems highly probable that referrals of children to home nurses are unduly low. An estimate of the demand for such a service would have to take into account this probability and the likely increase in referrals due to early discharge and day treatment from hospital. We have no firm data as to the size of this demand. Our own tentative estimate is that there might be some 95 cases of child home nursing annually among the 1,600 children assigned to an individual CHV. The amount of time required by each case would vary considerably but might average perhaps 2 or 3 visits. We hesitate therefore to make anything approaching a precise estimate of the number of child health nurses eventually required. We envisage their number as growing **pari passu** with the increase in the number of child health visitors, and we think that by the time the CHV staffing ratios reach the level we have proposed *it might be reasonable to think in terms of 1 child health nurse to 2 CHVs, ie a total strength equivalent to some 4,000 whole-time child health nurses.*

17.32 It is unlikely that all child health nurses would be able or need to work full-time, although they would need to work flexibly, sharing with the CHV the work that falls outside normal hours. There must be a considerable number of nurses with either a hospital or a community background who are not in employment but would be willing to keep up to date and to devote some time each week to children's nursing. We would emphasise however the need for research in this field and in Chapter 12 we have recommended that the development of nursing advice to sick children should be the subject of research aimed at establishing the most economical use of nursing skills.

School Nurses

17.33 If the target caseloads we have proposed for child health visitors and their parents are accepted, then two child health visitors would be responsible for the organisation of educational nursing services to five primary schools (with some 1,200 pupils) and one secondary school (with some 1,000 pupils). In Chapter 10 we have identified the tasks which the primary care nursing service would be required to provide for these schools. We have also attempted to calculate the amount of nurse time required to carry them out and we estimate that during term-time each primary school requires 6 hours of nurse time per week and each secondary school 15 hours, but again we would emphasise that this provides only an approximate target for planning purposes. *On this basis a planning unit of some 3,200 children aged 0–15 inclusive (the responsibility of two child health visitors) would require the equivalent of about 1.5 nurses during term-time to provide an educational nursing service to the children of school age (numbering some 2,200).*

17.34 We consider that this service could be provided on a day-to-day basis by school nurses who would be registered nurses with special training and skills in educational nursing. Child health visitors would retain overall responsibility for the service since it is they who are responsible for an overview of children at home and at school. It is moreover the child health visitor rather than the school nurse who would best be able to liaise when necessary with the primary health care team of those pupils registered with practices other than that providing health services to the school, and with the social services department. The precise pattern of staffing in any district would inevitably vary, depending on the location of schools in relation to practice areas, but typically one child health visitor might supervise one school nurse serving a secondary school and two primary schools and undertaking duties at special clinics held for school children. The time spent at schools would be subject to agreement between the head teacher and the CHV and SN but at the secondary school it should be sufficient to include counselling and health education as well as examinations. Wherever possible (Chapter 10, paragraph 58) authorities should aim to appoint a nurse to work full-time in the larger secondary schools.

17.35 Allowance has also to be made for nursing services required in special schools. In an average district of 60,000 children there might be one special school for physically handicapped children, two for severely mentally handicapped pupils, four for less severely handicapped ESN children and one for maladjusted children. These would require the equivalent of not less than four whole-time school nurses.

17.36 In total it would seem that the current requirement for school nurses would be of the order nationally of 7,000 whole-time equivalents during term-time (40 weeks)—(this would be equivalent to 5,400 wte per annum). At September 1974 there was 4,375 whole-time equivalent nurses employed in the school health service in England and Wales but 2,236 of them were trained health visitors who, as we have argued above, should be considered as a potential source of supply for child health visitors. If the whole-time equivalent of 2,236 was therefore deducted from the current school nursing strength, the additional need would be a whole-time equivalent of some 3,250 nurses.

Social Work Services and Primary Health Care

17.37 The changing rôle of the GP and the emphasis being placed upon chronic illness, handicap and the social and emotional problems associated with illness, brings into sharper focus the inter-relationship of health and social services. This relationship is a complex one and must not be viewed in the narrow terms of social work support for the health services if maximum benefit is to be gained. Changes in policy of the health services towards the care of physically and mentally handicapped children and their families, increased life expectancy, residential care and specialist services all have major financial implications for the social services in terms of buildings and staff. Both health and social services have inherited longstanding deficiencies from the past in the provision for physically and mentally handicapped children and pressing demands are also being made by other client groups. In a number of places in this report we have mentioned the need for sufficient and efficient local authority services. The local authorities themselves are fully aware of the deficiencies in their service, and are anxious to remedy them, but the severe financial constraints under which they are now working inevitably means that many cherished schemes will be deferred. It is essential, therefore, to make the best possible use of the joint resources of both health and social services and educational facilities, if improvements are to be made. Changes in attitude can be as important as production of new services. In the field of primary care the need is first to recognise the contribution that social workers and social service departments can make to health care, and then to build up effective arrangements for the staff of primary health care teams and social workers to work closely together.

17.38 The value placed by the primary health care team on such arrangements will depend in part upon their assessment of the unmet social needs of their patients. Studies have shown that such assessments vary between GPs,[1,2] between GPs and social workers,[3] and between GPs and the patients themselves.[4] Other studies show some of the ways in which patients' social needs are not being met.[5,6] Involvement of the social worker in the work of the practice makes it easier for both statutory and voluntary community services to be mobilised on patients' behalf and for patients to be offered the aids and benefits to which they are entitled. Social services are able to provide a wide range of services to all patients and families in need, home helps, transport, counselling, foster homes and residential care. They have special responsibilities also for the handicapped, and social service departments are particularly aware of the more severely disadvantaged families. Changes in attitude of professionals are

(1) Shepherd, D M et al (1964). Minor Mental Illness in London. Some Aspects of a General Practice Survey. Brit. Med. Jour. 2, 1359–1362.

(2) Harwin, B G et al (1970). Prospects for Social Work in General Practice. Lancet. 2, 559–561.

(3) Backett, E M et al (1968). Social Work in General Practice. Lancet. 2, 552–555.

(4) Collins, J (1965). Social Casework in a General Medical Practice. Pitman.

(5) Goldberg, E M, and Neill, J E (1972). Social Work in General Practice. National Institute of Social Services Library, No. 24.

(6) Willis, M (1973). Social Work. Health Bulletin. 31, 144–147.

also important in improving services to patients and full-time attachment of social workers to practices has enabled the GP to make a more accurate psychosocial diagnosis, placing the patient and his complaint more fully in the framework of family patterns of stress and interaction to illness, and to provide a wider range of treatment than might otherwise have been the case.[5,7]

17.39 In 1973, only eight instances were known of full-time attachment of a social worker to a general practice,[8] and in view of the very great pressures on social services departments it would be unrealistic to suppose this method of association between social workers and primary health care teams could be generally adopted. We have considered alternative patterns that are in operation and the liaison model appears to be the most practicable in the immediate future. Here, one social worker from the area team of social workers is linked to one (or a number of) practices within the geographical boundary of that team. The social worker spends a proportion of each week discussing with the GPs new referrals and the action taken on earlier referrals as well as holding sessions in practice premises and being available for self-referrals and referrals by the doctors. This social worker would not handle all referrals personally but in some cases act as an intermediary, introducing them to another member of the area team who could more appropriately provide the necessary help; but the social worker associated with the practice (or practices) would assume responsibility for reporting back to the GPs concerned on progress.

17.40 The liaison model has several advantages. The identification of nominated social workers with certain practices makes them accessible and without the stigma that a direct approach to the social services department still holds. At the same time, one social worker becomes familiar to the practice, and because she knows the doctors and their methods of working she is able to accept their estimation of need and avoid duplication of work and confusion to the patient. The social worker harnesses the resources of the whole social services department to the practice(s) and acts as a channel of information both ways. She is a consultant on social aspects of care, and because she does not handle all cases herself the GPs get to know the work methods and resources of a range of her colleagues; and she interprets the needs and actions of the doctors to the social services department, and acts as a consultant to colleagues on specific medico-social aspects in their own work. A recent study by the DHSS[9] has shown that the liaison model operating in a rural and a small town district increases the number of appropriate referrals from GPs to social service departments, and improves the quality of care of the patients. Each profession has modified some of its prejudices about the other and

---

(7) Forman, J A S, and Fairbarn, E M (1968). *Social Casework in General Practice*. Allen and Unwin.

(8) Ratoff, L (1973). More Social Work for General Practice. *J. Roy. Coll. Gen. Pract.* 23, 736.

(9) Meade, A (1974). The Actual and Potential Rôle of the Social Worker in the Primary Health Care Team: DHSS Feasibility Study, October 1973–September 1974.

learnt to use one another better. *We think this is the pattern of association that should be widely adopted at present between social workers and primary health care teams.* The social worker associated with a practice might also provide liaison with the schools for which the GPP is the school doctor and the CHV and school nurse provide educational nursing services.

17.41 The Social Services however are also the recipients of health services on behalf of the children for whom they act as parents, and as agents for other bodies such as the courts. They have particular and special problems in providing adequately for some of these children and their needs have not always been recognised and understood or met. Many of the children for whom they have direct responsibility come from the families about whom we have expressed concern elsewhere. Effective remedial services available to the Social Service departments is one way of helping some of the worst affected children. In addition, many children's homes in the community, reception centres and community homes contain a high proportion of children with emotional disorders and anti-social behaviour problems. The staff in these establishments require informed and specialised support from the primary health care services, and we have referred earlier in this chapter to some ways in which this might be provided.

Primary Care Health Services in Special Circumstances

17.42 Every child is entitled to receive health services and whether or not they do depends in the first instance upon whether their parents avail themselves of the services that are provided. There are two special kinds of circumstances which result in some children not receiving the professional health care they require: when their parents fail to make sufficient use of the services that exist and when these services are insufficient for the needs of a community. These circumstances commonly occur together.

17.43 In a number of places (see, for instance Chapters 1 and 9) we have referred to children who are socially disadvantaged. We realise the term is imprecise but studies agree on a cluster of personal and social variables which provide the working definition we have used (Chapter 1, paragraph 49). Amongst these children are many who have a greater than usual need for health services and parents with a tendency not to obtain them. Such children and families are to be found in every community, and in rural as well as urban areas. Some rural farm workers' children live in environments equally if not more disadvantaged, socially and economically, than those of children living in our worst city slums.[10] CHVs, working closely with social workers, are key personnel in the identification of these families and in recognising individual children who have special health service needs. When the concentration of such families is high, as it may be in the centres of large cities, we can think in practice of disadvantaged neighbourhoods. It is unfortunately a feature of these neighbourhoods, especially in the Midlands and in the North, that services are likely to be less numerous and of poorer quality than elsewhere and to be facing and often overwhelmed by an excess of illness, handicap, and psychiatric disorder in children and parents alike.

[10] Steele, E J. Personal Communication.

17.44 A just and rational distribution of health services not only implies an equitable provision throughout the country but also provision that is proportional not so much to the size of a given population as to its needs. To those whose responsibility it is to plan health services, the special needs of children living in disadvantaged families and neighbourhoods pose the question: should these be met by special services or a special concentration of ordinary services? Educational planners were recently faced with a similar problem[11] and we talked to some of those involved in the educational priority (EPA) movement over the last six years[12] to see whether the methodology of positive discrimination as applied to education could be applied or adapted for the health service. We see the logic of discrimination but foresee immense practical difficulties in drawing up criteria for designating health priority areas. Furthermore, this would be a relatively crude and inefficient procedure for reaching all individual children with special health service needs because there would be some children within such areas who do not have these special needs and others outside who do. There is always a risk that services for the poor may turn out to be poor services; besides which we do not think there is a single answer to the problem as it arises in different communities. Some neighbourhoods only need their fair share of resources, others need proportionally more; some need special arrangements, and yet others need both more of the ordinary services as well as special arrangements and the latter may vary from neighbourhood to neighbourhood. Some of these we now consider.

Nursing Services

17.45 CHVs have crucial rôle to play not only in the discovery of children and families with special health service needs but also in meeting these needs. The CHV is generally the first person to take the concept of a caring community into the homes of young families who find it hard to see any value in going out to find such services for themselves. Their subsequent use of services may depend on the quality of this first contact. The greater need for home visiting of these families, which is time-consuming, means that a more favourable allocation of CHVs than one per 1,500 children is necessary in areas where there are many such families. It also means that whilst attachment of the CHV to general practices should still be the rule, responsibility for geographically defined neighbourhoods would be equally important.

17.46 Recruitment of health visitors to work with these families has not been easy in the past, in part because of the lack of adequate accommodation within reach of the neighbourhood but also because the work is strenuous, often distressing and commonly requires to be carried out at unsocial hours. If in future more CHVs are to be encouraged to apply for such posts, these disadvantages will need compensation by special conditions of service (eg additional payment or car allowance).

---

[11] A Report of the Central Advisory Council for Education (England) on Children and Their Primary Schools (Chairman: Lady Plowden) (1967). HMSO, London.

[12] *Educational Priority:* Vol 1, *Problems and Policies* (1972); Vol 2, *Surveys and Statistics,* HMSO, London.

17.47 An increase in numbers may not be sufficient in itself in some areas. If CHVs are to find point and purpose in their work, and their morale sustained, they need to be able to play an active part in the practical aspects of health care. The extension of their health visiting rôle to include practical nursing will be an advantage to them as well as their patients. They must also fully understand the nature of the underlying social and domestic problems and to know exactly how they can help solve these with colleagues in other professions.

Medical Services

17.48 General practice in disadvantaged neighbourhoods can be very exacting but we know that in some, good primary medical care is being provided. An analysis of the ways in which it can be strengthened[13] has convinced us that the same could apply to other such neighbourhoods. Uncongenial living and working conditions act as disincentives and the use of deputising services (which is more common in urban than rural practices) is a solution that is not always as satisfactory for the children as it may be for the doctors.

17.49 The development of health centres, the amalgamation of small partnerships and single-handed practices into group practices, and the introduction of GPPs would go some way to overcome the problems. The GPPs increased contact with parents and greater involvement in the health care of their children, from undertaking preventive as well as therapeutic services is likely to be particularly beneficial. However, *we recommend that AHAs examine various ways of assisting GPPs, including help in providing good surgeries with on-duty sleeping accommodation.* Until there are sufficient numbers of GPPs in post, the appointment of trained and experienced CHPs as clinic and school doctors to neighbourhoods with working attachments to one or more general practices (see Chapter 19) would be a necessary measure.

Hospital Services

17.50 In the pattern of child health services that we have proposed, hospitals would continue to be the centre for supporting and consultant services, though we have urged that these should also be available more frequently outside the hospital. We have nevertheless recognised (Chapter 12) that in certain districts within large cities people will continue to use Accident and Emergency Departments of hospitals as an alternative to their general practitioner. We had particularly in mind the inner city neighbourhoods with a high concentration of disadvantaged families, whose members have for generations turned to A and E Departments for help in situations so often neglected, for a variety of reasons, until they have reached a crisis. The fact that for the foreseeable future A and E Departments will be used in this way as a source of primary care must be squarely faced by District and Area Health Authorities. They need to be more actively involved in coordinating this occasional component of primary care with that provided by general practice. Account must be taken both

(13) Wilks, E (1975). Lessons from bad general practice. *J. Roy. Coll. Gen. Pract.* 25, 82–91.

of the increased work load and the paediatric content of the work. This means that the staffing of such departments should include (whole-time or part-time) a consultant paediatrician and a clinical specialist in child health. The deputising services in respect of calls on behalf of children might well be based on the hospital using a rota which includes CHPs; other doctors wishing to take part should have had recent paediatric experience or be expected to obtain it. The high proportion of psycho-social problems underlying, and sometimes revealed for the first time by, a parent's bringing her child to an A and E Department, requires close liaison between these departments and social work departments. Social workers who work alongside doctors and nurses in this kind of primary care service need to be experienced in child care and well-informed about child health care.

17.51 *We recommend as a priority that SCM(CH)s, AN(CH)s and Joint Planning Teams should take steps to identify children living in socially dis-advantaged families (and particularly neighbourhoods in which there may be a high concentration of such families) and examine the possibility of implementing some of these suggestions for improving and supplementing primary health care services for these children.* Profiles of need should be worked out on a district basis that makes sense for subsequent planning.

17.52 It is equally essential that any such study should be comprehensive. Socially disadvantaged families are more than just a striking example of the need for health services for children to be closely coordinated with social and educational services; they demonstrate the need for a social policy for children that goes beyond primary health care services. To consider such a policy is outside our terms of reference but the impact of social and educational factors on the health of children, their consequences for health services and the potentialities they hold for preventing ill-health and developmental disorders are such that we venture to make the following observation.

17.53 The EPA enquiries created a notion of "local diagnosis"—that is, of the community itself with the help of professionals discovering its greatest needs and then drawing on its particular human physical resources to satisfy them. We think this idea has relevance for the present predicament of dis-advantaged families and especially for the contribution of health services towards its solution. We have emphasised many times in this report how we see child health services as more than the highly skilled work of professionals in a more or less technological setting. They have also to be a partnership between professionals and parents in which the professional encourages, sup-ports and educates the parents. But as for so much that we want to achieve we are puzzled about the way forward. The overall aims of health education and training in parenthood intertwine with the morale of a community but their practical application is conspicuously a field of activity in which current methods are necessary but not sufficient. The mobilisation of the community on a local and manageable scale as was so signally achieved by EPA experi-ments might be that way forward to more realistic, direct and effective programmes of health education and parentcraft. The community would be involved in its own health education—the creation of "a learning community" which must pragmatically be a sounder basis for continued success than total reliance on professionals; and ideally a better basis for life in communities. Community projects of this kind are likely to encourage people to be concerned about themselves in other ways. From a study of "Operation Headstart"[14] it was concluded that the involvement of a neighbourhood in its own community project (and not necessarily a health project) produces permanent change in that neighbourhood and, secondarily, change in its health behaviour.

17.54 Community projects would also offer rich opportunities for co-operation between health services and other services, especially education, where the development of nursery education is being seen as a movement aimed at creating a partnership between parents, children and teachers in understanding and providing for the needs of young children. Through the practical cooperation between education, health and social work services such provision might include more day care facilities. We have expressed the view (in Chapter 1) that such facilities are desirable in most neighbourhoods but they are essential in those with a high concentration of disadvantaged families.

[14] Yarrow, A (1970). The Training and practice of health educators in North America. *Health Bulletin, Scottish Home and Health Department.* Vol XXVIII, No 3, 5–11.

CHAPTER 18

SUPPORTING CARE

Definition

18.1 We first used the term *Supporting Care* in Chapter 7 and we examine it more fully here. Terminology in the health services has been changing for some time, and by usage rather than formal agreement. We have used "primary health care" and the "primary health care team" throughout in the belief that they are now generally understood and professionally acceptable. Until recently the general practitioner saw himself as a general physician providing first contact personal doctoring and continuity of care; when help was needed he consulted with a specialist in the home or referred his patient to the appropriate hospital department. In its search for a professional identity corresponding to present responsibilities and training general practice decided that it too was a specialty; that is, it possessed a distinct body of knowledge within medicine and professional standards appropriate to its application. The view that all the individual disciplines of medicine are "specialties" was recently endorsed by the Merrison Committee.[1] The aspects of the child health service with which we are concerned in this chapter can therefore no longer be called "specialist care". "Consultant care", though an important element, is incomplete because this second contact service is provided not only by a variety of doctors, but by nurses, therapists, social workers and other colleagues who are professionally independent of medicine. The term "consultant and hospital service" would cover much of what concerns us here but could imply the separation of hospital from community which we believe must be resolved. A logical progression from primary care would be "secondary" and "tertiary" care; but this again could imply a hierarchy which is contrary to the professional equality and unity necessary for true integration. For simplicity and brevity we have therefore used the general term supporting care to cover the work of the people described in this chapter: paediatricians, allied specialists involved in the care of children, paediatric nurses, and therapists. We have considered the reasons at some length but the essence is this: we seek well-trained and more comprehensive primary care with a range of special skills and wider experience to support it. The term has seemed useful to us; we have no wish to impose it but think it satisfactory until changing needs or professional convention decide otherwise.

Paediatricians

Consultant Paediatricians: Professional Responsibilities

18.2 In the previous chapter we defined the work of general practitioner paediatricians and we must be equally clear about the work of consultant paediatricians. This involves four main activities: clinical care, organisation, advice and teaching.

---

[1] Report of the Committee of Enquiry into the Regulation of the Medical Profession (Chairman: A Merrison) (1975). HMSO, London.

Clinical Care: This is personal responsibility for patient care and involves:

seeing children in consultation in hospital out-patient clinics, health centres, group practice premises or in their homes;

the care of children occupying paediatric beds or attending for paediatric day care in hospital and the oversight of junior paediatric staff;

the management of the newborn in the hospital maternity department, in particular those requiring special care;

consultation with colleagues about individual children in hospital;

sharing in the assessment and management in hospital, child development centre, home and school of infants and children with handicapping conditions.

Organisation: Here the paediatrician has three main responsibilities:

first organising within the hospital a comprehensive children's department, and the general oversight of all child patients including those attending the accident and emergency department;

second, in collaboration with the department of obstetrics and with general practitioners in GP maternity units, supervising perinatal care;

third, and this is taking more and more time, attending committees concerned with both his own and the general work of the hospital.

Advice: The areas where advice and consultation outside the hospital are most likely to be needed are these:

collaborating in the district arrangements for the health surveillance of children;

acting as consultant to GPPs or CHPs in their rôle as school doctors to primary and secondary schools;

maintaining good communication with the corresponding social service departments in matters affecting the health of children;

acting as paediatric adviser to Adoption Agencies and local authority fostering services.

Teaching: The paediatrician's teaching responsibilities are already heavy and our proposals will add to them. There are many professional needs to be met:

teaching the junior paediatric staff in hospital, especially in the course of their clinical work;

taking part in the vocational training of GPs, GPPs, CHPs, clinical specialists in paediatrics and of allied specialists;

taking part to a varying but generally increasing degree in undergraduate medical education;

contributing to the training of paediatric nurses, midwives, child health visitors, and nursery nurses;

participating in the training of therapists, social workers, especially those with a special responsibility for children, and teachers in normal and special schools and in hospital.

18.3 It is evident from this description of what is necessary and expected that the present complement of 393 consultant paediatricians cannot provide all the services required. The experience of the past 28 years has

306

shown that faced with the unceasing demands of the newborn and the acutely ill the majority of paediatricians have been compelled to restrict the preventive and social aspects of their work. They know that this type of paediatric care is as important as hospital care but limitations of manpower, time and training have made it very difficult to provide.

The Consultant Community Paediatrician

18.4 An answer, put forward with increasing insistence, is the development of a second type of general consultant paediatrician with community as well as hospital knowledge and skills.([2,3,4,5]) Many clinicians in the child and school health services have developed skills in the developmental, preventive, educational and social aspects of paediatrics, but this is personal competence rather than systematic knowledge. And though in the last 30 years national and local studies have steadily added to such knowledge it has only to a limited extent been incorporated in everyday practice.

18.5 Knowledge and skills in developmental, educational and social paediatrics are in short supply and unevenly distributed. We therefore see a new category of *Consultant Community Paediatrician* working in the following ways:

Care of the Handicapped: As a member of the district handicap team he would bring a paediatric contribution to the diagnosis, assessment and care of physically and mentally handicapped children and to research into prevention. In the care of such children within the family he would work closely with the GPP, a specialist Nursing Officer (HV) and a Specialist Social Worker.

Educational Medicine: He would be the consultant paediatrician to the primary and secondary schools in his district, available in the normal way to school doctors (GPP or CHP) and to school nurses, and would share, when required, in the teaching of personal health and other aspects of health education. He would himself act as the school doctor to the special schools in the district.

Social Paediatrics: Effective paediatric help to children with social needs requires a formal link with the LASS. "There has been little emphasis on the contribution paediatrics can make to the care of deprived, disadvantaged and delinquent children. Doctors with clinical ability as well as social understanding are needed."([4]) Such a link with social service departments would allow ready consultation in day and residential nurseries and for child minding services. Expert paediatric advice should also be available to all Adoption Agencies; we accept that this could be provided by an experienced GPP or by a consultant community paediatrician.

The Hospital Services: He would have full consultant status and specified duties in the district general hospital. These would vary

([2]) Mitchell, R E (1971). The Community Paediatrician. *Brit. Med. Jour.* 3, 95–98.

([3]) *Paediatrics in the Seventies* (1972). ed Court, S D M, and Jackson, A D M. OUP for Nuffield Provincial Hospitals Trust.

([4]) Davis, J A, and Banford, F W (1975). The Community Paediatrician in an Integrated Child Health Service. *Arch. Dis. Child.* 50, 1.

([5]) Steiner, H (1975). *Bridging in Health.* OUP for Nuffield Provincial Hospitals Trust.

with the needs of children's departments and the special interests of the individual consultant, and it would be unrealistic to attempt to define them here.

18.6 There are good grounds for the development of the concept of the consultant community paediatrician and there is broad agreement about his professional rôle. Integration means leaving behind false divisions between clinical and social paediatrics, treatment and prevention, hospital and community. But some consultant paediatricians will give their main attention to perinatal care and acute illness and others to handicap, educational medicine and to medical-social need; some will spend the major part of their time in hospital, others in the community. Since both will be consultant paediatricians in the full sense is a differentiating label really necessary? The answer will come with time and experience; we have decided that at this stage the need to develop the subject and to identify professional responsibility for its practice points to the use of the title Consultant Community Paediatrician. However, we believe the day will come when all consultant paediatricians will see these two aspects of their work as complementary, and when developmental and social ignorance will be as reprehensible as ignorance of clinical biochemistry and paediatric pharmacology.

18.7 This extension of the work of consultant paediatricians has important manpower implications. Only a general estimate of the total number of consultant paediatricians needed in the districts can be attempted. The actual figure will depend on present variations in the distribution of consultant paediatricians, the number who are still single-handed, the local need for the consultant community paediatricians we have just described, and the possible desire of some established paediatricians to move the emphasis in their work to community paediatrics. Analysis of unmet community needs indicates that a substantial increase in manpower at district level is necessary. *To cover all the necessary consultant needs of a district with a total population of 240,000 and a child and adolescent population of 60,000, three consultant paediatricians are required,* with the fullest use made of senior clinical medical officers from the child and school health service for whom we have suggested the title of *Clinical Specialists in Paediatrics.* (The period of transition is considered in Chapter 19.) We are anxious not to impair the professional flexibility and forbearance which will be needed. Yet until the developmental stage is over and the unity of hospital and community achieved *we recommend that the contract for one of the three consultant paediatricians in each district should specify the community component of the work, and the specific commitments to the AHA, LEA and the LASSD.* We make a fuller estimate of manpower when paediatric specialists and doctors in the training grades have been considered.

Training Grades
18.8 Doctors in training provide, under supervision, a large part of the service to patients, and are a source of trained doctors for all the

relevant specialties. Paediatric experience through junior hospital appointments should be provided for:

(i) all doctors intending to enter general practice and, more fully, for those who will become GPPs;

(ii) doctors intending to become consultant paediatricians or paediatric specialists;

(iii) doctors intending to become consultants in other specialties which require paediatric experience eg child psychiatry, paediatric surgery, orthopaedics, paedodontics, ophthalmology and community medicine.

In a 'model district' containing one District General Hospital with a comprehensive children's department, an associated maternity department, and an accident and emergency department, cover can be provided by 4 doctors in the SHO grade; or a total of 812 posts for England and Wales, an increase of 236. We believe this increase of 236 SHOs would be sufficient in present circumstances. We should remember however that the model district is the exception. Most districts contain several small children's units and isolated maternity units requiring paediatric cover, and this has the effect of sharply increasing the need for junior paediatric staff and of decreasing the quantity and quality of experience gained by them.

18.9 The restriction by the DHSS on the appointment of paediatric registrars at district level has created a serious deficiency in both service and training. The number of posts should be increased to correspond with the proposed increase in consultant paediatricians. Some paediatric registrars could then have experience in general practice, health clinics and schools as part of their training. *A minimum of 300 registrar posts is needed; an increase of 96 from the present 204.* There are at present 97 *Senior Registrar Posts* and *we have estimated the minimum need as being 182,* an increase of 85.

Paediatric Specialists

18.10 As in adult medicine complex investigatory and therapeutic techniques and the skills necessary to apply them have led to the development of paediatric specialties. This work is done at present by three groups of consultants: paediatricians with specialised training who give the whole of their time to a special area of paediatrics eg the fetus and newborn infant or to one of the major systems; general paediatricians with a special interest in an area or system specialty; and, to a decreasing extent, by adult system specialists who deal with some children.

18.11 Since paediatric specialists work and share facilities with adult specialists in the same discipline, why are they necessary? The answer is that the needs which justified the separation of paediatrics from adult medicine apply here with special force. Not only are the physiology and pathology of children different but the technical character of specialist investigations and treatment also calls for a special understanding of children in the way they are carried out. In many specialties too the treatment of children is taking place at a younger and younger age, and prevention is

309

moving into the prenatal period. While maintaining sophisticated technical skills, paediatric specialists must retain an approach to the child which only paediatric training can give.

18.12 Specialisation needs a minimum volume of special need to justify it and the number of specialists needs to be related to a child population which will provide this. However, with advances in diagnosis and treatment, levels of need change and call for regular revision. The numbers of children needing specialist care varies with the specialty. In perinatal paediatrics it is considerable and in large multi-district Areas may need to be developed at Area level. For complex handicaps a Child Development Centre in every Region is essential, and again in large regions additional centres for multi-district Areas may be necessary. For the system specialties uniform development in every region is not necessarily the right answer. In system specialties the prospects for the child's recovery or an improved quality of life are in general better in larger units. In some therefore greater concentration of resources than at present is desirable. Distant specialist hospitals conflict however with the desire of parents for local services. This tension is not easily resolved but provided that parents understand the advantages and feel they have the support of the general practitioner and the local paediatrician they will accept the difficulties. And the position becomes more tolerable if accommodation for the mother is available and assistance with travel provided. The need for specialist care is clear; its provision in individual specialties and in particular areas calls for joint professional, regional and central planning. Paediatric specialist services are geographically incomplete and professionally underdeveloped. Our suggested increases in whole-time appointments are restrained, and assume part-time support from consultant paediatricians with special interests. The availability of such support and the extent to which academic staff can contribute will vary in different specialties and in different regions, and can only be decided by local enquiry.

18.13 *The paediatric specialties which have developed to the stage when consultant posts should be established, maintained or increased and the necessary senior training posts provided are: perinatal paediatrics, complex handicap, cardiology, neurology, nephrology, endocrinology, gastro-enterology haematology and oncology:* The developing paediatric specialties of accidents and injury, infectious disease, respiratory medicine, nutritional and metabolic disorders are becoming of increasing importance and in allocating resources their needs should not be overlooked. Some 70 paediatricians are working in these specialties at the present time. Our suggestions for their individual development and staffing are summarised in the paragraphs which follow. They indicate the need for *a consultant strength for all paediatric specialties of the order of 137,* an increase of 67 and representing 17% of the total number of consultant paediatricians. The pattern of development is summarised in Appendix I.

18.14 *Perinatal Paediatrics:* In view of the extent of the need, and the slow rate of fall in perinatal mortality we recommend that this specialty should be organised at Area level. To enable the necessary consultants to be trained, the first stage should be the establishment of at least one full-time consultant in each University Centre. This would mean an increase of whole-time consultants from 11 to 17. "Special interest" consultant support is probably available, and trainee rotation already established or possible.

18.15 *Complex Handicap:* One whole-time consultant community paediatrician is needed to develop and coordinate the work of each Regional Child Development Centre. This is a key appointment in the services for handicapped children and should be an integral part of the related University Department of Child Health. The consultant will provide a combined District and Regional advisory and teaching service and conduct research. It requires an increase in full-time consultants from 9 to 17.

18.16 *Neurology:* It was put to us that between 20 and 30% of paediatrics is concerned with neurological disorders and that 5 to 10% may need specialist care from a paediatric neurologist. This would mean a ratio of 1 consultant paediatric neurologist for every 250,000 children, a total of 49 or an increase of 40 over the present establishment. We consider it would be wiser to staff the Regional and University Centres first. We are not convinced of the grounds for the larger increase; though this might be justified if paediatric neurology were to widen its outlook and training, and paediatric neurologists were then to replace consultant paediatricians dealing with complex handicap in the Regional Child Development Centres. By our estimate the first increase in full-time paediatric neurologists would be from 9 to 17.

18.17 *Cardiology:* For some time the accepted view has been that paediatric cardiology should develop in all University Centres. A review in 1974, and again in 1975, revealed an untidy situation. In 1974 there were 7 centres in London, 7 in provincial England and 1 in Wales. The staff consisted of 7 full-time paediatric cardiologists, 11 consultant paediatricians contributing from 3 to 7 sessions, 7 consultant paediatricians giving 1 to 2 sessions, 9 adult cardiologists giving between 3 and 6 sessions to children, and rather more adult cardiologists giving 1 or 2 sessions to children. Yet it would seem that services are not meeting needs. Many infants with heart disease are not receiving necessary care. The greater part of the mortality from heart disease in children occurs in the first two years of life. Technical advances are leading to earlier corrective surgery and, with present progress, most operations will in future be carried out before 5. These facts strengthen the need to develop paediatric cardiology. They also suggest its concentration in a smaller number of centres, well equipped, well staffed and with special expertise in the cardiology, cardiac surgery and personal care of the young child. Our estimates suggest the need for 5 centres for provincial England and Wales and 2 in London, with an increase in whole-time paediatric cardiologists from 12 to 21.

18.18 *Nephrology:* The staffing needs put to us were based on a ratio of one consultant paediatric nephrologist for every 850,000 children. Each regional centre would provide a comprehensive diagnostic, therapeutic and

311

advisory service for its region, the range depending on whether this was provided by a full-time paediatric nephrologist with adequate supporting staff and facilities or by a consultant paediatrician with a special interest giving a part-time service. A selected number of centres, in close association with adult renal units, would provide dialysis and transplantation for children with chronic renal failure. The suggested increase in whole-time paediatric nephrologists was from 5 to 13.

18.19 *Endocrinology:* The last decade has seen a rapid growth of specialist services in endocrinology for children, and Britain is now well behind the United States, Holland, Sweden and Switzerland in this field. Sensible development would be the establishment of paediatric endocrinology in a limited number of centres working closely with adult departments and the necessary laboratory facilities. The suggested number of centres is 6 in provincial England, 3 in London and 1 in Wales with an increase in consultant paediatric endocrinologists from 4 to 12. In view of the total lack of senior registrars in this subject at the moment a higher rate of senior registrar to consultant, 1:1.7, is suggested for the period of initial expansion.

18.20 *Gastro-enterology:* We accept the need for some expertise in this important aspect of paediatrics in all regional centres. This is available in 9 at present, though, with the exception of London and Birmingham, it is provided by part-time consultants with a special interest. Regional services need the support of 3 or 4 major centres with good laboratory services and facilities for research, close links with adult gastro-enterology, and staffed by well-trained full-time paediatric gastro-enterologists. We consider 2 such centres should be in London and 2 in provincial England. The initial increase in consultant paediatric gastro-enterologists would be from 7 to 11.

18.21 *Haematology:* Paediatric haematology is an established specialty within haematology and paediatrics. In each University centre there needs to be one whole-time consultant paediatric haematologist who is a member of both departments. This would call for an increase from 9 to 17.

18.22 *Oncology:* In England and Wales some 1,200 children develop malignant disease each year. The issue here is the degree of centralised care needed for optimum results and acceptable to child and parents. Emphasising family needs, some engaged in the specialty have suggested a paediatric oncology unit in every University centre. They also suggest that some clinical centres should be closely related to departments of cancer research. On balance this points, as in cardiology, to a smaller number of centres serving total populations of 4 to 5 million, possibly 8 in provincial England and 2 in London, with 2 of the English provincial centres serving Wales. The close links already developing with paediatric haematology should be maintained. Yet wherever the centres are sited, the service will need not less than 10 consultant paediatric oncologists.

Estimates for Paediatric Staffing
18.23 The following two tables show the present staffing pattern and

the numbers of consultants, specialists, and doctors in training we consider necessary to improve it.

TABLE 1
Present and Desirable Specialist and Training Manpower

	Consultant Paediatricians	Senior Registrars	Registrars	Senior House Officers
Present	393	97	204	576
Proposed	746	182	300	812
Increase	353	85	96	236

TABLE 2
Distribution of Consultant Paediatricians

Type	Consultant/ General	Consultant/ Community	Consultant/ Specialist
Number	406	203	137

18.24 The provision of an adequate number of consultant community paediatricians will take time. Some senior clinical doctors in child and school health, if necessary with additional training, will meet part of this consultant need. This will still leave a considerable gap and during the transitional period the services will be maintained by the appointment to the personal grade of clinical specialist in paediatrics of senior clinical medical officers. The administrative and training arrangements are considered in Chapters 19 and 20. *It is essential that transitional arrangements should not impede the development of trained consultant community paediatricians. Their provision in sufficient numbers will mean a re-appraisal of the priority given to child development and to social and educational paediatrics in every university; not only in Departments of Child Health but in departments of Social Medicine, Education and Social Work.*

Allied Specialists

18.25 Supporting care provided by consultants and hospitals involves a wide range of specialties. Child psychiatry is considered in Chapter 15 and dental health, to which services for children are the key, in Chapter 13. We are concerned here with specialties giving the major part of their time to adults but with a substantial, for many a very substantial, commitment to children. It was clear from the evidence they presented to us that these specialties are developing and anxious to develop further the paediatric aspects of their work. The extent and range of its services gives surgery a special place. Paediatric surgery, a growing specialty wholly concerned with children, shares a common approach with paediatrics. Most of the general surgery and certain forms of specialist surgery are carried out by general or specialist surgeons whose main work is with adults. Bearing in mind the variety of children's surgery and the unity of surgery

313

as a discipline, we have considered the surgery of childhood as a whole in this part of the chapter. For the other specialties we have gone as far as our information would take us; we have not attempted a detailed assessment of their professional needs and have avoided detailed recommendations, particularly on manpower, which our knowledge could not support.

The Surgery of Childhood

18.26 Half of the children admitted to general hospitals are admitted for surgery, and the major part of this is done by general or specialist surgeons whose main work is with adults. They may, but often do not, have sessions in their contracts specifically for children's work, and their interest in and understanding of the special needs of children varies widely. In some hospitals, a high standard is achieved, and this is more likely to happen where one or two, rather than all the surgeons, deal with the bulk of children's surgery. In many hospitals no such selection is attempted. *We recommend that at district level the majority of common surgical problems should be handled by a limited number of surgeons (not less than two) with a special interest in children's surgery.* Surgeons accepting this responsibility should have contractual sessions, including out-patient time, specifically for the work. When appointments are made which include paediatric sessions, some paediatric surgical training should be implied. These measures should accelerate an existing tendency towards partial child specialisation at district level.

18.27 In recent years growing numbers of surgeons are giving their whole time to paediatric surgery. In 1974 there were 25 paediatric surgeons and their regional distribution is shown in Table F7 in the Statistical Appendix†. They are developing important aspects of the subject, especially the surgery of malformations and the newborn. Experience, illustrated by Table 3 below, suggests that centres drawing from a population of two million will provide sufficient work for two surgeons devoting all their time to children. Paediatric surgeons work mainly in University Hospitals and Regional Centres, and even in the large conurbations with populations of more than four million, efficiency and economy require that centres should not be duplicated. *We accept the recommendation that at present, and apart from London, there should be thirteen Regional paediatric surgical centres for England and Wales.*

TABLE 3

Children's Admissions by Age for Paediatric Surgery in Six Centres 1972

Type	Age	Newcastle	Sheffield	B'ham	Carsh'ton	W'minst	GOS	Total
Emergency	< 1 mth	118	180	153	118	43	300	912
	1– 11 mths	50	178	135	128	274	46	811
	1 <4 yrs	41	359	259	264	625	139	1,667
Elective	– 1 mth	30	4	4	1	139	18	196
	1–11 mths	177	107	177	133	153	49	796
	1–4 yrs	475	416	655	499	436	294	2,775
TOTAL		891	1,244	1,383	1,143	1,670	846	7,177

† Subsequent appointments have increased this to 28.

18.28 The numbers in Table 3 apply only to children under 5, and they show that a major unit will treat about 1,200 in this age group every year 152 (13%) in the neonatal period. Spina bifida accounted for 12% of all children and for 20% of the newborn. The annual attendances for day cases were only available from five centres; the total was 1,862 and the average for a single centre 372.

18.29 Through developmental understanding and technical skill, paediatric surgeons (with paediatric anaesthetists) have pioneered neonatal and infant surgery. It would however be misleading to see their contribution limited to infants; they are involved throughout childhood in fields as diverse as malformations and oncology. What is equally important, their presence and approach can raise the level of children's surgery throughout a region. *We consider a ratio of one paediatric surgeon for every 250,000 children as appropriate and an increase in paediatric surgeons from 28 to 49 as therefore necessary.* System specialties also make an important contribution to the treatment of children, notably cardio-thoracic surgery, neurosurgery, urology and plastic surgery.

18.30 In many regions children's surgical services are fragmented, making sensible organisation and integration extremely difficult. Neonatal surgery may be in one hospital, trauma and orthopaedics in another, neuro-surgery and cardio-thoracic surgery elsewhere. We recommend that these be brought together in a number of regional or supra-regional centres where specialist surgical and nursing skills and anaesthetic and radiological services can be concentrated and where laboratory and other expensive technical facilities can be economically employed.

18.31 In the last twenty-five years paediatric surgery has made an outstanding contribution to the health of children and we are convinced that it should continue to develop. The larger part of the general and the specialist surgery of childhood will continue to be done by surgeons who also treat adults. This has two important implications: the need to maintain a degree of unity between the child and adult parts of system specialties to ensure that technical advances can be applied to all sections of the community and to promote the proper advance of the specialty as a whole; and the provision of this surgical care in a children's setting. *In our view paediatric experience should be a requirement in training for any system specialties that have an important commitment to children.*

Paediatric Anaesthesia
18.32 Paediatric anaesthesia demands special knowledge and skills. At present some 40 anaesthetists give all or a major part of their time to children. They work mainly in Regional Centres and University Hospitals, and paediatric surgery in such centres can usually obtain skilled anaesthetic support. Of equal concern is the quality of anaesthesia provided for relatively minor surgery, for example in accident and emergency departments or in dental treatment. Because the surgical problem is a simple one it is often incorrectly assumed that anaesthesia presents no problems and demands no special skills. It has been recommended to us that all children

315

requiring anaesthesia should have this administered by an anaesthetist who has had training and experience with children, a view which is particularly relevant with the increasing use of day surgery. Much of this surgery will also be considered minor, but it is important that the anaesthesia is not deputed to inexperienced doctors. The primary need is to provide training in paediatric anaesthesia for consultant anaesthetists dealing with children's surgery in district hospitals. This is already a requirement of the Faculty of Anaesthetists for general and for higher professional training; and there is a waiting list of senior registrars seeking it. The need will only be met when there are more University Centres capable of providing such training, and the research and teaching necessary to sustain it.

Paediatric Radiology

18.33 The need for a specialist service in radiology for children is generally accepted. To develop it in parts of the country where it is lacking will require the creation of more departments of paediatric radiology staffed by full-time paediatric radiologists. These would advance the knowledge and practice of the subject and, as there are insufficient training posts in existing departments, provide the necessary expansion of training facilities. There should be two types of senior registrar post available: the first for those intending to specialise in paediatric radiology; the second to provide experience in the paediatric field as part of general specialist training in radiology. Both patterns of training are of equal importance. The second type of senior registrar post is directly related to the need in all district hospitals for one of the consultant radiologists to have had training in paediatric radiology.

18.34 The facilities in district hospitals as in Regional Centres should include a specially equipped X-ray examination room or rooms, and professional support from radiographers trained in dealing with ill children.

Orthopaedics

18.35 There is a large children's component in this specialty. Many of the disorders dealt with are congenital, calling for early recognition and treatment at birth or early in infancy, and sometimes for continuing attention through adolescence into early adult life. Orthopaedic surgeons are also responsible for much of the management of accident and injury. Almost as many children of school age are admitted to orthopaedic as to paediatric beds. At present the majority are not nursed in children's departments, and the Committee urges that the Departmental guidance in this matter should be followed. There is opportunity for greater cooperation between orthopaedics and paediatrics in joint out-patient clinics and in improving the facilities for children in accident and emergency departments. We share the concern of the British Orthopaedic Association about the shortage of separate and suitable accommodation in hospital for adolescents, and the need for improved arrangements for the orthopaedic supervision of children with chronic disorders whether educated in normal or in special day or residential schools. We have suggested in relation to the general surgery of childhood that adult surgeons with a substantial commit-

316

ment to children should have paediatric experience in their training. The range and importance of the orthopaedic contribution suggests that orthopaedic surgeons with a special interest should have a similar training experience, and that some devote themselves wholly to children.

Otolaryngology and Audiology

18.36 This specialty compares with orthopaedics in the number of children in its care. Paediatric otolaryngology is accepted by the specialty as a necessary part of training. Present practice and future planning have been examined jointly by the British Association of Otolaryngology and the British Paediatric Association. The conclusions reached have been welcomed by the Department of Health and are available from the professional associations concerned. The BAOL regard it as desirable to test the hearing of school children annually. We would see this carried out by school nurses trained in the necessary skills, and where deafness is suspected referring the child to the Area audiology service. We have already drawn attention to the importance of assessment of hearing in the care of the handicapped child, paragraph 14.57. Medical audiology calls for special training, and a programme for doctors wishing to specialise in the non-surgical management of deafness is now available. Partnership between the disciplines concerned with hearing and language is developing and should be encouraged.

Ophthalmology

18.37 One in five of the patients coming to a department of ophthalmology is a child. A number of ophthalmologists are developing the paediatric aspect of the specialty though not to the exclusion of their work with adults. We agree with the suggestion made to us by the profession that this should increase. Such doctors would work mainly in University Hospitals and Regional Centres; and in appropriate appointments the terms could include the need for experience in paediatric ophthalmology. Separate ophthalmological out-patient clinics for children are desirable, and in spite of difficulties with accommodation and timing this should be the aim. Ophthalmologists are convinced of the advantage of working closely with other professional colleagues in assessment and care of handicapped children. The surgical treatment of squint now requires only a brief stay in hospital and the use of day surgery is increasing. The management of serious eye conditions in the wards of children's departments, as recommended in the Department of Health's memorandum, Hospital Facilities for Children, raises professional and administrative problems. We respect the professional concern felt by consultant ophthalmologists over this matter and understand that further consideration is being given to this by the Faculty of Ophthalmologists and the British Paediatric Association.

Dermatology

18.38 Skin diseases are the fourth reason for a child being brought to a general practitioner and the sixth for referral to a District Hospital out-patient department (Statistical Appendix, Table E.30). The majority coming to hospital are dealt with by out-patient consultation. Our evidence suggests that it is unusual for this to take place in special clinics for children. Children also attend for day treatment, but we have no information on whether separate facilities are provided or separate sessions held. Only a minority need admission and they can usually be accommodated in the children's ward but we have no evidence whether this is the general practice. In view of the frequency of skin disorders in children we believe that a part-time (in University Hospitals a whole-time) commitment to paediatric dermatology would be a rational development. In addition to advancing the subject, this would strengthen the vocational training of GPPs and consultant paediatricians in a subject important in itself and for its associations with so many general diseases.

Medical Genetics

18.39 The majority of clinical problems in this field relate to children and to parental concern about the potential risk of producing children with malformations or genetic diseases. The present position and the increasing opportunities for guidance and prevention were put clearly before us. It was suggested that provision for genetic counselling requires not less than two consultant medical geneticists in each Region, and by this standard the present regional distribution of medical geneticists with a total or major commitment to children and families is inadequate. For cytogenetics each Region needs one major cytogenetics laboratory. This should be equipped to handle both routine diagnostic procedures, and progressively, pre-natal screening which in the forseeable future may involve 10% of all pregnancies. Enzyme laboratories are in one sense part of the chemical pathology services but it is important that they should have a formal association with departments of medical genetics.

Laboratory Specialties

18.40 The specialties considered here are morbid anatomy and histo-pathology, chemical pathology and microbiology.

18.41. The provision of specialist paediatric morbid anatomy services is limited to University Centres and is provided by academic departments of pathology or by consultant paediatric pathologists in the NHS. Each University Centre should have at least one full-time paediatric morbid anatomist providing a routine service to the centre, a regional service for referred material, and involved in teaching and research; and a limited number of University Centres should accept responsibility for their training. There is no consistent provision of paediatric pathology services in district hospitals. While the appointment of paediatric pathologists to such hospitals is not called for, lack of paediatric experience by general pathologists can result in diagnostic delay and in failure to obtain appropriate specimens for referral to University Centres. The situation would be improved if sufficient general pathologists in training spent a period with a paediatric pathologist during their period as senior registrars.

18.42 The need for a specialist chemical pathology service for children is based on the special characteristics of their metabolism. The interpretation of many paediatric investigations differs from that of adults and certain complex estimations are required more frequently than in adults. In addition, special adaptations of standard techniques, such as balance studies and the use of micro-methods on blood, are necessary. There should be a department or section of paediatric chemical pathology in all University Hospitals or Regional Centres. The number of children in a district hospital requiring chemical pathology services is smaller, special techniques and micro-methods are often

318

not available and the quality of service may be lower than for adults. In such hospitals the director of the chemical pathology service should have some knowledge and experience of metabolic disorders in newborn and older children, and should ensure the use of micro-methods for blood sampling. The district hospital laboratory will undertake the common investigations and send specimens from unusual conditions to the regional paediatric laboratory. This practice is working well in some areas, but it is by no means general throughout the country. For rare disorders a greater measure of centralisation is required. It has been suggested to us that six "specialist centres" would meet these needs for England and Wales. We understand that the Royal College of Pathologists is well aware of the variation in the quantity and quality of service and of academic provision for children in different parts of the country. We ask it to review the need and to estimate the increase in specialist manpower needed especially in those university and regional centres which are less well provided for.

18.43 An increasing number of infective illnesses in children are now susceptible to rapid laboratory diagnosis and this makes the services of consultant paediatric microbiologists and supporting technical staff essential. There are a few consultant microbiologists working in children's hospitals who have had special training and experience in the microbiology of children. In University Departments and in large Children's Hospitals one or more consultants should give their whole time to the bacteriology or the virology of children. They are needed not only to improve the treatment of infectious disease but to intensify research in its prevention. In district general hospitals microbiology services for children will be provided by the general laboratory. It is important that the microbiologist should have had some training in paediatric microbiology. Regular consultation between paediatrician and microbiologist is increasing and has great advantages, for example in agreeing policies for the control of infection and for antibiotic therapy.

Nurses

Current Staffing Levels

18.44 *Sick children should be nursed by nurses who have been trained to do so.* This central conviction, repeatedly stated, has been reluctantly heeded. More nurses are needed in a children's ward than in a comparable ward for adults. Acutely ill children, especially infants, need more frequent observation and attention than adult patients for they can do little or nothing for themselves and are almost totally dependent upon the nurses. Even when recovering, infants need constant care and older children supervision and occupation. One third of all admissions to children's wards are under 5 years of age. Resident or visiting parents help in the care of their children but they also take up the nurse's time if she uses the opportunity provided for explanation, comfort and teaching. Teachers and play staff make an important contribution to general care, but there are many periods in the day and night when nurses are responsible for the total supervision of the children.

18.45 Our assessment of the present situation is derived from four sources. A sample survey carried out by the Department of Health and Social Security in 1975 of the nurse staffing of wards containing children in non-psychiatric

319

hospitals in England and Wales; a selective regional survey;[6] submissions to the Committee by nursing organisations; and visits to children's wards and hospitals.

18.46 In March 1975 there were 20,514 RSCNs recorded on the Register, but this figure gives no indication of the number actively nursing and the number nursing children, or in what type of ward or department and in what parts of the country they were working. The sample survey of the whole country (Statistical Appendix, Tables F14–16) shows that of a total of 3,663 registered nurses (whole and part-time) nursing in children's wards, 41% were qualified RSCN and out of a total of 1,763 enrolled nurses (whole and part-time) 22% had been trained in the paediatric field. Where children were nursed in adult wards with segregated children's beds, only 7% of the registered staff and 1% of the enrolled nurses were children trained.

18.47 The three sources of data together suggest that:

on children's wards between 20–50% of the trained staff are RSCN, with wide regional variations;

in special care newborn units between 10–20% of the trained staff are RSCN;

of all the children's wards in the 3 Regions surveyed in 1973[6], 15% were without children's trained staff by day, 50% by night and 11% at any time.

In the words of the regional survey, and we confirmed this on our visits, *"most children's wards are without a children's trained nurse for some of the time, many are without for much of the time and some are without at all times"*.

Estimates of Need

18.48 While the evidence we have supports the view that there is both an overall shortage and an unequal distribution of paediatric nurses, a realistic formula for the estimation of total and trained nurse staffing of children's departments has not been devised. Staffing ratios provided by DHSS can only be regarded as approximate: they are determined in part by financial implications, and in most situations the actual numbers are falling below the estimates. Any estimation of staffing needs must take into account:

(i) the age distribution of the children in the ward (young children take up a much greater proportion of nursing time);

(ii) the types and seasonal variations of illness, number of emergencies, amount of surgery and the number of operating sessions, bed occupancy, and mean length of stay;

(iii) the extent of nursing provision for intensive care, day care, out-patient clinics and Accident and Emergency departments;

(iv) the need for a complement of trained staff based on the hospital who will act as consultants to the child health visitors, especially when a child is discharged from hospital and requires the continuation for a limited time of special care and treatment;

(v) the current hours of duty, time for in-service training, holiday and absence through sickness.

(6) *Paediatric Nursing in Non-Psychiatric Hospitals*. Report of a joint working party of the British Paediatric Association and the British Association of Paediatric Surgeons. Unpublished.

18.49 Accepting the limitations of Departmental estimates, and until local assessments of needs and provision provide a more reliable measure, we give what guidance on nurse staffing we can. Recognising that the number of available beds and the size of wards varies enormously throughout the country we have used a 20-bed general children's ward in a children's department as our model. Experience suggests that 20 children are the maximum that can be cared for safely and adequately in one ward, and that this should be regarded as an optimum size. The staffing of such a ward, and of a 10-bedded day care unit, is shown in Table 4.

TABLE 4

Nurses Required for a Children's Ward of 20 Beds and an Associated Day Care Unit

Type of Unit	Sister	Staff Nurse	Enrolled Nurse	Learner	Nursery Nurse/ Nursing Auxil'y	Totals
20-Bed Ward	1	4	3	7	3	18
10-Bed Day Care Unit	—	1	1	1	1	4

If one ward is used as a five-day ward, the staffing requirements can be reduced by approximately one-third. General responsibility for the day care unit could be provided by one of the ward sisters. The estimate in Table 4 would provide 24 hour cover by trained staff for each 20-bedded ward, with a distribution of total staff of six in the morning, four in the evening and three for the night. This staffing requirement can be adapted to fit any size of peadiatric department in a district general hospital.

18.50 Paediatric nurse cover for Out-patient Departments and Accident and Emergency Departments will require additional staff.

TABLE 5

Additional Nursing Provision for Out-Patient and Accident and Emergency Departments

Type of Unit	Sister	Staff Nurse	Enrolled Nurse	Nursing Auxil'y
Out-Patient Clinic	1	2	1	1
Accident and Emergency Department	—	1	2	—

The additional staff suggested in Table 5 provide minimal cover as it is expected that additional help will be available from the staff of the children's department and the Accident and Emergency Department. The Night Sister (RSCN) in charge of the children's department at night would also be available for consultation by the Accident and Emergency Department. The total estimate must also include a complement of trained staff who will act as consultants to the child health visitors and allowance has been made for this in the estimate of

321

additional nurses needed for the out-patient clinic. Experience in Birmingham suggests that a minimum figure for a domiciliary consultant paediatric nursing service is one to every 60,000 children (ie one in the average district). Better staffing would allow more time for the continuing education of health visitors in children's nursing and would probably reduce the number of out-patient attendances and re-admissions to hospital.

18.51 *A named senior nurse with the RSCN qualification should be responsible for the overall supervision of the children's department* coordinate nursing relationships with other clinical and laboratory departments dealing with children, and represent a nursing view to senior management and in the division of child health.

TABLE 6

Mean Staffing of 20 Bedded Children's Wards in 3 Hospital Regions in 1973, compared with Minimum and Optimum Estimated Requirements
(Based on report of BPA/BAPS Working Party(6))

Nursing Staff	Mean for all Regions			Mean Excluding University Centres			Estimated Total Staff	
	D	N	24	D	N	24	Minimum	Optimum
Trained RSCN	1.7	0.7	2.4	1	0.5	1.5	1	4
SRN & SEN	3.4	1.2	4.6	3	1	4	4.5	8
TOTAL	5	2	7	4	1	5	5.5	12
Learners	6	1.3	7.3	4	1	5	8	15
Others	2	1	3	2	1	3	4	3
TOTAL	13	4	17	10	3.5	13.5	17.5	30

D = Day Staff
N = Night Staff
24 = Total Staff for 24 hours

18.52 In Table 6 are shown mean staffing levels in 1973 for a children's ward in three large hospital regions compared with an "optimum" which would ensure sufficient trained staff throughout the 24 hours and a "minimum" below which child safety and nursing morale are increasingly at risk. By these criteria the estimates given here in Table 4 and 5 are a minimum, below which safe and satisfactory care cannot be provided and for which the nursing service could not accept responsibility. We recognise the implications of current financial restraints, widening demands for women's labour and the rising needs of adults, *but we must stress again that in many children's departments for much of the time staffing falls well below our acceptable level.* The strains both on trained staff and learners when this happens can be very great, with danger to patients, especially acutely ill infants with their special risk of sudden deterioration, and adverse effects on the morale of nurses and their recruitment and retention in the paediatric field.

18.53 A higher ratio of staff to patients is necessary in University Hospitals and regional centres because of the increasing technical complexity of many diagnostic investigations and the concentrated and often continuous care required by children with severe and complex illness or recovering from specialist surgery. Each unit needs an RSCN of Nursing Officer status, with a Senior Nursing Officer in charge of the whole children's hospital or department. As the size of these centres and the distribution of paediatric specialties varies from region to region no attempt has been made to provide a precise estimate of nursing needs. The ratio would certainly not be less than one nurse to one child, and in certain specialist units the ratio would be higher. Of greater importance is a greater proportion of trained staff.

18.54 Our staffing base line is uncomfortably near the frontier of safety. On visits and in conversation, experienced nurses and doctors repeatedly used the word "precarious" (sometimes "perilous") to describe the present situation. Nursing acutely ill children is an anxious, trying business and we were impressed by the skill and resourcefulness with which nursing staff are responding to the changing and ever increasing demands made on them in children's wards.

18.55 An essential condition for making the best use of scarce nursing (and medical) resources is the concentration of all sick children in children's departments within district hospitals, *and a necessary first step to the maintenance of nursing establishments which do not fall below the level we propose.*

18.56 *Within this establishment our first priority would be a Sister/charge nurse with RSCN qualification in charge of each ward.* In England and Wales at present there are a total of 1,824 sisters (whole and part-time) caring for children in children's wards, of whom 1,130 are RSCN. There is therefore an immediate need for a further 694 RSCNs to meet our priority. There are also 25 RSCNs in charge of adult wards with segregated children's beds; and if these were willing to return to children's nursing the deficiency would be reduced to 669. The amount of time necessary for these additional RSCNs to achieve registration will vary with individual previous experiences. There are at present two types of course available: secondment for 6 months post-registration training (one course only at Sheffield at present); and more numerous 13 months post-registration courses.

18.57 1,839* staff nurses, of whom 1,062 are RSCN, and 1,763* enrolled nurses, with 440 trained in the paediatric field, are at present employed in children's wards. It is unrealistic to assume that financial resources are available at present for the secondment for post-registration and post-enrolment training of all of the above staff who are not paediatrically qualified. However, in-service training by day release might well be possible, and it would establish the principle and go some way to meet the need.

18.58 *In the longer term the maintenance of a satisfactory nursing establishment with RSCNs and paediatric SENs will require an increase in the number of nurses in children's nursing.* One study estimated that to provide a minimum of two RSCNs on each children's ward, with an additional number for tutorial and administrative staff and specialist advisory services, the number entering

---

*Whole and part-time.

training each year should be almost twice the present number.(6) A corresponding increase is estimated for pupil nurse training. When financial resources improve such an increase should be given high priority. An increase in learners would also need some increase in clinical teachers and tutors. This too is not possible in the short term because of the persistent shortage of tutorial staff and the financial implications of secondment for tutor training.

Recruitment

18.59 Aware of the wider problem of recruitment to the profession as a whole and the claims of others, beside children, our concern is to encourage paediatric nursing. Many find they are naturally attracted to children's nursing, and this is confirmed by the conspicuous use of pictures of children in the brochures of nurse training schools and in the careers advisory publications of the Department. Although some school leavers may have an unrealistic idea of what children's nursing involves, there is also a wealth of genuine interest waiting to be fully used. The realisation of this depends on three things—information, encouragement and opportunity.

18.60 The existing schemes for training in children's nursing are not widely known, and the Department of Health's publications are not always as informative as they might be. For example ,"Someone Special" (1971) featured a nurse with a sick child on the front cover but made no reference in the text to children's nursing. And "A Girl Like you" (1971), which was concerned with SEN training, referred to the specialised parts of the roll but did not mention that in training for the general roll 18 months of the two years can be spent with children. There has been a welcome improvement in recent publications, but paediatric SEN courses are still poorly publicised. We hope the Department and the College of Nursing will ensure that careers advisers in schools are kept up-to-date with information about the openings for children's nurses.

18.61 In many schools there still appears to be considerable prejudice against nursing. The development of cadet schemes at 16 and full entry at 17 would allow a direct transition from school to profession. And at the end of training, nurses who hold additional qualifications should receive adequate recognition. The principle of additional payments for such qualifications should be restated, with amounts related to present-day values. The position for paediatric SENs is more complex. At present those who do the "paediatric" course take the same examination as those training with adults, and successful candidates are listed in the general part of the roll. There are in addition "special courses" (eg in mental subnormality nursing) with different examinations leading to entry into specialised parts of the roll. Such "specialist" SENs are not qualified to undertake nursing duties outside their special sphere. We do not advocate a special paediatric roll of this limited kind. *But we recommend that those who have spent 12 months or more of their two years with children should be given the opportunity to take, in addition to the general SEN examination, a paediatric examination,* with the entry of successful candidates on a paediatric as well as on the general roll, and with additional payment for the double qualification.

18.62 The present career structure and its consequences are also relevant here. This should allow a nurse to pursue a comparable career in either clinical nursing, teaching, or administration. In spite of recent changes there is still a tendency to devalue clinical in comparison with some administrative nursing. Opportunities for children's-trained nurses to progress beyond the level of ward sister without leaving the paediatric field are very limited. There are some administrative opportunities in the new remaining children's hospitals and larger units: and there are teaching opportunities in the 27 schools offering paediatric courses. But able and ambitious young nurses would be deluding themselves if they did not see that a career in clinical children's nursing comes to an abrupt halt at the top of the sister's salary scale. The Committee on Nursing[7] felt that recognition should be accorded to exceptional abilities and multiple responsibilities and recommended that ward sisters by virtue of professional expertise linked with other responsibilities, such as teaching and a consultancy function, should be accorded increases in status and reward within the like structure. We consider that these proposals merit consideration by the nursing profession.

Nursery Nurses

18.63 The inclusion of nursery nurses in the pattern of ward staffing expresses our conviction that they have a real and specific contribution to make to the care of children in hospital. They have an important and versatile rôle; providing help with feeding, dressing, toileting and play, and to help to meet the needs for solace and support when parents are not there. Because the majority of them work in day and residential nurseries and in nursery schools and classes it is often forgotten that some 414 are working with children in hospital. We hope that the development of different patterns of training for those working in the local authority social services will not undermine their recruitment and training. *When the new pattern of nurse training is established the rôle of nursery nurses should be re-examined with a view to allowing their training and experience to count towards nurse training.* Indeed those wishing to work in hospitals should be fully integrated into nursing and the ward team.

Therapists

18.64 We have in mind physiotherapists, occupational therapists, speech therapists, dietitians, ophthalmic opticians, orthoptists and dental auxiliaries. To list them in this way is not to suggest that they are a homogeneous group or in some way ancillary to medicine. They are independent professions and one, speech therapy, has recently been the subject of an independent enquiry.[8] Our observations are derived from the varied but limited information we have received. Although change is in the air it is clear that for some of the special therapies the need to examine the paediatric requirements of their discipline has only just begun.

Physiotherapists

18.65 Physiotherapists play an essential part in the care and treatment of many ill, injured and handicapped children. During the last two years those wholly or mainly working with children have formed the Association of Paediatric Chartered Physiotherapists. Its purpose is to promote the study of paedi-

---

[7] Report of the Committee on Nursing (Chairman: Asa Briggs) (1972). Cmnd 5115. HMSO, London.

[8] Report of a Committee on Speech Therapy Services (Chairman: R Quirk) (1972). Department of Health and Social Security. HMSO, London.

atric physiotherapy and to improve the training, education and professional standing of paediatric physiotherapists, including the establishment of a specialist diploma. There is a present membership of 500 and support from the parent society. This is a welcome development.

Occupational Therapists

18.66 Some 111 of the occupational therapists employed by health and local authorities in England work mainly with children but we have no corresponding figure for Wales. The development of a paediatric interest group is being considered within their professional organisation. Occupational therapists working mainly with children are eligible for associate membership of the Association of Paediatric Chartered Physiotherapists and this suggests the possibility of closer professional association in work and training. We believe such a development would have advantages for child and parents as well as the professions concerned.

Speech Therapists

18.67 The training and professional development of speech therapists has recently been reviewed. Speech therapists work with both children and adults, but figures are not available to show what proportion of their work is with children or the number dealing only with children. There were 1,062 speech therapists (wte) employed in the NHS in England and Wales in 1974. Numbers are increasing, but there is still a good way to go before the 20-year target of 2,500 is reached. Total training capacity has risen, however, to some 310 places for England and Wales and this exceeds the Quirk Committee's 1982 target by about 50 places. Submissions from many organisations and individuals showed how widespread is the concern for more help for children with problems of language and speech and this was cogently supported by observations from audiologists and speech therapists. It was suggested to us that as a child's over-riding need is the development of language it would be realistic to consider language disorder as the primary disability in deafness, and that the care of deaf children in the first five years should be the responsibility of a specially trained person, teacher of the deaf or speech therapist, with particular emphasis on family guidance. If this view commands wide support it should lead, as in the United States, to professional unity and shared training between speech therapists and teachers of the deaf.

Dietitians

18.68 In 1973 there were 424 dietitians in England and Wales. An unpublished survey by the British Paediatric Association in that year covering 11 hospital regions, including 4 in London, reached the following conclusions. Dietetic services are available in most hospitals and their help is valued. The proportion of dietitians with substantial training in the dietetics of childhood is very small, probably not more than 4%. Paradoxically the University Centres where the more complex nutritional and metabolic problems are concentrated are less well staffed than some districts. Since NHS reorganisation, District Dietitians have been appointed to extend the dietetic services in hospitals to the outside community and to coordinate any existing services. They are available to advise local authority social services departments, education authorities and other bodies on nutrition. There is only one consistent training centre for paediatric dietitians in England—at the Hospital for Sick Children, London. The lack of training facilities and of any financial incentive to obtain specialist qualifications in paediatric dietetics are the main deterrents to a necessary advance in the best interests of children and the profession. We understand that a society for paediatric dietitians has recently been formed and this is a welcome step.

Ophthalmic Opticians

18.69 This is an established profession with more than 5,000 members. They provided the Committee with a clear account of their training, the services they provide and their wish to contribute more fully to the visual care of school children. We are aware of the closer professional association between consultant ophthalmologists, ophthalmic medical practitioners and ophthalmic opticians which is taking place and hope that in the light of our general recommendations a comprehensive policy for the visual care of all children will be examined and appropriate recommendations made.

Orthoptists

18.70 Orthoptists work with ophthalmologists in the diagnosis and treatment of patients with defective binocular vision or abnormal eye movement. Under the general supervision of a doctor, they share in the treatment of squints and certain forms of double vision, and undertake clinical measurements which assist in the management of conditions requiring surgery. The greater part of their work is concerned with children. In 1974 there were 334 orthoptists (wte) employed in the NHS in England and Wales, most of whom were working in hospitals or in school clinics. Orthoptists provide a necessary service for children. The Committee of Inquiry into the pay and conditions for all the "professions supplementary to medicine" estimated that present needs justified a 20% increase in the total number of orthoptists. No figures for their regional distribution, and the areas of greatest need, were available to us.

Dental Auxiliaries

18.71 Our proposals for this group of therapists are given in Chapter 13.

Social Workers

18.72 The report of the Working Party on Social Work Support for the Health Services[9] has dealt comprehensively with the present situation, the problems arising from it and possible future developments. We are in general agreement with the conclusions of that working party as they affect supporting care. The integration of the social work services in hospitals with the local authority Social Services will call first of all for considerable rethinking as to what is, or should be the precise function of the hospital based social worker, what pattern of organisational structure best suits this work and how to effect this. We hope that local authorities will not interpret their responsibilities narrowly. Whilst there will be undoubtedly problems of accountability, communication and scarcity of resources, nevertheless the opportunity arises for additional strength and support to be given to improving the social and personal conditions of children in hospital. We have drawn attention to the failure of some hospitals to implement some of the recommendations of the Platt Report

---

[9] Department of Health and Social Security and Welsh Office (1974). Report of the Working Party on Social Work Support for the Health Service. HMSO, London.

relating to the setting in which children are cared for in hospital. We would hope that the Social Services department and the social workers in hospital would increasingly concern themselves with the wider social issues involved in caring for children in hospital, and that the experience gained in the field of residential child care would be drawn upon.

CHAPTER 19

THE TRANSITION TO THE NEW SERVICE

Primary Medical Care

19.1 We are concerned that the pattern of staffing we have proposed for primary child health services should become a reality as quickly as possible. When the amalgamation of the preventive and therapeutic services was first proposed in 1920, the Dawson Committee recognised that this would not happen overnight:

"The scheme of services we have outlined may on superficial reflection be deemed by some people to be so ambitious as to be impracticable. We are well aware that the realisation must be slow and, from the difficulty of adapting existing institutions and methods, may be imperfect. Apart from the lack of material equipment, trained personnel in adequate numbers is not at present available, though the acceptance and approval of this scheme by the profession and the public should give the educational stimulus to its production. To construct any part well, and to avoid mistakes in local effort, the whole design must be before the mind. This is an undertaking which can be at once begun and steadily proceeded with, and at a rate proportional to the enlightenment and determination of local public opinion—lay and medical".[1]

Forty six years later the Sheldon Committee, reviewing the functions and medical staffing of child welfare centres, was equally cautious about the likely rate of progress:

"The acceptance by family doctors of clinical responsibility for the Child Health Services at a national level must inevitably be a gradual process".[2]

We trust that our recommendations which we see as completing those of previous reports, will not suffer the same delay. We can no longer be content with the hope that some day preventive and therapeutic services for children will drift into the unity that pioneers were seeking and we believe that the recent developments in primary care make the necessary changes possible.

19.2 Moreover, reorganisation has introduced an element of urgency into the situation today which was not present even 10 years ago. The preventive child health services built up over a century by local health and education authorities, and maintained by AHAs since 1974 at a level which those who provide them are painfully aware is less than adequate, face increasing problems of medical recruitment. A decade of uncertainty about the future of the services, and a mounting feeling of frustration among clinical medical officers who after years of professional isolation still find themselves separated from their clinical colleagues by their attachment to administrative health departments, have taken their toll and staffing levels are dangerously low. *The preventive health services for children cannot be allowed to wither away*. It will be to the advantage

[1] Consultative Council on Medical and Allied Services: Interim Report on the Future Provision of Medical and Allied Services (Chairman: Lord Dawson of Penn) (1920). HMSO, London.

[2] Central Health Services Council, Report of a Sub-Committee of the Standing Medical Advisory Committee on Child Welfare Centres (Chairman: Sir Wilfrid Sheldon) (1967). HMSO, London.

of all concerned that they should become an integral part of the primary care services. If the present opportunity to achieve this is not taken the preventive child health services will need to be retained and strengthened.

19.3 The problem is how to keep the preventive services functioning satisfactorily while they are being incorporated within another service. GPP posts should be established as quickly as possible but this will take time. This means that during the transition the service will rely on the efforts and expertise of existing clinical medical officers and their numbers are declining. Their interests must therefore be protected and recruitment safeguarded. This will mean providing appropriate training and a proper career structure for an interim period of uncertain length. Yet to do so may delay the establishment of the new pattern of services by seeming to cling to the old.

19.4 How can this real dilemma be resolved? There are a number of steps which could be taken immediately to launch the GPP pattern of staffing and to sustain and improve the preventive services in ways which would facilitate a gradually widening adoption of the pattern.

Appointment of GPs to GPP Posts

19.5 During the initial phase there should be criteria for the accreditation as GPPs of GPs at present in practice which are based primarily on practical experience rather than formal instruction; this will avoid a situation in which the hoped for best becomes the enemy of the potentially satisfactory. Where GPs are interested in paediatrics and are willing to develop the GPP pattern in their own practices we recommend that they should be accredited without delay if:

   (i) they have had at least 3 years' experience as a principal in general practice;

   (ii) they have had at least 6 months' post-registration experience in paediatrics;

   (iii) they agree to undergo training (either in the form of short, intensive courses or appropriate part-time equivalents) in developmental and educational medicine and the care of handicapped children. Any previous experience in the school health service would be taken into account in determining the level of training required in individual cases.

These arrangements would be operative for 5 years and then would be reviewed. This would allow the training and professional bodies concerned to reach a decision on long-term conditions for accreditation and enable young doctors in vocational training to complete acceptable courses for becoming GPPs.

Appointment of Clinical Medical Officers to GPP Posts

19.6 Clinical medical officers wishing to enter general practice as GPPs should be regarded as eligible for immediate accreditation if:

   (i) they have had a total of 3 years' whole-time equivalent experience in the child health and school health services;

   (ii) they have had at least 6 months' post-registration experience in paediatrics;

(iii) they agree to undergo the whole-time equivalent of one year as a trainee in general practice, unless they can show that they have such experience already.

19.7 In addition to the above, *we recommend that clinical medical officers who wish to become GPPs should also attend short courses of training (on a full-time or part-time basis) in clinical paediatrics and preventive child health, unless they can show that they have had such training in the recent past.* This is necessary because of the general absence of required and appropriate training for appointment as a clinical medical officer to an AHA.

19.8 We see clinical medical officers as an important potential source of GPPs but they will need to obtain entry to general practice as a principal following accreditation. We realise this presents problems, but retrained staff from the AHAs could make a valuable contribution to group practice and there is no reason to think that they would not be very acceptable.

19.9 The present system of remuneration in general practice would probably provide adequate financial reward where these doctors become full-time principals and undertake child health work as GPPs. This may not be so where they make only a part-time contribution to the work of the practice. *We recommend the profession and the DHSS examine this point and negotiate suitable arrangements because we hope that in other respects it will prove possible for appropriately trained clinical medical officers to be accepted into group practices as part-time GPP partners.* This would be an important factor in launching and maintaining the GPP pattern of staffing. (80% of all clinical medical officers are at present employed on a sessional or part-time basis.)

19.10 The distribution of work between practitioners accepting a full-time commitment in general practice and those available only for part-time work would be a matter for agreement within each practice, though the SCM(CH) would need to be kept informed since it would have implications for providing health surveillance and educational health services in the neighbourhood. However, part-time GPPs like those in full-time partnership, would be expected to spend a substantial amount of time working in the preventive services. The details will need to be negotiated with the profession but it would not be in the interests of either the services for children or the doctors themselves if they were allowed to undertake commitments in primary care that are smaller than those prevailing elsewhere in the NHS. For this reason it would not be desirable for the minimum commitment of 20 hours per week required to qualify for the full basic practice allowance to be relaxed for part-time GPPs.

19.11 The overall medical manpower situation is unlikely to improve substantially until towards the end of the next decade and the best use has therefore to be made of existing personnel, especially of the increasing number of women medical graduates many of whom will for much of their lives be unable to devote themselves full-time to professional work. (Two-thirds of clinical medical officers are women.) Many such women will be well qualified by inclination and training to undertake the work of a GPP. For this reason *the remuneration structure should not be such as to discourage partnerships in group practices from including part-time GPPs.*

Clinical Medical Officers as Child Health Practitioners

19.12 We are convinced that in the long term a future for clinical medical officers in the child health services that is both professionally satisfying and compatible with the service children need, only exists for them either as members of primary health care teams or as part of the supporting consultant paediatric services. In the primary care field there will at first be relatively few general practitioners and clinical medical officers who would be eligible immediately for accreditation as GPPs and while we anticipate that more will accept immediate training for accreditation, there will be some GPs who will not want to undertake preventive work and some clinical medical officers who will not want to undertake curative work or to join a group practice. Thus, for some time to come many neighbourhoods will be without GPPs and the task of providing a service in health surveillance and educational medicine will be continued by clinical medical officers not wanting or not eligible to be GPPs. The rôle of the clinical medical officer in primary care should be recognised by a change of title to Child Health Practitioner. Their work will be exclusively concerned with the developmental and preventive aspects of child health. In their clinical preventive work including immediate treatment where necessary, they should be responsible for the children they see.

19.13 In view of the importance of the work it is essential that they should be trained for their rôle and it will be necessary therefore to provide opportunities for short, intensive training for these doctors. Training must be followed by acceptable career prospects and work that carries challenge and responsibility, and there must be a re-thinking of the ways in which the clinical preventive services are organised until such time as they are fully provided by GPPs.

Attachment of Child Health Practitioners to General Practice

19.14 Child health practitioners will need to work closely with GPs and CHVs and to have well established and definitive lines of communication with the primary care team. This will be of special importance when providing for the ongoing treatment of children, the referral of treatment to the supporting services and in the case of handicapped children. A satisfactory working relationship can only be achieved when a CHP is working in relation to a limited number of primary care teams who themselves do not yet have a GPP. The SCM(CH) should have the responsibility for arranging the attachment of CHPs in an area to individual practices (see paragraph 21.16).

19.15 *Child health practitioners would continue in the main to be employed by AHAs* but whereas at present they are attached to the staff of the AMO, *in future they would have an independent "personal" professional status within the primary care field.* They will need, however, a professional group with whom they can relate in their day to day work. This is distinct from a professional base from which to function, and here we see them working from group practice premises, health centres, clinics and schools. It is different also from the need to belong to a professional association appropriate for their discipline. It is akin to the sense of "belonging" to a hospital enjoyed by consultants or to a school by teachers. Since the work of child health practitioners is essentially primary care, even though it may be exclusively in child health, *we hope that each practitioner will become associated with one or two group practices. For some the form of association might be employment by a group practice as a part-time assistant.*

19.16 During the first few years of our pattern of services we would expect to see an increasing number of clinical medical officers join group practices as GPPs and a diminishing number remaining as child health practitioners. The rate at which this took place would be one measure of the success of our proposals, and a sensitive indicator of the willingness of child health practitioners to make the approach and of the readiness of general practice to respond. We believe the association between GPs and child health practitioners that we have advocated here will encourage new interests and a change in attitudes that would materially assist the change we wish to see. We appreciate that it will have consequences for the staffing of other services which AHAs provide, eg family planning.

Supporting Medical Care

19.17 Our proposals for the organisation of supporting consultant paediatric care for children include the creation of a consultant community paediatrician post in each district carrying major responsibilities for handicapped children and health services in schools. The need to fill these posts as quickly as possible is no less urgent than the need to fill the GPP posts. Eventually all consultant community paediatricians will have followed approved training programmes and will apply in the usual way for consultant posts as these are established or become vacant. It is with the interim period, during which consultant community paediatrics is being developed, that we are concerned here.

Appointment of Paediatricians to Consultant Posts in Community Paediatrics
19.18 Some consultant paediatricians already have the interest and experience with handicapped children and in educational medicine which would qualify them for consultant community paediatrician posts. We hope many of them will apply for these posts as they become established. They are needed not only to man the proposed service but to shape its future as the specialty develops. For research and training reasons priority should be given in the first place to making such appointments in Areas that contain university hospitals.

19.19 We believe also that there are senior registrars in paediatric training who already have the interest and some of the expertise and experience needed for consultancy in community paediatrics. *Adjustment of training and experience may be all that is required for them to become eligible for appointment as community paediatricians.* We hope too that registrar training will include this aspect of paediatrics so that, knowing there is a career ahead, more will pursue this when they become senior registrars.

Appointment of Senior Clinical Medical Officers to Consultant Posts in Community Paediatrics
19.20 On the basis of their training and experience in paediatrics, in the care of handicapped children, and in educational medicine, some senior clinical medical officers would also be eligible from the outset to become consultant

community paediatricians. In this starting phase, a balance must be struck between the unattainable (ie the possession by all candidates of MRCP and full paediatric hospital training in addition to special experience in the work) and the conferral of consultant status on terms that might be unacceptable to consultant colleagues in conventional circumstances. We hope that the lack of what would be usually regarded as the necessary academic qualification will not debar these doctors from applying for, and being appointed to, these new consultant posts during this interim period. There are precedents for this, for example in geriatrics. *The new service must get off the ground;* the level must of course be satisfactory but the proposed raising of standards will take time.

19.21 There may be some senior clinical medical officers who lack general paediatric training although having a wide practical experience of the care of handicapped children and of educational health services. *They should be given the opportunity to become eligible for appointment to consultant posts in community paediatrics following the successful completion of short, intensive courses in paediatrics.* There will also be some medical assistants highly skilled in acute paediatric care who will need corresponding training in the social and educational aspects.

Appointment of Senior Clinical Medical Officers as Clinical Specialists in Paediatrics

19.22 However only a minority of senior clinical medical officers are likely to be appointed quickly to these consultant posts, with or without further training in paediatrics. Many may be neither willing nor able to fulfil the training requirements for consultant work. Promotion for them in the clinical field has in the past not been available. Within the reorganised NHS they are acknowledged as clinicians but lack a suitable career grade. The only career grades in the NHS are those of principal in general practice and consultant in the hospital service, neither of which is appropriate for these "senior" clinicians in the health and preventive services. It would be even more inappropriate for them to remain indefinitely in a training grade, eg as senior registrars. The transfer of these doctors from local health authority services to the unified NHS has created a situation which was neither present nor allowed for when the staffing structure of the NHS was drawn up in 1946. Our proposals for the establishment of GPP posts in the primary care services and consultant community paediatric posts in the supporting services will eventually resolve this difficulty but that will take time.

19.23 It is clear therefore that *a need exists within the proposed integrated child health service for a specialist career grade in paediatrics, carrying responsibilities in both the community and the hospital that parallel those undertaken by consultants. We suggest that doctors in this category could appropriately be called Clinical Specialists in Paediatrics* and they would work, full-time or part-time, mainly in the community or mainly in hospital. This is an essential element in any realistic solution to the problem of staffing the supporting services during the interim years in a way that strengthens the services for children and satisfies the professional aspirations of the senior doctors concerned.

19.24 *The interim nature of the clinical specialist grade would be indicated by appointments being "personal" to selected doctors.* On their relinquishing the posts, the need to make further personal appointments should be carefully considered in the hope that a trained consultant would be available. The personal character of those appointments makes it clear that we are not seeking an established sub-consultant grade. *We suggest that appointments to this specialist grade should be made by a special appointment committee* which would include the SCM(CH), a clinical specialist in paediatrics and a consultant community paediatrician.

Nursing Care

19.25 *There will be a need for special inpost training courses in paediatric nursing for health visitors wishing to become CHVs.* Also during the early stages of the transition, *it will be necessary to ensure that the introduction of CHVs and NO/CHVs with a special responsibility for handicapped children, does not leave too thin a spread of health visiting services for other age groups,* especially the elderly to whom the services have a heavy commitment. Beyond this we see no serious difficulties in the implementation of our proposals for the CHV pattern of staffing for the child health services.

Progress Review

19.26 It would be naive to suppose that nationwide changes on the lines proposed could be accomplished quickly or could be imposed by central direction. We have no means of knowing in advance how many or how quickly GPPs could be appointed from among existing general practitioners and clinical medical officers, or consultant community paediatricians from among paediatricians and senior clinical medical officers. The rate of progress will inevitably vary from district to district. It is essential therefore that the introduction of the GPP, CHV and CCP scheme should be fully recorded and assessed.

19.27 *We recommend that AHAs should be formally asked to review the situation five years from the date of commencement* to discover whether any additional measures or incentives are needed to accelerate implementation of our proposals. This would be a matter in the first instance for the SCM(CH) and the AN(CH) to undertake.

CHAPTER 20

IMPLICATIONS FOR TRAINING

A New Emphasis

20.1 A good system is one in which all know what is required of them and feel they have been adequately trained for the work they are expected to do. Our proposals for a better service cannot be realised without an extension of training involving children, parents, and professionals alike. We have no intention of telling teachers how to teach but since we are asking for change we must justify the request. The reasons run through the report. They are of particular significance for children's services, but at the same time we recognise that they are relevant to the education and training of health service professionals over a much wider field. The changing pattern of ill-health and with it the importance for the future of finding ways to persuade people to change their behaviour mean that skills in communication must assume increased emphasis in professional training. In particular ways have to be found to communicate more successfully with those who at present make little use of services. Equally because many ill and handicapped children will require a multi-professional approach, so communication between professionals assumes a new importance. One way to foster this would be through common core training, and multi-professional in-service training schemes. We are aware that many professional groups already appreciate these points and are beginning to develop programmes which reflect the importance of communication; and we have noted particularly in this respect what has been said in "The Future General: Practitioner Learning and Teaching".[1] We welcome these developments and we hope that others will follow. We believe however that there is also a more fundamental need, for research aimed at establishing how best to communicate health advice in ways which make it easy to understand and to remember. It is against this background that we have put forward the concept of training which the new service requires and for which in this chapter we ask.

20.2 Our proposals for staffing the child health services require changes in the rôles of some doctors, nurses and social workers. They come at a time when the reports of the Committee on Nursing[2] and the Committee of Inquiry into the Regulation of the Medical Profession[3] are under consideration. We have kept in mind the wider changes in professional training foreseen in these reports. We see many advantages in the pattern of nurse training that has been recommended and assume it will be implemented. We accept the concepts of undergraduate, general professional and vocational stages in medical training and welcome the efforts of the Universities and the Royal Colleges to work out detailed arrangements. We have also taken into account the commitment that has been made to "harmonise" medical training within the member states of the European Community. *New programmes of training will clearly be needed in many fields, but the initial emphasis should be on supplementary training for those who are doing the work at present.*

[1] Royal College of General Practitioners (1972). The Future General Practitioner: Learning and Teaching. *Brit. Med. Jour.*

[2] Report of the Committee on Nursing (Chairman: Asa Briggs) (1972). Cmnd 5115. HMSO, London.

[3] Report of the Committee of Enquiry into the Regulation of the Medical Profession (Chairman: A Merrison) (1975). HMSO, London.

Primary Care

General Practitioners, GPPs and Child Health Practitioners

20.3 It is now accepted that all principals in general practice require a period of formal vocational training. The paediatric content has been examined by a working party of the RCGP and the BPA. Their recommendations, accepted by the Councils of both bodies, are so relevant to our immediate proposals and to our essential philosophy of child care that they are given in full in Appendix J. Their general implementation would fulfil our first training objective—an increase in the paediatric knowledge of all general practitioners. Here we quote the essence of their recommendations from the summary of their report:

"All vocational training schemes for general practice should include formal training in paedriatics.

This training should take place in junior hospital posts, in the community health services, and in teaching practices; either by whole-time courses or on day or half-day release.

Junior hospital training posts should last not less than four months. They should usually be in acute non-specialised paediatric units and should include experience in neo-natal paediatrics. While in hospital, trainees should have experience of general paediatric surgery and of those surgical specialties which are particularly relevant to general practice ie orthopaedics and ENT.

Developmental paediatrics and the early detection of handicap are essential subjects for general practitioners. Since they must be taught partly in teaching practices, these could with advantage run special sessions for screening well-babies and toddlers. Alternatively, a local arrangement will need to be made with a child health clinic.

Emotional disturbance in children needs to be considered at all stages of training. Child psychiatrists, who are too few in number, can spread their influence by teaching general practitioners to take increasing responsibility in this field. More academic departments of child psychiatry are needed to produce such teachers. It is important to teach about the impact of children's needs on practice organisation—especially the need for easy contact, quick appointments and satisfactory emergency coverage."[4]

20.4 This joint report also examined the knowledge of children's development and disorders in the social and the practice context and the attitudes and skills which general practitioners should possess at the completion of vocational training. The objectives are far-reaching and would require longer than the intended six months training followed by continuing education to achieve and maintain them. It also suggested a number of different ways in which the paediatric contribution to primary care could be made, and again we quote (our italics):

"We believe that there are bound to be some general practitioners who have a special interest in children and who will wish to increase their training and experience. We believe this is desirable. It might take the form of hospital attachment or more detailed work in developmental assessment or work in the school health service. We believe that some general practitioners will

---

[4] *J. Roy. Coll. Gen. Pract.* (1976). 26, 128–136.

be required and will wish to work in the school health service. This is likely to deal in the future with medical conditions limiting a child's ability to take advantage of normal education or requiring special education. (Illnesses and injuries presenting at school are likely to be dealt with through the ordinary practice arrangements.) In so far as this work is different from the paediatric work done by every general practitioner in his own practice setting, they will need special training. This must be provided by paediatricians, child psychiatrists, psychologists, general practitioners with appropriate training, or clinicians at present working in the community service."

General practitioners who accepted these wider responsibilities in relation to children and with the suggested additional training in developmental paediatrics and educational medicine would correspond to the General Practitioner Paediatricians we see developing within general practice. (In Chapter 17 we have recommended that the RCGP and BPA should be asked to advise more specifically on the training and experience required by the GPP.)

20.5 Within the four years following qualification it should be possible for the first generation of GPPs to spend 18 months to 2 years in the main areas of paediatrics described in the joint report, working in hospital, with the community services, and in appropriate general practices. It is suggested that eventually vocational training will be increased to 5 years in all and if experience supported the need, the paediatric component might increase to $2\frac{1}{2}$ or 3 years, an appropriate part of which would be in general practice.

20.6 Up to this point training proposals have applied to men and women proceeding by choice, from the pre-registration year or soon after, to vocational training. We are equally concerned with those already in general practice who have a special interest in children, some with previous, sometimes considerable, paediatric experience, generally acquired in hospital. The gaps in their knowledge are likely to be in child development and health surveillance and educational medicine, and it will be necessary to arrange short intensive courses or appropriate part-time equivalents in the experience they lack. With clear objectives and well planned courses experienced people can learn more rapidly than is commonly believed. We have already suggested (Chapter 19, paragraph 6) that clinical medical officers wishing to become GPPs would need to agree to undergo the whole-time equivalent of one year as a trainee in general practice, unless they can show that they have such experience. In addition they should attend short courses in clinical paediatrics and preventive child health.

20.7 Some clinical medical officers will prefer to contribute as *child health practitioners* to the developmental preventive and school health elements only of the child health services, though we hope they will do so increasingly in relation to general practice and within the framework of the primary child health care team (Chapter 19, paragraph 14). These doctors will need to attend concentrated or day-release courses in clinical paediatrics and preventive child health.

20.8 *The courses for GPs and clinical medical officers wishing to become GPPs should be integrated as far as possible and provided through general practice vocational training schemes.* Examinations as a sign of relevant training are a matter for training bodies to decide. Paediatrics already forms part of the examination for the MRCGP; it might be an advantage if there was in addition an optional paediatric section. In recent years, the Diploma in Child Health has become more relevant to the work of GPs and clinical medical officers; with further amendment it could become a useful diploma for doctors interested in the paediatrics of primary health care. The RCGP and BPA could usefully look at the place of both examinations in the training of GPPs and CHPs.

Child Health Visitors

20.9 The introduction of the comprehensive training programme described in the Report of the Committee on Nursing would be compatible with the preparation of nurses skilled in the care of children both in and out of hospital. The programme is based on:

an initial basic education in nursing (18 months) leading to a Statutory Certificate in Nursing Practice, common to all nurse training;

a post certificate 18 month course leading to Statutory Registration;

a 6 month course leading to the Higher Certificate in Nursing Practice which can be taken when preparing for, or after, registration; and a variety of post registration courses to extend training into specialist fields.

In what follows immediately and later in 20.23 *et seq* we have indicated training requirements in terms of this new pattern.

20.10 A close professional partnership between general practitioner and health visitor is the essence of the primary health care team. The GPP will increase the range and quality of paediatric medicine in general practice and the child health visitor will do the same for paediatric nursing. Her work is described in Chapter 17. If our proposals are accepted, within the overall scheme of training outlined above *the Child Health Visitor would be a registered nurse who has completed a suitably designed post-registration course leading to a Higher Certificate in Health Visiting. A prerequisite for entry to the Child Health Visiting Service would be some paediatric nurse training which would usually be obtained through modules in the training for basic certification and registration.* Admission to the course should be open to registered nurses with this type of experience. At present only those having the statutory Certificate in Health Visiting can be employed by health authorities as health visitors. Under the new proposals, health visitor training would no longer lead to a statutory qualification. To safeguard standards of practice an administrative *requirement should be imposed on authorities to employ in the* CHILD HEALTH VISITING SERVICE *only those accredited with post registration Health Visitor training or health visitors already qualified.*

20.11 The training in sick children's nursing required by health visitors already in post could be organised within the context of the new programme when that is implemented. *For the present, special courses in paediatric nursing for 4–6 weeks full-time, or the equivalent by day release, would need to be planned,* bearing in mind local training facilities and the previous experience of the health visitor. This would be much less than the training undergone by her hospital counterpart, the paediatric ward sister. Some health visitors are already Registered Sick Children's nurses and will require no more than an appropriate refresher course. With appropriate in-service training, the HV should feel adequate to fulfil her new responsibilities for treatment as well as for prevention within an integrated nursing service.

Child Health Nurses

20.12 Under the Briggs Committee proposals, the minimum qualification of CHNs would be that *they had obtained their Certificate in Nursing Practice, with experience in paediatric nursing, and had taken an option or an additional module in community nursing.*

School Nurses

20.13 The rôle, training and status of the school nurse are not uniformly defined, and consequently they vary between one Area Health Authority and another. We see the school nurse as essential to good primary care, working closely with the GPP in his rôle as school doctor and looking for professional guidance to the CHV from his practice. We have defined her work in Chapter 10. The Briggs Committee on Nursing did not give clear guidance for this important field of nursing and we offer our proposals for training. The previous experience of those attracted to school nursing will vary and training must be related to individual needs. *For Registered nurses with paediatric experience there should be a post registration certificate in "educational nursing".* We are not aware that such a course has been designed and tested. However, the Committee on Nursing favour "special courses" and, in view of the distinctive character of the work, one leading to a higher certificate in educational nursing should prove attractive. Registered nurses who have had little previous paediatric training would need additional experience with well and ill children as well as the course in educational nursing. *We ask the Council for the Training and Education of Health Visitors, (or any educational body who may carry this responsibility in future), in association with the appropriate Teacher Training Body to design such a course, indicating the arrangements for implementing it and the conditions of certification.*

20.14 School nurses working in special day or residential schools will have specific needs to meet and many will need additional experience of particular types of handicap. Arrangements for such training are the responsibility of the Area Health Authority and should be related to the individual nurses' needs.

20.15 We have been particularly concerned with the care of handicapped children living in the community. Normal primary care will be provided by the GP or GPP and the CHV, but every family with a handicapped child should have one experienced person to whom they can turn for guidance and support. One such person would be the NO/CHV in the district handicap team. The varied previous experience of persons undertaking this work again calls for individual training arrangements. The formal responsibility for this rests with the AHA, but much of it will be acquired through working with the consultant community paediatrician and as a member of the district handicap team. Experience could be further strengthened by attachment in appropriate ways to the Regional Child Development Centre. Such specialist consultant nurses should be encouraged to attend conferences on various aspects of handicap and should be encouraged to keep themselves informed in every possible way on new aspects of care.

340

Supporting Care

Consultant Paediatricians

20.16 We see consultant paediatricians working in four main fields: in the general medicine of childhood, mainly in hospital; in developmental, educational and social paediatrics, mainly in the community; providing intensive care for the newborn; and working wholly or mainly in one of the system specialties. The patterns of training are given in summary in the Second Report of the Joint Committee on Higher Medical Training (1975) and in detail in the Recommendations of its Specialist Advisory Committee on Paediatrics (1973). It is important in this context to note that *paediatrics is not represented, as we believe it should be, on the Central Council for Post Graduate Medical Education.*

20.17 The main service needs are: sufficient consultant paediatricians throughout the country to cope with the special care of the newborn and with children's illnesses; sufficient, properly distributed, paediatric specialists; and a steady increase in consultant community paediatricians. This might suggest a separation in training and that is the reverse of what we want to see. All are paediatricians and their training must provide that common body of knowledge and practice which is the basis of paediatrics. Changes are taking place in the training of the first two groups, and we are satisfied that these will strengthen the services they provide. Our main concern is with the third group, where needs are many and men and women trained to meet them few. We have described the work to be done in Chapter 18. Some aspects of their training can be found in the advice from the JCHMT, but no coherent programme has yet appeared. In one sense, as with all new advances, the pioneers must discover what needs to be done before what is necessary for training can be clearly defined. The needs however are so urgent that training routes must be opened up without delay. And they will not attract the right people or lead to the kind of consultant we need unless all paediatric education, including undergraduate education, includes experience of family and community paediatrics.

20.18 We are in no doubt that if the posts and the training were available a growing number of young paediatricians would enter this field. If the needs are to be met and training responsibilities accepted *University Departments of Child Health working with Departments of Social and Community Medicine, General Practice, Child Psychiatry, Education, and Social Work should initiate or expand post-graduate training programmes now.* And while these will apply immediately only to interested senior registrars, experience in this area of paediatrics should become a natural part of rotational training schemes for all registrars and senior house officers. The development of this new pattern of consultant paediatrics is the central challenge to academic paediatrics today. We are confident that with some increase in academic staff, by using the resources of Area and Region as well as of the University and by learning from those already working in this field, a start could be made now. *The initiative would best come from the Association of Clinical Professors and Heads of Paediatric Departments, and we ask them to estimate the increase in staff needed and pursue its implementation with the University Grants Committee.*

Allied Specialists

20.19 The medical care of children depends on a wide range of professional services. Paediatricians have their own job to do but they can only do it in cooperation with other specialists. We have noted in Chapter 18 the changes in attitude and practice which are taking place in relation to the paediatric aspects of the work of allied specialties. These indicate an increasing contribution by these specialties to the health of children which should be reflected in their training: we regard the implications for training as the concern of the appropriate colleges, faculties and associations.

Clinical Specialists in Paediatrics

20.20 The traditional concept of supporting medical services is that they should be staffed by consultants and by doctors preparing to be consultants. The increasing unreality of this situation is evident from our critical dependence in the lower training grades in this country on doctors from overseas, and the inescapable demand for a comparability of training and status for doctors acceptable to our European colleagues. These issues have been recently reviewed.[5] Their full consideration is a matter for the profession as a whole; they go beyond the limits of our brief, which is to consider the health services for children. It would be improper to derive a general answer to them from a particular need. Nevertheless, they are issues which are particularly significant for paediatrics because of the need for consultant paediatric care in the community, the range of such care, the limitation imposed on the necessary increased manpower by present and projected financial constraints, and the time it will take to develop new training programmes for consultant community paediatricians. Yet the needs of families and schools which justify these training programmes for additional consultant paediatricians are everywhere and urgently present. This means that the fullest use has to be made of the skills and experience of the present senior clinical medical officers. Some could assume consultant responsibilities now and others could do so with appropriate training. Some, however, (and possibly most of them) may prefer to practise as clinical specialists in paediatrics (see Chapter 19) and we think it likely that such clinical specialists will be a necessary feature of the paediatric services for some time to come. Many of them will require further in-service training, and this needs to be developed in a systematic way and linked with the training of consultant paediatricians.

20.21 The nature of this specialist training has a bearing on the wider issues of professional reciprocity with Europe. The Specialist Advisory Committee in Paediatrics of the JCHMT has for some time been wrestling with these compelling yet conflicting demands. They have suggested a pattern of training which could prove acceptable, here and in Europe, as the basis of "specialist status", and, if it is introduced, of "specialist registration". It would not meet present requirements for "specialist accreditation" and therefore a consultant appointment. We have been informed of their approach and we hope what follows is a fair summary.

A certificate of "specialist status" would be granted to registered medical practitioners who have had at least four years training in paediatrics on the satisfactory completion of a programme built up from the following areas of experience:

---

(5) *Brit. Med. Jour.* (1976). 1, 546.

a resident post of at least 6 months duration in a children's hospital or the children's department of a general hospital.

a further year of general paediatrics, including residence in a neonatal unit and experience in the child development and handicap services.

a final period of two and a half years involving experience of two or more of the following: general paediatrics; handicapped, including mentally handicapped, children; child and adolescent psychiatry; educational medicine; general practice; one of the paediatric system specialties.

20.22 This illustrates how a general paediatric training could be acquired in four years, the period favoured by most of the member states of the European community. The right combination of common and chosen experience could produce a "clinical specialist in paediatrics" capable of working alongside the consultant both inside and outside the hospital, and a substantial part of the training of both could be taken together. A flexible training programme of this kind has wider possibilities: 2 years training with the right components could equip a man or woman to be a GPP and 4 years to be a clinical specialist in paediatrics; 4 years, plus further prescribed training, could lead to specialist accreditation and eligibility for a consultant appointment. This seems to offer a rational framework for GPP, as well as specialist and consultant training and *we hope the Specialist Advisory Committee in Paediatrics of the JCHMT will examine this with the RCGP in the expectation that a way forward can be found.*

Paediatric Nurses

20.23 We are encouraged by the evident awareness of the Committee on Nursing of children's nursing needs and its clear expression in their Report (Paragraph 283):

"One special field which we regard as particularly important is paediatric nursing. Such nursing calls for special skill and we have been impressed by the evidence presented to us which suggests that some young people enter the profession with a particular motivation towards this kind of nursing."

The Committee's approach to training would advance our proposals in a more straightforward way than the existing system. (The present arrangements are considered in Appendix K.)

20.24 Convinced of the central importance of clinical experience in basic nurse training, we are glad to know that a major part of that experience, both for the Certificate and the Register, can be with ill and handicapped children in hospital and in the community. With the flexibility which a modular system provides, the Certificate, with this substantial paediatric component, could take the place of the present paediatric SEN course; and similarly preparation for the Register and Higher Certificate provide the equivalent of SRN/RSCN status. Post registration courses could lead to diplomas in special aspects of paediatrics, including the new-born.

20.25 In this new pattern of nurse training senior clinical nurses, the paediatric ward sisters, would have the Higher Certificate in Paediatric Nursing, and this would be obtained in a large children's department or hospital. In addition to post-registration diplomas eg in neo-natal or other specialist fields of children's nursing, it would be valuable for some to have training in clinical teaching. The paediatric ward sister is the natural clinical teacher of junior nursing and medical staff and a course of this kind would increase her ability and her confidence. This would supplement the work of the clinical nursing instructor. There is also need for a consultant paediatric nursing service based in hospital to be available to the child health visitor in the home. *The nurses providing this who would hold a Higher Certificate in Paediatric Nursing might usefully obtain in addition the Higher Certificate in Health Visiting.*

Specialists in Community Medicine (Child Health)

20.26 With their expertise in epidemiology, assessment of the health needs of populations and the planning and evaluation of health services, members of this new professional group can make a vital contribution to the integration and improvement of health services for children. We describe their functions and responsibilities as we see them in Chapter 21. The question of appropriate training for their exacting job is the responsibility of the Faculty of Community Medicine, but we believe this will need to include experience in clinical paediatrics, child development and educational medicine and probably some experience in general practice and child psychiatry. As senior registrars their research project for Part II of the MFCM will naturally be in the field of child health. *We recommend that the contribution of paediatrics to their training should be the subject of joint consultation between the Faculty of Community Medicine, the Royal College of General Practitioners and the British Paediatric Association.*

Area Nurses (Child Health)

20.27 These senior nurses will need a training and experience which will fit them for the important planning and coordinating rôle they have to fill. In present terms they should be RSCN and HV. When the new pattern is operating they will need Higher Certificates in Paediatric Nursing and in Health Visiting.

University Departments of Paediatrics

20.28 The training requirements of our proposals make it essential to take into account the present strength of University Departments of Paediatrics and related academic departments. The success or failure of our proposals will depend on their combined ability to provide and coordinate a range of graduate training programmes for a variety of professional groups. A precise estimate of the paediatric manpower needs has not been attempted. In 1970 there were 40 whole-time clinical paediatric teachers in England and Wales holding consultant contracts in the NHS, and an additional 45 were considered necessary[6] to cope with the increase in undergraduate numbers and graduate teaching. The demands for graduate teaching have risen steeply in the past five years. With the added training requirements of this report an establishment of not less than 100 full-time paediatric academic staff will be needed. Their national distribution will depend on present levels. *The position should be examined now by the Association of Clinical Professors and Heads of Paediatric Departments, the SAC in Paediatrics of the JCHMT and the University Grants Committee so that during*

(6) *Paediatrics in the Seventies* (1972). Ed Court, S D M, and Jackson, A D M. OUP for Nuffield Provincial Hospitals Trust.

the present period of severe restrictions a policy can be worked out for the time
when improvement is possible.

Women Doctors in Paediatrics

20.29 Paediatrics is a discipline to which women are naturally attracted, and to which they have much to give. Their contribution, however, is hindered by present training and career structures which affect all women doctors and which we consider in Appendix L. As in other branches of medicine some women will complete their higher medical training before marriage and family, but many will not. Some will become consultants in one stage, others in two, and if the suggested four-year training programme is established the second group could remain for a time at the "clinical specialist" stage. There are some who do not seek consultant responsibility and they do invaluable work in general practice, in the child and school health services, in children's departments in district hospitals and in accident and emergency departments in children's hospitals. In the common situation where the consultant paediatrician has to provide services at several hospitals they contribute a valuable stability to the main department, or, in the associated hospitals, they provide consistent support to isolated and often inexperienced junior staff. *We see realistic part-time training schemes for women doctors in paediatrics as the most urgent question facing the SAC in Paediatrics of the JCHMT and the RCGP. We suggest that they should examine this question jointly with the Women's Medical Federation and with the DHSS so that posts and training for women in paediatrics can be developed sensibly together.* While we appreciate that such a review would have to be carried out within the broader context of opportunities for women in medicine as a whole, the proposals we have made for increasing medical manpower in paediatrics make it particularly necessary to make full use of this important source.

Social Work Training

20.30 The unification of the Local Authority Social Services in 1971 was followed by the integration of formerly separate training councils. The Central Council for Education and Training in Social Work (CCETSW) is now responsible for all forms of social work training, and the basic qualification for all social workers is the Certificate of Qualification in Social Work (CQSW). Although the training courses leading to this qualification vary in duration and type of student they are all generic in character. They aim to fit students to work in departments dealing with a multiplicity of social problems with increasing community involvement and the range of subjects and skills which must be covered in the basic training inevitably limits the time which can be given to studying any one aspect in depth. However, specialisation is necessary in any profession if the quality of work is to improve and knowledge to be advanced.

20.31 This need was recognised in 1968 in the Seebohm Report[7] and the CCETSW is encouraging the growth of post qualifying courses in specialist fields. It is hoped that these courses will be arranged both nationally and

---

(7) Report of the Committee on Local Authority and Allied Personal Social Services (Chairman: Baron Seebohm) (1968). Cmnd 3703. HMSO, London.

regionally, and at both further and advanced levels of study. We have noted too that the Working Party on Social Work Support for the Health Services referred to the need for social workers to have not only a broad knowledge of a range of related social problems but thereafter to have opportunities for developing specialised knowledge and skills in different branches of social work. *We consider that specialisation within social work is essential if children and families are to receive the skilled services they need.* We consider that social workers who are concerned with sick children and their families should initially be familiar with the range of work associated with "child care" and not less skilled in this work than the former child care officers. From this base they would develop further expert knowledge in the needs of different groups of children and families or in the requirements of different settings. We have for example recommended the development of post qualification training in the field of child handicap. We welcome the news that CCETSW has set up a group to study the question of direct work with children at both basic and advanced levels and look forward with interest and concern to their findings.

20.32 Specialisation is of particular importance in work with children and their families. Social workers need opportunities to observe and be with children and to learn how to relate and communicate with them. The acquisition of such skills depends largely on good supervision of direct practice in the field from someone experienced in the work. We have already mentioned our fear that the expertise at present available may diminish because of the system of rewarding experience by promotion to administrative positions within the social work profession. We emphasise here the importance for future social work practice with children of a sufficient number of experienced and skilled practitioners to train newcomers in children's work, to supervise the work and further education of those already in practice, and to develop research from a practice base. The involvement of such senior social workers in teaching on social work training courses about the needs of children from the basis of their own experience would further improve the quality of training available for social work trainees. A strengthened tie of this kind between field and training course would help to ensure that those aspects of the law most relevant to work with children and families was part of the knowledge of all social workers.

CHAPTER 21

ADMINISTRATION

21.1 In this chapter we look at certain aspects of the reorganisation and administration of the NHS as they affect health services for children. The background to reorganisation and an outline of the new administrative structure of the NHS are contained in Appendix M.

Collaboration between Health and Local Authorities

21.2 The need for the closest collaboration between health and local authorities in the provision of services for children has been a recurring theme throughout our report. Personal social services, education, housing and the environmental services are, in some respects, as important for the health of children as the health services themselves. However, the concurrent reorganisation of both the NHS and Local Government has set up a number of administrative hurdles in the way of progress towards full coordination of all services for children. Whereas previously boundaries were blurred, now health services for children lie within the administrative framework of the NHS and outside Local Government; and the local authority services mentioned above lie outside the NHS and within the orbit of the separate administrative structure of Local Government. To compound the problem, outside the metropolitan areas, social and education services are county responsibilities whereas housing and environmental services are district responsibilities and local government districts and health authority districts are by no means always coterminous. Local authority educational and social services are organised at County level. This is also true for the planning of health services, and the boundaries of the Counties and the Area Health Authorities are coterminous. But health services are actually delivered at district level, and this is where cooperation between health personnel and social and educational professionals is mostly needed. Social services are also delivered locally at "area" level but social services areas and health districts are also not coterminous. And whereas NHS planning is developing along the lines of client groups (and our concern in this report is with children as a client group), the creation of Social Services Departments has meant the breaking down of the traditional barriers between social workers in Children's Departments, Welfare Departments and Mental Health, the development of the concept of the generic social worker and the view that clients can best be helped by recognising the needs they have in common with the rest of humanity rather than by categorising them into client groups.

21.3 The issues are complex, and they have been discussed in the three Reports of the Working Party on Collaboration Between Health and Local Authorities. Their recommendation for the setting up of Joint Consultative Committees at County and Area level has been implemented but the Working Party were unable to formulate a clear and neat pattern of collaboration at district level because of this lack of correspondence between management functions and responsibilities, except in the single district health areas. The coordination of all three services is therefore dependent upon the activities of the Joint Consultative Committees, Joint Care Planning Teams at Area level

347

and District Planning Teams at district level, and the senior medical, nursing and dental administrative officers of AHAs.

Joint Consultative Committees

21.4 Section 10 of the NHS Reorganisation Act requires the establishment of Joint Consultative Committees for ensuring collaboration between each Area Health Authority and the County and District Councils whose areas match or fall within the AHA boundaries. Decisions about membership of the committees have been left to the AHAs on the one side and the associated local government authorities on the other, and the Committees themselves, when established, have been free to explore the ways in which they will work together and to devise the arrangements and procedures most suitable to their local circumstances. The purpose of the JCC is first to advise the two sets of constituent authorities on the performance of their statutory duties to cooperate (for example in the fields of school health, the provision of social work support for primary care teams and hospitals, and the provision of health services for children in care). Second it is to further the collaborative planning and operation of services of common concern. For example health, education and social services have each developed within their own organisations systems for diagnosing the problems and assessing and meeting the needs of children and their families and, to a greater or lesser degree, they need and receive help from each other to achieve their objectives. While the focus of concern of the three services is different and is reflected in the facilities they provide, there is considerable overlap in what they are trying to do and collaborative planning is necessary.

21.5 *We see Joint Consultative Committees as an important forum from which to encourage local authority members to promote the recommendations in our report for better cooperation in child health.* In Chapter 16 we have recommended that Joint Consultative Committees should consider how best to ensure that the particular needs of children receive due priority and attention. In this context, *they may wish to appoint a subcommittee of members of health and local authorities to advise on the development of services for children,* including children who are mentally or physically handicapped.

Joint Planning Teams

21.6 Both the NHS planning system introduced in England in April 1976 and the DHSS Consultative Circular "Joint Care Planning: Health and Local Authorities"[1] recognise that AHAs are responsible for defining area strategies covering a 10–15 year period in collaboration with local authorities for services of common concern. To assist in these planning tasks the Circular recommends the establishment of a Joint Care Planning Team (JCPT) at Area level to develop strategic proposals, and of District Planning Teams (DPT) in Health Districts to advise on the operational planning of services carrying the highest priority. The AHA and matching Local Authority will receive proposals on the strategy for services requiring a joint health/LA approach from the Joint Care Planning Team, acting under the general direction of the JCC. Officers of the AHA and Local Authority will carry their knowledge of their respective authorities' policies into their work as members of the JCPT. If either authority does not agree with particular recommendations from the JCPT, these matters will be referred back to the JCC for further consideration.

---

[1] HC(76)18.

21.7 The concept of planning teams for client groups is an important one. It is however for AHAs to decide, in consultation with the JCC, where the need for DPTs is most urgent and could be most beneficial. We therefore welcome the statement in HC(76)18 that in England Departmental planning will concentrate on services for children in 1976/77, for *we hope that in the light of this, and of our recommendations, high priority will be given to the establishment of District Planning Teams for Children's Services. Their remit should include services for mentally ill children, and those who are mentally or physically handicapped.*

21.8 In Wales, where the NHS planning system was introduced in April 1975, strategic and operational planning are both primarily an area responsibility, with input from districts. Health care planning teams for priority client groups, including children, are already operating—mainly at area level but with district participation. Membership includes social work officers and other local authority officers as appropriate from time to time; health advice is reciprocally available to personal social service departments. As in England, Joint Consultative Committees are responsible for overall collaboration between health and local authorities and they are supported by joint teams of senior officers. A variety of patterns of collaboration has emerged. The Welsh Office is currently reviewing with health and local authorities the effectiveness of existing arrangements and the possible need for modification.

21.9 The composition of Joint Care Planning and District Planning Teams will no doubt vary according to local circumstances, but *when services for children are under consideration the composition should reflect the need to see their provision and operation as a joint exercise involving health, education and social services at every level.*

The Specialty of Community Medicine

21.10 The new specialty of community medicine is described in detail in the Hunter Report([2]) and its rôle in the reorganised health service is spelled out in "Management Arrangements for the Reorganised NHS"([3]) and the Welsh Office's "Management Arrangements for the Reorganised Health Service in Wales".([4]) Despite these publications many clinicians are still uncertain about the functions of community medicine and the responsibilities of community physicians. We therefore provide a summary of this before discussing in more detail the rôle of the Specialist in Community Medicine (Child Health).

21.11 The specialty of community medicine is concerned with the health of populations rather than with the clinical care of individual patients. It comprises measuring the level and distribution of mortality and morbidity in communities, determining the needs for preventive and health care services in those communities, evaluating and monitoring existing services, and health service planning.

([2]) Department of Health and Social Security (1972). Report of the Working Party on Medical Administrators. HMSO, London.

([3]) Department of Health and Social Security (1972). Management Arrangements for the Reorganised Health Service. HMSO, London.

([4]) Welsh Office (1972). Management Arrangements for the Reorganised Health Service in Wales. HMSO, Cardiff.

Community physicians are full-time medical officers of regional and area health authorities. Those based at the headquarters of these authorities are called specialists in community medicine. Most of those in post were previously either medical officers of health, their deputies or senior medical officers with local authorities, or were administrative medical officers with regional hospital boards. Each area health authority is served by an Area Medical Officer (AMO) who is a member of the Area Team of Officers (ATO), and a variable number of other community physicians, one of whom is the Specialist in Community Medicine (Child Health) (SCM (CH)). Each health district, other than those in single district areas has a District Community Physician (DCP), who is a member of the District Management Team (DMT). Community physicians working in the National Health Service have four main functions: to provide epidemiological advice on the health of the population served by their authorities, ascertain the effectiveness of existing health services and identify priorities and alternative ways of delivering health care; to serve as members of regional, area and district multidisciplinary teams where they make their specialist contribution to the formulation of health-care plans, the development of information systems and the monitoring of health and the effectiveness of services; to coordinate preventive measures such as family planning, vaccination, immunisation, screening and health education; and to provide medical advice and services to matching local authorities in the fields of child health (including school health), the personal social services and environmental health and housing.

Specialists in Community Medicine (Child Health)

21.12 Specialists in Community Medicine (Child Health) are community physicians with special knowledge of the epidemiology of child health and of the health and related services for children. Their responsibilities have been fully set out in DHSS Circular HRC(74)5, where they are described under three headings. First, they have NHS responsibilities for the planning and organisation of integrated child health services in the community and in hospitals. These responsibilities are undertaken in conjunction with DCPs and with general practitioners and consultants. They include developing preventive services for children, arranging resources for the medical inspection and treatment of school children and supervising the organisation of the work of clinical medical officers (this latter function may by agreement be delegated to a DCP in multi-district health areas). For all these NHS responsibilities the SCM(CH) is accountable through the AMO to the AHA.

21.13 Second, they have responsibilities in relation to certain functions LEAs have for which they require medical advice and/or action. These responsibilities are both advisory and executive. They have to provide health advice to LEAs; and they have executive responsibility for ensuring that medical and other health staff are available to advise head teachers about pupils' health and to assist the LEA in carrying out their duties under Section 34 of the 1944 Education Act (concerning the ascertainment of handicapped pupils); they are also responsible for the health of teachers in school and environmental hygiene and safety in maintained schools and colleges. For these responsibilities the SCM(CH) is directly accountable to the LEA.

21.14 Third, they have a general responsibility for assisting Joint Consultative Committees in carrying out their functions in relation to child health and education services.

21.15 In Wales the Specialists in Community Medicine (Child Health) also carry responsibility for the Special Needs Group (the mentally ill, mentally handicapped and physically handicapped adults, and old people). This is in contrast to England where a Specialist in Community Medicine (Social Services) has this responsibility.

21.16 The great majority of the Specialists in Community Medicine (Child Health) now in post have a wide experience of child health. After paediatric hospital training posts and perhaps some experience in general practice most of them worked for a number of years as clinicians in the Local Authority Child and School Health Services, acquiring the Diploma in Public Health and special-ised knowledge from courses in audiology, child development and the ascertain-ment of handicap. This experience is now their strength. In the future, they will for the most part be recruited from the ranks of community medicine and their expertise will lie in the fields of epidemiology and the planning and monitoring of child health services; the consultant community paediatrician will provide the clinical expertise and advice for LEAs in relation to individual children, eg handicapped pupils who may need special education. However, in our view (see Chapter 20, paragraph 26) *doctors in training to become SCM(CH)s will still need experience in clinical paediatrics, developmental paediatrics and educational medicine and probably some experience in general practice and child psychiatry.* For whilst we do not see the SCM(CH) in future supervising the organisation of the work of GPPs and CHPs in the same way as they do that of clinical medical officers at present—we have previously recommended CHPs should acquire an independent status (Chapter 19, paragraphs 12–16)—he will need to advise them and coordinate their appointments if he is to play his part in ensuring that the health services to which all children are entitled are available. To do this satisfactorily *the SCM(CH)s will also need more administrative support than they are now getting.*

21.17 There is one aspect of the SCM(CH)'s work which is not given the recognition we consider it merits: this is the opportunity it provides to speak for the community as well as the hospital aspects of child health at a high level in the counsels of the AHA where there is always competition for limited resources. The preventive child health services are an essential but unobtrusive need, easily over-shadowed by the extensive demand for adult hospital services. And in this respect we wish to draw attention to the SCM(CH)'s special relationship with the LEA. He has not only advisory but also executive responsibilities for the health services the Authority may require. Moreover, he is in the unique position of being directly accountable to the LEA for these services although he is not a member of the Area Team of Officers (ATO). *It is imperative that the SCM(CH) should be entitled to direct access to the ATO on all matters relating to child health services* (as the Area Dental Officer is for dental services).

21.18 It also seems to us to be anomalous that LASSD's do not routinely have the benefit of the expertise of the SCM(CH) in respect of children for whom they

351

provide day and residential services. At present liaison between health authorities and social service departments on all matters affecting children and adults alike, handicapped or not, is the responsibility in England of the SCM (Social Services). *We recommend that in England the SCM(CH) should be responsible for liaison with social service departments of local authorities in all matters relating to the health of children. In Wales we consider that the responsibilities of the SCM (Child Health and Special Needs Groups) are too heavy and should similarly be divided between an SCM(CH) and an SCM (Adult Social Services).*

Medical Advisory Machinery

21.19 The administrative structure of the reorganised NHS recognises that in order to formulate and implement necessary and acceptable health care policies there must be a partnership and interaction between four elements: the health authorities themselves; their full-time officers (including of course medical, nursing, dental and other professionals); members of the health professions who are providing the clinical services; and the consumers. (We give a simplified account of the complex administrative machinery that has been devised to meet that demand in Appendix M.) At the present critical stage in the development of child health services, the need for coordination, integration and mutual understanding between the four groups or bodies mentioned above is paramount. We consider in some detail elsewhere in this chapter the rôles of Specialists in Community Medicine, Joint Planning Teams, Joint Consultative Committees and Community Health Councils. Here we consider whether the professional advisory machinery at local level needs to be modified to effect a more satisfactory coordination of services for children inside and outside hospital, and in particular whether any new advisory bodies need to be set up specifically for that purpose.

21.20 The need for such consideration arises from our concern that whilst there is provision(5) for specialist paediatric subcommittees to provide advice directly to regional health authorities no machinery exists for paediatric advice to be made available directly to area authorities. We recognise two important constraints. The effectiveness of an advisory committee, however ingeniously contrived, depends on the expertise, dedication and enthusiasm of its component members and any proposal to set up a new body must balance possible benefits against the certain disadvantage of increasing the already excessive erosion of the clinical time of the professionals on it by giving them further advisory and administrative commitments. (It is worth recalling here that this erosion of clinical time by management responsibilities has been brought about, at least in part, through political pressures applied by the professions themselves.) The second constraint is that the new health service districts and Areas are extremely diverse in size, structure and function. Thus an area may contain one district or several, and one district may be served by a single consultant paediatrician or by the staff of a children's hospital. Consequently, different districts are evolving different advisory structures for their child health services. Experience to date does not suggest that any one pattern is substantially more effective than the others.

---

(5) Department of Health and Social Security Circular HRC(74)9, Local Advisory Committees.

21.21 In single-district Areas the Cogwheel division provides a channel for paediatric advice to the authority (see below). *In multi-district Areas we recommend that the SCM(CH) should establish a small paediatric advisory group, with representation from the constituent districts and, in teaching areas, from the Academic Department of Child Health.* The membership of this group might be solely medical, with members of other disciplines coopted from time to time as appropriate but in the early period it would be wise not to extend membership too widely in an attempt to further the aim of integrating the approach to health needs. However, this is something which may vary from one area to another. Where such groups have been established, experience suggests that monthly meetings are justified and that valuable advice can be made available to the SCM(CH) and through him to the ATO on matters such as, for example, the inter-relation of district plans for paediatric services.

21.22 We have considered the question whether a separate division of child health within the Cogwheel structure is either desirable or universally applicable. Taking the district general hospitals as the basic unit, the three "Cogwheel" reports[6] have developed the concept of grouping together related hospital specialties into "divisions" with a small Medical Executive Committee composed of representatives of the divisions. This arrangement is designed to provide a representative system through which hospital medical staff can coordinate their work and make a more effective contribution to the management of medical care in their hospitals. The Cogwheel system has purposely been kept fluid. By 1972 of the 281 large general groups of hospitals 114 had implemented the Cogwheel proposals and a great variety of divisional arrangements had developed. The main divisions that have been formed include the medical specialties, the surgical specialties, pathology (the laboratory services), anaesthetics, obstetrics and gynaecology, radiology and psychiatry, but there are many more. The allocation of specialties to particular divisions is variable and derives in part from specific developments in particular hospitals and in part from the enthusiasms and beliefs of the specialists themselves. Child health appears most frequently in the division of medicine, but in about one quarter of cases it is in the division of obstetrics and gynaecology and in the remaining quarter in a division of its own. The third Cogwheel report recommended that membership of divisions should be enlarged to include consultants and other permanent medical staff, non-medical scientists of equivalent standing, senior registrars, representatives of junior medical staff and representatives from other divisions as necessary. The appropriate administrator, nursing officers and specialists in community medicine, and a spokesman for general practitioners should also have a standing invitation to attend and participate. The over-riding need for coordination of hospital and community services for child health was recognised but the recommendation was that the Cogwheel system should be left free to concentrate on organising the work of the doctors who man the hospital services for children.

21.23 In relation to the question of a separate division of child health we can begin by stating firmly that in two situations there can be no doubt about the need for this. One of these is where there is a separate children's hospital or a

---

[6] Department of Health and Social Security (1967, 1972, 1974). Reports of the Joint Working Party on the Organisation of Medical Work in Hospitals. HMSO, London.

large paediatric service in a district general hospital; the other is when the Area Health Authority includes only a single health district. In the remaining situations, because of the importance of achieving professional collaboration between hospital-based and community-based staff and of inculcating in both a sense of working within a single child health service, *we endorse in principle and wish to encourage the trend towards the establishment of Divisions of Child Health within the Cogwheel system*, but we recognise that, for the present, decisions about this will be determined one way or the other by local circumstances. Where such divisions are established, it is impracticable, except in small districts, to extend membership to all the professionals who might have claims to it (eg every GPP, every CHV and every social worker concerned with children). Nevertheless, as well as senior and junior doctors from the hospital paediatric department and the SCM(CH), *we recommend that membership should include representatives of other disciplines involved in the health care of children* (CHPs not attached to group practices, senior nursing officers, appropriate medical administrators, DCPs, social workers in the community as well as hospital social workers). Also, the Local Medical Committee should nominate a GPP, or where there are none in post, representatives of CHPs attached to group practice and of GPs.

21.24 We have also examined the question of the professional identity of medical staff in the child health services and consider the CHPs should be regarded as belonging to the primary health care services. *We recommend, therefore, that CHPs who are attached to group practices should be represented on the Local Medical Committee.* We understand that they would be eligible for associate membership of the Royal College of General Practitioners and hope they will avail themselves of the facilities and opportunities this offers.

Nursing Services

21.25 The Salmon and Mayston Reports both recommended a hierarchical structure for the nursing services. Their recommendations were accepted and have been built into the framework of the reorganised NHS.

Area Level

21.26 At area level, an Area Nurse (Child Health) AN(CH) is responsible to the Area Nursing Officer (ANO) for all aspects of the nursing services for children throughout the area. Unlike the SCM(CH), she does not have a direct responsibility to the local education authority for providing the nursing services it may require. We think she should, and accordingly *we recommend that the ANO's responsibility for providing comprehensive nursing services and advice to local education authorities should be delegated to the Area Nurse (Child Health).*

21.27 *We also consider that, like the SCM(CH), the AN(CH) should be entitled to direct access to the Area Team of Officers on all matters relating to nursing aspects of the child health services.* (We have referred in Chapter 20 to the training she will need to equip her for this rôle.)

21.28 Among her supporting staff at Area level the ANO may also have an Area Nurse responsible for liaison with the local authority social services department. We recommend that, in line with our recommendations relating to the SCM(CH) and the SCM(SS), *the AN(CH) should have delegated to her responsibility for liaison with the social services department of the local authority in nursing matters where social services for children are concerned.*

District Level

21.29 The District Nursing Officer (DNO) is a member of the District Management Team, alongside the District Community Physician, Administrator, Treasurer and two medical members from the District Medical Committee. She has reporting to her a number of divisional nursing officers, who have administrative responsibility for particular clinical areas of work and are supported by Senior Nursing Officers. Within the primary care division there is usually a Senior Nursing Officer responsible for coordinating health visiting and home nursing services. She works through Nursing Officers who have a rôle which is that of clinical consultant combined with day to day management responsibility for a group of staff, either HVs or district nursing sisters. With the concept of health visitors having responsibility either as CHVs for children and their families or as HVs for the rest of the practice population, *we recommend that Nursing Officers should similarly have responsibility for services for children and families or for others.* In addition to their responsibilities to their own group of nurses, *we recommend that the Nursing Officers should have a further responsibility for providing a link with hospital and social services and for advice up the line for a specific feature of nursing services* (eg for handicapped children, schools, or children in day and residential care of social service departments). This responsibility should extend to advising and supporting health visitors and where necessary families. The Nursing Officer with a responsibility for handicapped children (see Chapter 14, paragraph 28) would be a member of the district handicap team.

21.30 In the hospital services, SENIOR NURSING OFFICERS may cover a number of units and, with the relatively rare exceptions of the children's hospitals, seldom find themselves solely responsible for children. *We recommend however that there should always be a senior nurse (of at least grade 8 of the Salmon scale) responsible for ensuring that children's needs are met and understood wherever there are children under hospital care,* including inpatients (long-stay and short-stay), outpatients and day patients and that, even if this senior nurse has additional responsibilities not related to children, *she should be a registered sick children's nurse.*

21.31 We have considered whether it would be desirable to recommend the establishment of a division of children's nursing, covering both primary and specialist services. We think, however, that there are arguments against such a course because it would divide responsibility for primary care nursing when the primary care team is still at an evolutionary stage, and also because child health visitors would have responsibilities towards families and not just to children. It is important, however, that there should be a nurse at district level with a responsibility for seeing that the special needs of sick children are met throughout the district, and *we recommend that the senior nurse with RSCN training referred to in paragraph 21.30 above should have this responsibility.* She would, in respect of her hospital work, be in a line management relationship to her divisional

355

nursing officer, but she would, by virtue of her training and experience, have an advisory rôle in aspects of the nursing care of sick children in other nursing divisions (eg maternity, mental health, primary care) which require her particular expertise. She should be able to report direct to the District Nursing Officer on any problems she encountered and the Area Nurse (Child Health) would depend on her for assistance in policy making and for advice on the extent to which the nursing needs of children were being met.

Dental Services

21.32 In the present situation the Area Dental Officer is the key administrator and fulfils the following functions related to the dental care of children:

    (i) provides advice on dental services to the Area Health Authority;

    (ii) manages the School Dental Service;

    (iii) liaises with consultant hospital dental staff and the General Dental Service;

    (iv) coordinates the hospital dental service, general dental service and community dental services;

    (v) is responsible for the dental health education programme.

It will be through the Area Dental Officer's efforts that many of the suggestions detailed in Chapter 13 will, it is hoped, be implemented, with the support of the Area Dental Committee (Advisory). We do not under-rate this task, for as a result of the lack of Regional Dental Officers and the shortage of District Dental Officers, the Area Dental Officers are over-burdened, may not be well informed about regional matters, and may find communication with the district levels difficult, although they are entitled to attend meetings of the Area Team of Officers and the District Management Teams, when appropriate.

Community Health Councils

21.33 The setting up of Community Health Councils, one for each of an area's health districts, marks an important new development in the National Health Service: a formal arrangement at district level for representing the consumer's interests in the health services to those responsible for managing them. It is as yet early days to assess their effectiveness but we look to them to inject a fresh democratic note into health service planning. That they have a rôle to play is clear. Efficient administrative practice may not satisfy the total needs of a community and what appears rational to the administrator may not always meet the needs of those who use the health service. In the foundation of the CHCs the National Health Service Reorganisation Act (1973) has deliberately separated the functions of consumer representation from the functions of management in that they lie outside the formal management structure of the service. The purpose of this separation is to ensure that CHCs take an independent view of the services provided. Although they have no executive powers, they have rights of access to NHS plans and to the AHA and its officers; they can visit hospitals and other health services premises and the AHA has a duty to consult them about any substantial development of the health services in their district and in particular about any important variations in services affecting the public such as the opening of new services and the closure of hospitals or other services.

21.34 CHCs have from 18 to 33 members, of whom half are appointed by the local authorities covering the district they represent, at least one-third by voluntary bodies concerned locally with the NHS and the remainder by the RHA after consultation with appropriate local authorities and other organisations. In a postal survey we undertook we found that between 8% and 15% of CHC members were members of voluntary organisations concerned with children's needs and we feel confident that they will press children's interests. However, evidence[7] suggests that the average age of CHC members tends to be high and although many of them are parents, we believe that to represent fully the views of children and parents, *membership should include mothers of young children.* We recognise the difficulties mothers with young children face in finding time to devote to community work and we recommend that *authorities should be able not only to pay travel and subsistence allowances, but also to reimburse non-working mothers for financial loss,* eg cost of babysitters, incurred through attendance at the meetings and involvement in other CHC activities. Only if health authorities meet such expenses can we expect a full representation of the interests of mothers and young children on the CHCs. *We recommend too that CHCs should include in their membership some young persons,* as their views on their recent experiences of the child health services could be revealing. However, if young working people are to give their time in this way, it is important that *the terms of the Employment Protection Act 1976 should be extended to cover CHC members.*

21.35 It is too early to get a clear picture of the directions in which the CHCs' interests are moving, but we hope that the major recommendations in our report will be taken up by them with informed enthusiasm. We welcome the recommendation given in the Department of Health's Circular, HRC(76)25 that members of CHCs should live or work in their health district, and thus acquire at first hand a "feel" for its needs. We believe it is of great importance that *CHCs should investigate the needs of client groups in their districts and the extent to which those needs are being met.* The least articulate are often the most disadvantaged members of the community and are therefore in greater need of a consumer voice to speak for them, for they are unable to speak for themselves. Such members include children in long-stay hospitals, mentally handicapped children, mothers with large families and low incomes, and immigrant families. We have already recommended in Chapter 16 (paragraphs 16.32 and 16.36) that CHCs should be given a full opportunity to consider and comment on all health services, including primary care services, and that to fulfil their monitoring function, they should be supplied with copies of all relevant circulars, reports and memoranda issued by the DHSS.

21.36 It will be some time before we shall know whether CHCs can effect a shift in the allocation of resources. As we have seen, their function is advisory and consultative: they can comment and advise on needs and on policy decisions but have no direct rôle in the management of the services. CHCs may publish reports and statements about their views at any time, as they see fit, but they are required to present an annual report to the RHA on their activities.This is published and their AHA must in turn publish its response to the report, including

---

(7) Klein, R, and Lewis, J (1974). Community Health Councils: The Early Days. *Health and Social Services Journal.* No 2812.

any steps taken in consequence of the proposals made by the Council.[8] CHCs will depend for their effectiveness on the publicity given to their views and the extent to which those views are based upon acceptable statistics and reputable surveys of services needed and provided. We believe that the *CHCs could make much more effective use than at present of consultation with the District Community Physician and of the Area Medical Officer and Specialists in Community Medicine as a means of obtaining the needed epidemiological and health services data. We also strongly support the suggestion that CHCs should enlist the support of University Departments and Polytechnics in their investigations.*[9] We hope that the National Association of CHCs, whose terms of reference are now being decided, will help to meet the needs of CHCs for research and information as well as giving a national voice to their views of consumer's interests.

Child Health Records

21.37 A good system of recording clinical information is essential if a high standard of care is to be achieved in the child health services. The first function of clinical records is to help doctors to care for their patients. They also act as a means of communication between two or more doctors treating the same child, facilitate the evaluation of medical treatment, provide morbidity and other data for epidemiological and operational purposes and are a source of medico-legal evidence.

21.38 The present state of clinical records reflects the divided history of the child health services. The main types are records used by general practitioners and hospitals, pre-school and school medical and dental records, and records for children in day nurseries, residential nurseries and other children under the care of the local authority social services. There are also several closely allied records, such as immunisation, physical measurement charts and a variety of developmental progress charts. In addition numerous forms are used for managerial, epidemiological and data collection purposes related to children's health. Examples are those for the notification of births under Section 46 of the National Health Service Reorganisation Act 1973, form SD56 issued by the Office of Population Censuses and Surveys for notification of congenital malformations and form HMR1 (IP)—a combined identification data collection sheet—for all age patients in connection with the Hospital Activity Analysis. Although a large number of widely diverse types of clinical records exist, only those in the pre-school and school health service were specifically designed for children (standard national cards 10M and 11M).

21.39 It is true that there have been moves generally towards more standardisation and coordination of records but progress has been slow. Within the hospital field the Tunbridge Report[10] pointed out that the diversity of hospital clinical records caused their importance to be under-rated and recommended

(8) Department of Health and Social Security (1974). Democracy in the National Health Service. HMSO, London.

(9) Department of Health and Social Security (1975). Final Report of the Advisers on Community Health Councils.

(10) Central Health Services Council: Standing Medical Advisory Committee. Report of the Sub-Committee on the Standardisation of Hospital Medical Records (Chairman: R Tunbridge) (1965). HMSO, London.

their standardisation. The Department of Health's Circular, HSC(IS)197 again encouraged health authorities to use standard hospital clinical records and forms devised by the Advisory Committee on Hospital Records under the Chairmanship of Sir Francis Avery-Jones. These include a basic clinical record for all ages and forms which fall into two groups: those for communication between hospital and general practitioner and those for communication within the hospital. In addition a number of experiments in unifying clinical records used in different parts of the service have taken place; in one area the neonatal clinical record initiated in the hospital becomes the pre-school clinical record and other areas have combined pre- and school health clinical records. A number of early attempts at improving records within general practice were hampered by the small size of the general practitioner envelope and clinical record card, and the decision to adopt the A4 size was a first step towards better design and legibility. In addition an ad hoc working group set up by a joint BMA/DHSS Working Party has devised a "paediatric development sheet", which includes head circumference and weight charts, to assist those general practitioners who are taking an increasing interest in child health work. We are also aware that a Departmental Steering Committee is at present advising on the development of a standard computer-based pre-school recording system as part of a programme aimed at provision of a national computer-based multipurpose recording of certain aspects of the health of children. The aim of the project is to assist in an effective and economic way the planning and organisation of preventive and curative child health services. Although this project is still at a very early stage, it is a further development which is likely to have implications for clinical records. The DHSS is also currently considering the introduction of a national record card for health visitors to use in their domiciliary work with families with pre-school children.

21.40 Our findings are therefore that there are far too many different types of clinical records used in the child health services and that this is an obstacle to integrating child care in the way that we are proposing. In particular records used by hospitals and general practitioners are not designed to monitor child development or cater for the special circumstances of the growing child. There are also serious omissions, such as the absence of a separate record for every newborn baby. (At present, by tradition, a baby born in hospital is not counted as a separate in-patient or as a separate clinical record unless admitted to a special care nursery.) This omission is important in view of the recommendations of the Peel Committee, which we have endorsed, that the immediate post-natal care of every infant irrespective of where it is born should include a full clinical examination and that this screening medical examination should be fully recorded and act as a basis for the future health record of the child. Equally the current diversity of records does little to assist the development of comprehensive assessment of handicapped children, a service of considerable complexity, where competent clinical recording is essential.

21.41 We have not felt that we are qualified to consider these questions in greater detail. *We recommend therefore that a suitably constituted committee, with representatives from the Advisory Committee on Hospital Medical Records, should be set up to consider the question of clinical records for children in hospital and in the community, including those under the care of the local authority social services department.* An important aspect of their work should be to publicise among doctors the contribution which good clinical recording makes to medical care. While we would leave detailed matters to the discretion of the Committee, our view is that the merit should be examined of a standard basic clinical record card encompassing both preventive and curative medicine from birth to school leaving age.

21.42 This matter of children's clinical records is exceedingly complex and the development of a single record is bound to be slow. *We recommend that in the meantime the DHSS should consider the introduction and design of a health record book,* similar to the Carnet de Santé, issued to mothers in France.

21.43 We have not thought it appropriate to discuss the complex issues involved in the confidentiality of clinical records. We would however wish to state, as a matter of principle, that we believe the exchange of information within and between different professions to be essential for the health care of children, and that this should not lightly be forgone on the grounds of confidentiality.

Research

21.44 We considered it outside our terms of reference to undertake a detailed examination of the need for research in child health or to plan any programme in this wide field. However, at appropriate points in the chapters of Part II we have attempted to indicate the degree of established knowledge on which our recommendations are based and the consequent research implications. For example, the recommendation on fluoridation of drinking water is supported by extensive researches but the recommended programme of surveillance has only limited research support and a great deal remains to be done in evaluating the effectiveness of various surveillance procedures and in measuring their cost and the benefit that accrues from them. In this section we can do no more than provide an outline of the national framework for research, indicate the place of child health in that framework and comment on the research budget. A great deal of money for child health research comes from non-government sources—Trusts, Foundations, etc—but here we shall concern ourselves only with government sponsored research and development.

21.45 A new strategy for government research was laid down in the White Paper "Framework for Government Research and Development"[11]. The new strategy demands that government research and development should be managed on a customer/contractor basis, that certain Departments (including DHSS) should set up Chief Scientist's Organisations, and that there should be some transfer of the various Research Council's funds to customer Departments, with the expectation that the money will be used to commission applied research from those Research Councils as contractors.

21.46 *The Customer/Contractor Approach* implies that those responsible for defining departmental objectives should also be responsible for commissioning the research and development work needed to achieve them. To do so departmental "customers" must work in partnership with their research "contractors" inside and outside their Department. Departments as customers are responsible

---

[11] Cmnd 5046. HMSO, London.

for defining their requirements, contractors advise on the feasibility of satisfying them and undertake the work. Within DHSS the "customers" are the administrative divisions of the Services Development Group (See Appendix M, paragraph 13). The allocation of responsibility for child health research between the administrative divisions is arbitrary and confusing. For instance although the Children's Division is concerned with the prevention of handicap in children, the Mental Health Division has responsibility for children who are mentally handicapped and the Social Handicap Division for children who are physically handicapped. Outside the Department the Home Office has responsibility for juvenile courts, Borstals and other aspects of the treatment of juvenile delinquency, while the responsibilities of the DHSS and the DES intermingle and overlap in the case of children from the age of three upwards.

21.47 The *Chief Scientist, DHSS,* is responsible to the Secretary of State for Social Services for England and the Secretary of State for Wales for ensuring that scientific advice is brought to bear on all relevant parts of the Department's work. The Chief Scientist is supported by scientists of many disciplines from outside the Department who give advice on scientific aspects of the planning and execution of the Department's research and development programme. They do this by considering together matters referred to them by the Chief Scientist; discussion within the Department about research objectives, managing the research programme and specific projects; by visits to research teams to assess capabilities and programmes; and by considering and advising on proposals for new research units. The Chief Scientist's Research Committee considers and gives advice on the research and development programme and makes annual recommendations to the Planning Committee of DHSS on research priorities and on the adequacy of arrangements for the management, evaluation and implementation of the results of the research programme. Supporting the Chief Scientist in the whole range of his tasks is a Research Management Team which consists of all the Department's most senior professional and administrative staff engaged in the research field with representation on the Chief Scientist's Research Committee.

21.48 The cornerstones of the research structure are the research liaison groups which bring together members of the Chief Scientist's organisation, research management and the appropriate client group to plan and agree policy for that particular group and to see that it is carried out as effectively as possible. The focus of the *Children's Research Liaison Group* is on services provided for children and families with children. It makes recommendations on research objectives relevant to child health services, child care, intermediate treatment and other DHSS aspects of juvenile delinquency, the support of children and families with children in their homes, the protection of children and adoption and related services. There is also a Mental Health RLG which covers services for the mentally handicapped and we consider it particularly important that the needs of mentally handicapped children should not be overlooked because they are in the fields of interest of two RLGs. Among the membership of the Group, the Children's Division is responsible for formulating research objectives which will assist the development of policy objectives and for reviewing and acting on the results of research; research management is responsible for promoting research to meet the approved objectives and for securing decisions on and monitoring individual projects and programmes; the scientific advisers are responsible for the scientific merit and feasibility of the research programme and of individual projects.

21.49 The Chief Scientist chairs a *Small Grants Committee,* which includes scientists drawn from outside the Department, to consider unsolicited applications for grants of less than £30,000 to carry out research which will last for less than three years. Client groups and Research Liaison Groups are not consulted unless it is known that the proposal fits in with the research objectives and priorities of particular client groups.

21.50 As well as financing applied research to meet departmental objectives the Government also supports research through Councils to help develop the Sciences, to maintain a capacity for fundamental research and to support higher education. As mentioned in 21.44 some of the funds allocated to the Research Councils through the Department of Education and Science are being transferred to customer Departments. In the case of the two Research Councils with which DHSS is most closely linked, something less than a quarter of the funds provided for the Medical Research Council are to be transferred to the DHSS, while responsibility for funding the Social Sciences Research Council remains wholly with the Department of Education and Science. Links between the Department and the two Research Councils are being developed and full use will be made of both as departmental contractors.

21.51 In the Medical Research Council there is no separate statement of policy for research related to child health. The Council's policies and priorities are determined in relation to fields which are characterised by scientific coherence. The needs of client groups such as children tend to involve many separate fields of research and come under consideration during the process of policy development as part of the review of each scientific field relevant to them rather than as separate subjects. Responsibility for child health problems is therefore divided between the four MRC Boards (Neurosciences Board, Cell Biology and Disorders Board, Physiological Systems and Disorders Board, and Tropical Medicine Research Board) and its Environmental Research Policy Committee. Grants supported by the MRC are mainly of two kinds. Once off *Project grants* with a tenure usually of three years; and *Programme grants* to establish teams to meet the Council's objectives, awarded for an initial period of five years with an expectation of renewal subject to satisfactory progress. We consider it unfortunate that the Research Councils do not produce a statement of their activities on a client group basis. We recommend that *the children's RLG should ask the MRC and SSRC to provide an annual statement of those parts of their research programmes that are relevant to the needs of children so that there is nationally a comprehensive picture of the work being done in this field.*

21.52 We have obtained information on the proportion of the DHSS total budget for research and development given to projects relevant to child health. The table below gives a breakdown between Child Health and the remainder of the Children's Research Liaison Group of present and projected expenditure on existing commitments. The figures exclude expenditure through the Small Grants Scheme and Special Medical Developments, the costs of in-house research, and minor expenditure incurred by other divisions in the Department (eg Supplies Division).

				£000s		
		1975–76	1976–77	1977–78	1978–79	1979–80
(I)	Child Health	157.1	190.6	118.2	90.4	50.0
(II)	Remainder CHRLG	339.1	364.4	327.2	263.7	230.8
(III)	Total	496.2	555.0	445.4	354.1	280.8
(IV)	Total R+D Commitment	5,466.0	6,403.0	5,859.0	4,579.0	3,299.0
(V)	(III) as % (IV)	9.1	8.7	7.6	7.7	8.5

21.53 The share of the budget allocated to children's research will apparently remain static at around 8% over the next four years. However, the table does no more than project expenditure on existing commitments. The apparent falling off in the total figures from 1977-78 onwards reflects the rate at which existing research projects are expected to be completed, and will in due course be made good to the extent that new research is commissioned in their place. Thus additional money has been allocated provisionally, for 1977-78 amounting to £30,000 for the Children's RLG as a whole and £410,000 for other RLGs. At the time of writing it is impossible to say how much will be available for subsequent years or how it will be divided under the above headings. *In the course of our report we have recommended a substantial amount of research, and we hope that in the light of this, as additional resources are allocated for research there will be a significant increase in the share devoted to the children.*

21.54 *We should like to point to the need for more research into consumer attitudes to be undertaken.* As we have made clear throughout our report, improved health care for children will depend in some measure on better take up of services and greater cooperation between parents and professionals. Surveys of consumers' opinions are therefore of value, even though they may not always be rigorously scientific in approach; the fact that a number of parents are discontented with or reluctant to use services available is important in its own right. Studies of this kind might profitably be initiated both by DHSS and by voluntary bodies, CHCs etc. Further we are keen that independent research into all aspects of child health services should be undertaken by voluntary bodies, consumers groups and CHCs. Funds for this purpose should be provided by DHSS without conditions about publication of the results. If such research is carried out by good researchers on properly evaluated principles, then there is no reason why the results should not be accepted as valid.

21.55 Finally we would hope that in the field of research as in other areas the proposed new Joint Committee for Children would have an important rôle to play in ensuring that the needs of children were satisfactorily provided for.

CHAPTER 22
PRIORITIES

The Problem

22.1 From our first meeting we have been aware of the problem of relating the improvements and changes in the child health services we consider desirable, or even essential, to their financial implications. Even at the best of times, when resources are abundant, the expressed demand by the general public and the health professions for expenditure on more and better health and personal social services inevitably exceeds what can be afforded out of public funds. We have been working throughout our deliberations against a background of mounting inflation and increasingly severe constraints on public expenditure.

22.2 Finance is not the only constraint. There are also constraints in respect of human resources. These are particularly important where medical staff are concerned. The training programme is long and the output of doctors over the next 10 years is already fixed by the past and present intake of medical students. That intake has been and will be increasing, but we are aware that any great increase in the time spent by doctors in the child health services will be bought in part at the expense of doctors' time in other parts of the services. And similar, but shorter-term, considerations apply to increases in the number of qualified nurses caring for children.

22.3 There is also a constraint in relation to the changes necessary for the establishment of more highly trained or new kinds of professional staff. Such changes inevitably call for consultation with a wide range of interests, and even when accepted a great deal of work needs to be done in the formulation, location and staffing of the new training programmes before the training can be provided.

22.4 Despite these rather stultifying considerations, we decided that in the body of the report we would recommend without inhibitions what changes and improvements in the health and social services we believed to be necessary if the health needs of the country's children were to be met. We would also provide as careful an estimate as possible of the resource implications of these recommendations in the knowledge that many of them would have to be seen as long-term objectives to be achieved perhaps over the next 15–20 years as the financial crisis through which we are passing is contained and once again there is sustained growth in available resources and public expenditure. We also decided to limit our estimates of resource implications largely to questions of increases in manpower. An economically sophisticated approach to the cost of our recommendations was not possible, for we found that we were unable to quantify the benefit likely to accrue from the implementation of our recommendations even at the crude level of expected improvements in the control of morbidity and mortality in childhood. And since most of our proposals must constitute a long-term programme we also decided that it would probably not be very helpful to include estimates of even the manpower costs in financial terms.

22.5 Nevertheless, despite these difficulties, we decided that at the end of our report we should make as clear a statement as possible about where our priorities lie. A list of all our proposals in some agreed rank order would not be very helpful for it is clear that there will be insufficient resources to implement all our recommendations for a long time to come. And what are the decision makers then to do? Should they spend all the available revenue on achieving the first few objectives, or would it be preferable to spend some revenue on all the objectives, achieving none of them completely (and how much should then be spent on each)? In what follows first we make a statement about what, if our report is accepted, we regard as a matter of the greatest urgency, next we give the nine resource-consuming recommendations which we consider of the highest priority, and then we give four other important recommendations which do not carry such heavy resource implications.

A Matter of Urgency

22.6 *We urge the Government to reach a decision about our recommendations for the reorganisation and staffing of the primary care services for children at the earliest possible moment. This is of the utmost importance.* First because, if our recommendation to develop these services on the basis of the concept of general practitioner paediatricians and child health visitors is accepted, the decision to implement it will call for consultations with interested professional bodies and this will take time, and for the child health services time is running out. Second, the decision, when made, will end the present disturbing uncertainty surrounding the future of the pre-school and school health services and the position of the doctors working in them. Third, because the decision will influence the pattern of development of child health services for a long time to come, it has a bearing upon and will influence decisions about a number of our other recommendations.

High Priority Recommendations with Major Resource Implications

Child Health Visitors

22.7 This is a very high priority not only because child health visitors will be key figures in the reorganised primary care services for children, but because the number of health visitors in the country even now needs to be increased by 50% to reach the levels recommended by the Jameson Committee in 1956, whether or not our concept of a child health visitor is accepted. (Paragraphs 17.24–17.27).

General Practitioner Paediatricians

22.8 We consider early implementation of our recommendations about the establishment of general practitioner paediatricians to be of the utmost import-ance. Although the training implications are large, the extra manpower needed to implement the concept is not prohibitive when the doctors at present working in the pre-school and school health services are taken into account. (Paragraphs 17.19–17.23).

Consultant Community Paediatricians

22.9 We are also most anxious to see a progressive provision of Consultant Community Paediatricians in all Districts, combined with the full use of present senior medical officers, some becoming Consultant Community Paediatricians, others with the professional status of Clinical Specialists in Paediatrics. (Paragraphs 18.4–18.7).

365

Children's Nurses in Hospital

22.10 We have set out minimum requirements for a children's department in a district hospital providing out-patient consultation, paediatric advice for the accident and emergency department, day care, ward admission and consultant nursing advice in the community. All children's departments should achieve this level of staffing as soon as possible as the present levels of staffing are unacceptably near the frontiers of safety. The first step should be the appointment of a sister/charge nurse with the RSCN qualification to each children's ward. (Paragraphs 18.49–18.56).

Care of the Newborn

22.11 We attach high priority to the improvement of services for the newborn, and in particular to the implementation of our recommendations for the organisation of intensive care, and for the resuscitation and clinical examination of the newborn. (Paragraphs 8.27–8 and 8.34 and 8.39). We welcome the Department of Health's new Circular asking authorities to review facilities for the newborn.

Increase in Child Psychiatrists

22.12 In the country as a whole the number of child psychiatrists remains substantially below the level recommended by the Royal Medico-Psychological Association as long ago as 1960. This situation must be remedied, and the aim should be to provide over the next decade at least one child psychiatrist per 35,000 children. (Paragraphs 15.34–5).

Mental Handicap Services

22.13 There is an urgent need to improve the services for mentally retarded children and their families. The most pressing requirements are improved and expanded community services, much greater provision of local authority hostels and children's homes, better facilities for short-term residential care and the more rational use of valuable psychiatric and paediatric expertise. (Paragraphs 14.66–91).

Fluoridation

22.14 We are sure of the value, safety and effectiveness of fluoridation in the prevention of dental decay in children and the recent report of the Royal College of Physicians has endorsed the validity of the evidence on which this conviction is based. We understand that although revenue costs are relatively small, the initial capital costs are significant and we are glad to see that the Government has now earmarked £0.5 million pa to assist authorities in meeting them. This is an encouraging start which should lead progressively to fluoridation on a national scale.

School Nursing Service

22.15 We attach particular importance to the need to provide a trained school nursing service, ideally at the levels we have recommended in Chapter 10 (paragraph 48) particularly during the transitional period when some of the health visitors in the school health service may be retraining to work as child health visitors.

High Priority Recommendations Without Major Resource Implications

District Handicap Teams

22.16 The establishment of a handicap team in every district, coupled with the development, in districts lacking it, of necessary accommodation (particularly in small residential units) for handicapped children who cannot be cared for at home. (Paragraphs 14.22–14.44).

Joint Committee for Children

22.17 We would like to see early implementation of our recommendation that the present Children and Family Life Group should be reconstituted as a Joint Committee for Children responsible to the Personal Social Services Council and the Central Health Services Council to keep under continuous review the needs of children and the services provided to meet them. This would provide the machinery to ensure that the accepted recommendations of reports such as ours are implemented satisfactorily and at an acceptable rate.

Children's Departments

22.18 We urge an acceleration of the slow process of redeploying beds and staff in general hospitals to enable children to be nursed together by properly trained staff in children's departments (Paragraph 12.18).

Training and Career Opportunities for Married Women Doctors

22.19 In view of the importance of making the best possible use of available manpower for the child health services we would like the Specialist Advisory Committee in Paediatrics of the Joint Committee on Higher Medical Training and the Royal College of General Practitioners to examine the question of part-time training schemes for women doctors in paediatrics jointly with the Women's Medical Federation and the Department of Health so that posts and training for them can be developed together. (Paragraph 20.27).

The Consultative Documents on Priorities

22.20 The Secretary of State for Social Services has recently issued a Consultative Document, "Priorities for Health and Personal Social Services in England" and the Welsh Office has published a comparable document for Wales. These documents give the level of resources which will be available over the next few years and outline a strategy to provide the health and local authorities with a basis for their planning work in the face of the difficult choices which will have to be made. We were pleased to find that our priority recommendations are in line with proposals in the document relative to the expansion of health visiting services, vocational training for family doctors, special care facilities for newborn babies and services for handicapped children and for giving high priority to the development of primary health care teams. We believe therefore that there is a sound basis from which to proceed with the implementation of our major recommendations.

PART IV

SUMMARY OF MAJOR RECOMMENDATIONS

We can summarise our objectives quite simply: we want to see a child and family centred service; in which skilled help is readily available and accessible; which is integrated in as much as it sees the child as a whole, and as a continuously developing person. We want to see a service which ensures that this paediatric skill and knowledge are applied in the care of every child whatever his age or disability, and wherever he lives, and we want a service which is increasingly oriented to prevention. Our recommendations are directed to these ends.

CHAPTER 7

AN INTEGRATED CHILD HEALTH SERVICE

1. The organisational structure of the child health services should be changed to provide an integrated 2-tier system based on comprehensive primary care firmly linked with supporting consultant and hospital care.

2. Within general practice there should be a number of general practitioners, who would have a "special interest" in paediatrics whom we call general practitioner paediatricians, GPPs.

3. To be eligible to practise as a "general practitioner paediatrician" a doctor should have successfully completed appropriate training leading to accreditation.

4. A GPP should normally have responsibility, in his capacity as GPP for
    (i) ensuring the provision of full developmental surveillance and preventive services to the children registered with the practice;
    (ii) providing a minimum sessional commitment to the Area Health Authority to meet the requirements of the LEA and LASSD for medical services in respect of children;
    (iii) taking the lead in ensuring continuing education and maintenance of standards in child health care within the practice as a whole;
    (iv) acting as a link between the primary care services for children and the child health services in hospital.

5. Within the community nursing services there should be a distinct group of nurses, called child health visitors, who combine preventive and curative nursing responsibility for children, and advisory responsibility in respect of their parents, and who would work in close professional association with the GPPs.

6. Nursing duties in schools should be carried out by specially trained school nurses who would look to the CHV for guidance in their work.

7. The CHV should be assisted with her work in surgeries, health centres and home nursing by a child health nurse who would have paediatric training.

8. The nursing officer who coordinates the activities of a number of CHVs should ensure that as best befits local circumstances the attachment of each CHV to a general practice obliges her to have a clear responsibility for a geographically defined "patch".

9. There should be a new type of consultant paediatrician (the consultant community paediatrician), who would be the specialist counterpart of the GPP with special skills in developmental, educational and social paediatrics. There should be at least one consultant community paediatrician in each health district.

10. In each health district there should be a multiprofessional team to provide a special diagnostic, assessment and treatment service for handicapped children.

11. There should be a single supporting child psychiatric service covering the functions of both the child guidance service and the hospital based child psychiatric services.

12. The guidance given by the DHSS in 1971 that the nurse in charge of each non-psychiatric ward of the children's department and of the outpatient services for children should be a paediatric nurse should be fully implemented.

13. The training of the registered children's nurse should be broadened to include community as well as hospital experience.

CHAPTER 8

THE UNBORN AND NEWBORN BABY

1. There should be further study aimed at providing those involved with clearer guidance on what advice parents need during the antenatal period and how best to give it to them.

2. Research into and development of methods for prenatal diagnosis should be continued and the specialised facilities required for this should be carefully planned.

3. Further research should be encouraged into ways by which the prenatal well-being of the fetus can be monitored by methods which can be routinely applied and which do not cause distress to the mother.

4. Mothers should be encouraged to take a larger part in the post-natal care of their babies and the maternity and neonatal departments should be sensitive to their social and psychological needs during this period.

5. Every newborn baby should be evaluated immediately after delivery and should have a full post-natal examination between the age of 6-10 days. This postnatal screening examination should be the basis of the child's health record.

6. The facilities for the transport of immature and seriously ill babies should be reviewed.

7. Nurseries providing intensive care should be centralised with at least one in each Region which is of adequate size, appropriately equipped and staffed, and directed by a consultant in neonatal paediatrics.

8. A substantial proportion of the nursing staff in special and intensive care nurseries should hold the certificate in special and intensive care for babies awarded by the Joint Board of Clinical Nursing Studies.

9. The child health visitor should have contact with the expectant mother during pregnancy, and with mother and baby during the first few days of the baby's life.

10. Further encouragement should be given to the training of midwives in the care of the newborn, and the social and emotional aspects of childbirth.

11. High priority should be given to research into the aetiology of handicapping conditions, and into the regional and social class variations in perinatal mortality and morbidity.

Postscript: Family Planning

1. There should be more extensive and better education on family planning.

2. Professional workers other than doctors should play a greater rôle in family planning.

3. Community workers should be well informed about the services and the kinds of help they provide.

4. More active steps need to be taken to bring these services to particularly needy groups.

5. There is need for greater cooperation between different groups of professional workers concerned with family planning, both inside and outside the NHS.

CHAPTER 9

HEALTH AND DEVELOPMENT IN THE EARLY YEARS

1. A basic programme of health surveillance should be offered to all children.

2. Any doctor who undertakes the serial observation of health and physical growth and the monitoring of developmental progress of children should also be in a position to prescribe any medical treatment that he may consider necessary and to seek consultant opinion if he so desires.

3. Additional health surveillance should be arranged for those children who need it, particularly for children who are "developmentally vulnerable" or "disadvantaged".

4. Health surveillance should be shared between CHV and GPP and the CHV should herself undertake some developmental examinations.

5. As an aid to achieving whole child population health surveillance:
   (i) Nursing Officers (child health visiting) should have an explicit responsibility for arranging that CHVs who are members of primary health care teams are also assigned a geographically defined community with whom they should ensure that the child health services keep in touch.
   (ii) An effective system should be devised for recording a family's "transfer in" and "transfer out" of a defined neighbourhood.
   (iii) Parents should be required to notify a change of address when applying for family allowances.
   (iv) CHVs should have a right to apply for legally enforceable medical examinations of young children whose health and welfare they fear may be jeopardised by the failure of their parents to make use of available child health services.

6. The use of risk and observation registers should be abandoned.

7. Domiciliary visiting should continue to be a feature of the functions of CHVs.

8. The timing of clinic sessions should take account of the commitments of working parents.

9. When clinic sessions are provided at unsocial hours, the staff should be appropriately paid, and given compensatory time off-duty.

10. Clinics should be provided in premises that are appropriate to their function which should have a social as well as a health component.

11. Serious consideration should be given to the sessional employment of social workers in clinics.

12. AHAs should adopt computer-linked schemes for immunisation appointments and records, as a means of improving the level of immunisation among children.

13. Consideration should be given to devising standard health records for all children aged 0–15, in relation to both preventive and therapeutic health care.

14. The possibility and advantages of such a standardised health record being computer-managed should be studied.

15. CHVs should sometimes undertake health surveillance of children in nursery and play groups, in cooperation with social workers, child care staff and nursery teachers.

16. Research should be undertaken into the short-term and long-term efficacy of health surveillance programmes.

CHAPTER 10

HEALTH FOR EDUCATION

1. Health surveillance of school children should be planned as a continuation of that for pre-school children.

2. The medical examination in relation to entry to school should be made statutory.

3. Subsequent medical examinations of individual children should be carried out only when required.

4. Every pupil should have an annual health care interview with the school nurse.

5. All 13-year old boys and girls should have an interview with the school doctor.

6. The school doctor should hold regular clinics in secondary schools for adolescent pupils to attend, if they choose, independently and in confidence.

7. A school doctor should have the right to examine a child, if necessary without the parents' consent, if there is in the opinion of the headteacher reasonable ground for concern as to his health and safety.

8. Direct responsibility for a school or schools within a district should be the underlying principle in the organisation of medical and nursing services to schools, as an aid to continuity of care and inter-professional collaboration.

9. Every ordinary school should have a nominated school doctor.

10. Primary schools should as a rule have not less than one medical session per fortnight, and secondary schools not less than two sessions per week.

11. GPPs should provide these sessions, under contract to the AHA.

12. Every ordinary school should have a nominated school nurse.

13. Primary schools should as a rule have not less than 6 hours of nurse-time per week, and secondary schools not less than 15 hours and preferably 30 hours (full-time).

14. These nursing services should be provided by specially trained school nurses, who would be members of the same primary health care team as the school doctor (GPP) though the CHV would retain overall responsibility for them and provide professional support.

15. Every special school should have a nominated school doctor who should be a consultant community paediatrician.

16. A sufficient number of nurses should be appointed to each special school to meet its individual requirements, taking account both of the actual nursing involved and the need for nurses to participate in assessment and counselling.

17. Doctors and nurses providing health services in school should be required to have undertaken the appropriate training.

18. Health records should be maintained for every pupil and relevant information be made available to the education services.

19. The views of parents and pupils should at all times be taken into consideration by health care staff working in schools.

20. The present legal limitation upon the power of LEAs to provide special education for children before the age of 2 years should be removed.

CHAPTER 11

ADOLESCENTS

1. Adolescents warrant consideration as a distinct group for health care provision.

2. Total specialisation in adolescent care is not recommended; the aim should be for all professionals with a special interest to have better training and more experience. The training of GPPs, CHVs and School Nurses should include an understanding of the particular needs and development of adolescents. Close collaboration should be maintained between paediatricians and child psychiatrists, and, as necessary, with other appropriate specialists.

3. Consideration should be given to the provision of adolescent in-patient units in acute hospitals.

4. If informal vigilance in school is to be successful, teachers must be better trained in health, especially psychiatric, problems and have ready access to expert advice. Adolescents should have the opportunity of self-referral to school doctors and nurses.

5. Further epidemiological study of the pathology of adolescents should be undertaken and a pilot "walk-in" counselling service (on the lines of the student health service) mounted for scientific evaluation.

6. Advice to young people on sex education should be available in various forms from a variety of sources including schools, the health services and voluntary bodies. All sex education for young people but particularly that in schools should include information on the transmission and detection of sexually transmitted diseases. Health education and counselling services should be available in all adolescent std clinics and publicity campaigns should be concentrated on the at-risk groups.

7. When abortion is under consideration skilled counselling should be available to the girl and, wherever possible and appropriate, to the boyfriend and family in advance of any decision. Girls in care should be given the opportunity of discussing abortion with someone not administratively concerned with their care. There is need for further research into the physical, psychological and social effects of abortion or the failure to obtain it.

8. The needs of adolescents with psychiatric disorder include greater facilities for counselling over a range of problems; the provision of psychiatric help in "walk-in" clinics; collaboration between child/adolescent psychiatrists and "adult" colleagues; and increase in the facilities for residential care and treatment; and the evaluation of treatment of the chronically socially disruptive adolescent.

9. Much wider recognition should be given to handicapped adolescents' need for psychiatric, genetic and psycho-sexual counselling. They should be able and encouraged to seek help and guidance on their own initiative and should therefore have direct access to the professionals involved in their treatment.

10. Close liaison should be maintained between child- and adult-oriented services for the handicapped, although the responsibility for overall care of the individual should at all times be clear. Local education authorities should keep in close touch with the career of a handicapped adolescent for at least 2 years after leaving school.

CHAPTER 12

ILLNESS

1. Studies should be carried out with the aim of supplementing national and regional statistics with local data on childhood illness which is "patient" as well as "disease" oriented. Such data should provide a basis for the rational planning of services, in particular hospital facilities.

2. Health authorities should be asked to explore the possibility of providing a mechanism whereby a parent seeking primary medical help for a sick child could be put in touch with whoever is providing the service.

3. The development of nursing advice and support for sick children in the community by child health visitors and child health nurses should be evaluated to determine the most economic and efficient use of nursing skills.

4. The guidance given in the Department of Health's memorandum, HM(71)22 and the paper for Regional Medical Officers (1975) on the organisation of hospital facilities for children should be fully implemented.

5. With the expansion of numbers of paediatricians, regular paediatric consultation clinics in health centres and group practices should be developed for the benefit of children and parents and as an essential prerequisite for the more selective use of district and regional hospital facilities.

6. The Department of Health and Social Security, in conjunction with professional and parent associations should carry out a study of out-patient clinics for children in England, comparable to that carried out in Wales by the Welsh Hospital Board.

7. District Planning Teams for children's services should as a high priority review the use of Accident and Emergency departments by children and make recommendations for the development of a more rational working relationship between these departments and primary care and out-patient services.

8. In view of the apparent overlap in the categories of illness coming to different hospital departments, there should be combined study in a variety of hospitals and communities of children coming to out-patient and Accident and Emergency departments, and a similar comparative evaluation of children treated by day care and admission.

CHAPTER 13

THE PATH TO DENTAL HEALTH

1. Immediate steps should be taken to introduce the fluoridation of the community water supply at a level of one part per million on a national scale.

2. A model should be set up to investigate and evaluate a primary care service for children based on the General Dental Service with a system of remuneration provided by a capitation fee.

3. There should be a review of the manpower needed for the provision of a satisfactory dental service which accords priority to children, taking into account the implications for undergraduate and postgraduate education.

4. The School and Priority Service should be increased to a level which would allow: a minimum of one dental inspection per year; treatment to be offered to every child from the age of 5 years, and where the manpower permitted, to every child from the age of $2\frac{1}{2}$ years; a special service for handicapped children; the organisation of dental health education in the community.

5. Consideration should be given to the incentives needed to attract practitioners to those regions which are seriously understaffed. These would include better facilities, especially in Health Centres, and a system of preferential remuneration acceptable to the profession and the DHSS.

6. Consultancies in Paediatric Dentistry should be established. When available there should in the starting phase be at least one in each region. They would have a special responsibility for the dental care of the severely handicapped and a close association with Regional Child Development Units.

7. The establishment of orthodontic consultants responsible for the treatment of children should be increased in terms of regional need. The proposed norm is one consultant orthodonist per 100,000 children:

8. Two additional training schools for dental auxiliaries should be set up as soon as possible in association with provincial dental schools.

9. The dental care of mentally and/or physically handicapped children should be brought up to the level of that provided for other children. This calls for a partnership between consultants in children's dentistry and members of the school and general dental services with special interest in and training for this work. The responsibility for implementing and maintaining this development will lie with the Area Dental Officer and the Specialists in Community Medicine (Child Health).

10. Postgraduate training facilities in the field of children's dentistry should be considerably extended, special attention being given to the handicapped and to pre-school children.

379

11. Consideration should be given to the revision of dental records with a view to rationalising and harmonising the statistics of dental care in the general dental service and the school dental service so that individual children and all types of attention can be identified.

12. Experiment should be encouraged in the evaluation of different methods of dental health education. As effective methods are found they should become part of the education of children, and the special education of expectant mothers and the parents of young children, and of all professionals concerned with the care of children.

13. We believe that television and the press could play a more positive rôle in promoting dental health and that greater responsibility could be shown in the content and timing of advertising. The Health Education Council should continuously transmit up-to-date information to the media on the subject of dental health.

14. The value and cost effectiveness of different supplementary preventive procedures aimed at individuals and groups should be evaluated.

15. The effectiveness of orthodontic surveillance of all children in their tenth year should be evaluated.

CHAPTER 14

HANDICAP

1. AHAs should conduct periodic local surveys of the epidemiology of handicap in order to obtain appropriate data on which to base services to meet local need.

2. Primary health care teams should provide the main health service contribution in quantitative terms to the diagnosis, assessment and treatment of handicapped children.

3. A district handicap team should be established in each district based on the DGH, the basic staff to comprise a consultant community paediatrician, a nursing officer for handicapped children, a specialist social worker, a principal psychologist and a teacher with wide experience of handicapped children, together with supporting administrative staff.

4. The district handicap team should be regarded as a common service to which health, education and social service authorities contribute professional staff through whom they have direct access to the team.

5. The unit in the DGH on which the district handicap team is based should be described as "a child development centre".

6. Regional handicap teams should be established in paediatric departments of university teaching hospitals under the direction of a consultant paediatrician with special experience of handicapped children.

7. Parents should have the right of direct access to the district handicap team and others concerned with the treatment of their child.

8. Each health, education and social services authority should assume responsibility for ensuring that transport is, if necessary, provided for handicapped children and their parents when attending their respective services.

9. As recommended in the Quirk Report there should be a large expansion in the number of speech therapists and a substantial force of aides.

10. An experienced and senior speech therapist should be appointed to each child development centre and a full-time speech therapist to the area audiology service.

11. There should be an area audiology service in each area, with strong functional links with the child development centre of the district in which it is situated; the consultant community paediatrician and the teacher of the deaf should have joint appointments to the child development centre and area audiology clinic.

12. Arrangements for the investigation and assessment of children with visual handicaps should be made at both area and regional level.

13. Physiotherapists, occupational therapists and remedial gymnasts working with children should be specially trained to do so.

14. DHSS should as a matter of urgency examine the manner in which

various aids are supplied to children, and devise ways to ensure that they are supplied promptly; each district handicap team should keep a constant watch on the supply of all aids and appliances to children in their district.

15. The health and social services required by mildly mentally handicapped children should be met by the general services provided for the child population as a whole.

16. Consultant paediatric and child psychiatric services should assume responsibility for providing supporting health services for severely mentally handicapped children.

17. When specialist psychiatric advice and treatment are required by severely mentally handicapped children they should be provided through the child psychiatric service by child psychiatrists with a special interest and experience in mental retardation.

18. District handicap teams should ensure that help for parents in dealing with problems of management of severely retarded children at home is provided through visits of individual team members to the family, as well as through clinic attendance. This necessitates a considerable expansion in community services for this group of children.

19. About 35 day places are required in an average-sized district for severely retarded children aged 0–4 years.

20. About 10 beds in an average-sized district should be provided for the short-stay residential treatment and care of severely retarded children with psychiatric problems.

21. Severely mentally handicapped children requiring short-stay hospital care for other reasons should normally be admitted to the ordinary paediatric wards in the DGH.

22. Long-stay residential accommodation should be provided for about 80 severely retarded children in each average-sized district; not less than 40 of these places should be in local authority children's homes. This necessitates a major expansion in local authority provision.

23. Up to 20 places may be required in each district for the long-term psychiatric inpatient treatment of severely retarded children with psychiatric disorders.

24. Long-stay hospital accommodation for severely retarded children should generally be in units forming part of the children's department of the DGH.

25. The feasibility should be examined of providing "technical" nursing in units for the severely retarded that are as far as possible residential homes.

26. The frequency of medical examinations of severely mentally handicapped children placed by LASSDs in voluntary and private homes should be a matter for the professional discretion of GPPs, who should be appointed to provide primary medical care for such children.

27. LASSDs placing severely retarded children in voluntary and private homes should require a report following the annual review of these children.

28. Wider and repeated publicity should be given to a paper issued by the DHSS in 1974 in which excellent suggestions were made whereby hospitals could provide "home care" for long-stay children.

CHAPTER 15

PSYCHIATRIC DISORDER

1. Both innovation and research are needed in the area of preventive services together with further research into treatment and systematic study and evaluation of therapeutic techniques.

2. The nature and extent of psychiatric disorder necessitates the use of professionals from a wide range of disciplines—psychologists, social workers, child health visitors, GPPs both in general practice and as school doctors, child psychotherapists, counsellors in schools, teachers, paediatricians, child psychiatrists and child psychiatric nurses. Collaboration and communication should be facilitated by joint working arrangements and by joint elements in both basic and in-service training.

3. All workers with children with psychiatric disorders should have some knowledge of normal and abnormal child development, family pathology and interaction, the effect of parental personal problems and a range of treatment techniques. They should receive further training throughout their careers; employing authorities should have an obligation to enable people to undertake it. Training involving therapeutic skills must include supervised clinical work, followed by some form of clinical attachment in which consultation, advice and supervision is available.

4. There should be continuous monitoring to determine how far the development of new and possibly more effective services alters the demand for longer established services. If professionals from the range of disciplines given in Recommendation 2 are to be utilised, their numbers must be increased. For child psychiatrists the aim should be to provide a staffing level of at least 1 per 35,000 children over the next decade. Career structures and financial rewards should encourage workers of all disciplines to remain in active clinical/field work.

5. Child Guidance Clinics and Psychiatric Hospital Services should be recognised as an integrated Child and Adolescent Psychiatry Service. Child Psychiatric Clinics should be developed on the basis of a well-integrated interdisciplinary team with a regular commitment to the clinic providing a coordinated service.

6. Given the planned expansion of other services, psychiatric in-patient provision for short-stay, pre-adolescent children should probably be of the order of 20 beds per 250,000 child population. The need for long-stay hospital units for severely disturbed children with chronic psychiatric conditions should be assessed and appropriate units established.

7. Day services should provide facilities for the attendance of children and groups of parents with children and should also work with families at home. 20–30 day places per 60,000 child population would seem a reasonable estimate but this provision should be reassessed in the light of experience.

8. In order to provide help to more young people, local education authorities should support the provision of counselling in schools and

384

teachers should have greater access to the consultative services of psychologists and child psychiatrists. Services in schools should have good functional links with other services, and especially with child psychiatric clinics, the school psychological service and social services.

9. Consultative support from psychiatric clinic personnel is needed in both community homes and special schools for help with individual children, for advising staff, and for planning services.

10. Greater attention must in future be paid to the provision of psychiatric services for children of pre-school age, with more training for GPPs, child health visitors and community paediatricians to enable them to recognise psychiatric disorders in this age group. Support and consultative advice from psychiatric clinic personnel should be freely available.

11. The psychiatric care of younger adolescents should be part of child and adolescent psychiatry while most services for older adolescents can be considered in relation to those provided for young adults, provided that training in general psychiatry includes knowledge of developmental issues and that services for this age group are strengthened and expanded. Facilities such as walk-in clinics should be evaluated for their effectiveness in helping adolescents to seek psychiatric help.

12. There should be a greatly increased provision of residential facilities such as hostels, schools and hospital units. Given adequate facilities and sufficient places, in-patient units should be able to provide sufficient security for the severely disturbed adolescents whose problems stem from an acute mental illness. Adolescents should not be inappropriately placed in adult wards; where such a placement is appropriate adequate schooling should be provided and a consultant psychiatrist with special experience in adolescent disorder should advise when necessary.

13. Child psychiatrists should provide the psychiatric care needed by mentally handicapped children; the mildly retarded can generally be served adequately by existing in-patient, day patient and out-patient services but the severely retarded require special provision. Training in psychiatric work with mentally handicapped children should routinely be included in child psychiatry programmes. A marked increase is needed in psychiatrists with expertise and interest in working with severely mentally handicapped children and their families.

14. There should be long-stay residential provision for just over a third of all severely mentally handicapped children, of whom at least half could adequately be cared for in local authority hostels. At present there appears to be a need for approximately 25–30 psychiatric in-patient beds for 60,000 children; of these approximately one third should be for short-term admissions. Hospital units should have the necessary facilities to admit severely handicapped children who may often have associated behavioural problems.

CHAPTER 16

A VOICE FOR CHILDREN

1. There should be a statutory medical examination of all children at school entry.

2. Where surveillance services are not taken up or where there is suspicion of serious ill-health for which medical help is not being sought the CHV should seek access to the child by persuasion; in the event of failure, she should have the right to apply for a legally enforceable medical examination.

3. Head teachers should have the right, on reasonable grounds for concern, to request the medical examination of a child in their charge, if necessary without the consent of the parents.

4. In cases of suspected abuse or neglect, Local Authorities should have the power to seek a legally enforceable medical examination separately from a removal order.

5. A majority of the Committee endorse the present practice of permitting children under 16 to receive medical advice and treatment without parental knowledge in sensitive cases such as for sexually transmitted diseases or contraception.

6. No research investigations involving children should be undertaken without approval from the appropriate ethical committee.

7. Consideration should be given to how best to ensure that the well-being and needs of children in long-stay hospitals are adequately reviewed at appropriate intervals and particular attention given to the possibility of loss of parental contact.

8. There is need for continuous review of the needs of children and the services provided to meet them; for better coordination amongst existing bodies; for the stimulation of public opinion; and for the dissemination of advice, committee recommendations, research results etc together with the monitoring of their implementation. The present Children and Family Life Group should be reconstituted as a sub-committee jointly of the Personal Social Services Council and the Central Health Services Council and asked to undertake these responsibilities at national level. The man-power resources of the PSSC should be strengthened to enable it to service this new Joint Committee for Children.

9. The Secretary of State for Social Services in England and in Wales the Secretary of State for Wales should have a statutory duty to lay before Parliament, from 1979 on, a triennial report on all aspects of their responsibilities for children, together with relevant aspects of DES and Home Office interests.

10. Joint Consultative Committees should be given responsibility at local level for ensuring that the particular needs of children receive due priority and attention. They may wish to appoint a standing children's

sub-committee or to consider the matter themselves not less than once a year.

11. Community Health Councils should seek opportunities for discussion with members of the primary care team, if necessary in the practice premises. The proposed Joint Committee for Children should in due course review the effectiveness of these arrangements.

12. The remit of the new children's team of the Health Advisory Service should cover hospital and related services for all children other than the mentally handicapped.

13. CHCs should receive copies of all relevant circulars, reports and memoranda issued by the DHSS.

CHAPTER 17
ORGANISATION AND STAFFING OF PRIMARY CARE

1. To be eligible for appointment as a GPP a doctor will need to have successfully completed a more extensive training in child health than is at present included in most programmes of vocational training for general practice.

2. The RCGP and the BPA should be asked to advise more specifically on the training and experience required, and to consider whether some form of assessment is desirable at the conclusion of training.

3. A GPP will need to have a contract with the AHA for the services he provides in educational medicine for the pupils and teaching staff in specified schools.

4. While there is a case for the GPP having a single contract with the AHA for all his preventive work as a GPP (ie both within the practice and in the school), the number and form of contracts should be left to negotiation between the profession and the Department of Health.

5. In order to practise as a GPP within the practice, a GP should also have a contract with an AHA for the medical services they require to meet the needs of local authority education and social services departments in respect of children. Such contracts should normally be for not less than two sessions a week.

6. As a general rule a GPP should be involved both in developmental medicine within the practice and educational medicine in the community, and this should be the aim in establishing GPP posts.

7. The need for GPP services should be based on an estimated requirement of some eight sessions per week (in term-time) for 3,200 children aged 0–15 inclusive.

8. Each AHA should establish a sub-committee including representatives of the FPC which would have the responsibility for approving GPP posts, so that they meet the criteria proposed.

9. Financial recognition of the extra responsibilities of the GPP will be necessary, but it should be for the Department of Health and the representatives of general practitioners to negotiate how much should be paid and in what way.

10. There should be a minimum of one CHV per 1,600 children aged 0–15, and ideally, one per 1,500.

11. The numbers of child health nurses should grow in parallel with the development of child health visitors. The aim should be to have one wholetime equivalent child health nurse in support of two child health visitors.

12. The equivalent of about 1½ school nurses should be appointed to provide educational nursing services for a school population of 2,200 children aged 5–15.

13. A social worker from the local authority social services department should be nominated to liaise with one or more specified general practices.

14. SCM(CH)s, AN(CH)s and Joint Planning Teams should take steps to identify children living in socially disadvantaged families (and particularly neighbourhoods in which there may be a high concentration of such families) and examine the possibility of improving and supplementing primary health care services for these children.

CHAPTER 18

SUPPORTING CARE

1. The number of consultant paediatricians should be increased to an estimated total of 746, requiring the creation of 353 posts additional to those in 1974.

2. An estimated 203 posts should be for consultant community paediatricians. Until the unity of hospital and community services is achieved, the contract for one of the proposed three consultant paediatricians in an average health district should specify the community component of the work, and the specific commitments to the LEA and LASSD.

3. In order to provide
   (i) essential "resident" paediatric cover to children's and maternity departments,
   (ii) basic paediatric experience for all GPs and longer training for GPPs,
   (iii) paediatric experience for medical graduates during general professional training and especially those intending to go into paediatric surgery, child psychiatry and other allied specialties and the child health component of community medicine,
   (iv) initial training of doctors intending to adopt a career in paediatrics,
   the number of posts at registrar level should be increased by 96 to 300, and at SHO level by 236 to 812.

4. To provide for the proposed increases in consultant paediatricians, including consultant community paediatricians and consultants in the paediatric specialties, the number of paediatric senior registrar posts should be increased by 85 to 182.

5. The specialties of perinatal paediatrics, complex handicap, cardiology, neurology, nephrology, endocrinology, gastro-enterology, haematology, and oncology have developed to the stage at which they should be formally recognised and the necessary consultant and senior training posts provided.

6. The number of consultant posts in the paediatric specialties should be increased, from the present 70 to an overall total of 137.

7. At district level the majority of common surgical problems should be handled by a limited number of adult surgeons, (not less than 2) with a special interest in children's surgery.

8. There should be a ratio of one paediatric surgeon for every 250,000 children, making an increase from the present 25 to 49.

9. All sick children admitted to hospital should be nursed in children's wards and cared for by nurses with special knowledge of their needs and special training to meet them.

10. As an essential condition for making the best use of scarce nursing resources sick children in hospital should be nursed together in children's departments in district hospitals.

11. The level of nurse staffing for children's departments should not be allowed to fall below the minimum levels we have proposed. Within this establishment the first priority should be the appointment of sister/charge nurse with RSCN qualification in charge of each ward.

12. A named senior nurse with RSCN qualification should be responsible for the overall supervision of the children's department.

13. Those State Enrolled Nurses who have spent 12 months or more of their two years with children should be given the opportunity to take, in addition to the general SEN examination, a paediatric examination, with successful candidates having their names entered on a paediatric as well as a general roll.

14. When the new pattern of nurse training is established the rôle of nursery nurses should be reexamined with a view to allowing their training and experience to count towards nurse training.

15. In University and Regional centres there should be a higher ratio of nursing staff (compared with district departments), of not less than 1 nurse to 1 child.

CHAPTER 19

THE TRANSITION TO THE NEW SERVICE

1. GPs should be eligible for accreditation as GPPs without delay if:

    (i) they have had at least 3 years' experience as a principal in general practice;

    (ii) they have had at least 6 months' post registration experience in paediatrics;

    (iii) they agree to undergo training in developmental and educational medicine and the care of handicapped children.

2. Clinical medical officers wishing to enter general practice as GPPs should be eligible for immediate accreditation if:

    (i) they have had a total of 3 years' whole-time equivalent experience in the child and school health services;

    (ii) they have had at least 6 months' post registration experience in paediatrics;

    (iii) they agree to undergo the whole-time equivalent of 1 year as a trainee in general practice; unless they can show that they have had such experience already. They should also attend short courses of training in clinical paediatrics and preventive child health if they have not had such training in the recent past.

3. The profession and the DHSS should seek to negotiate suitable financial arrangements for the situation where clinical medical officers practising as GPPs can only make a part-time contribution to the work of the practice.

4. Clinical doctors not wishing or eligible to be GPPs should work exclusively in the developmental and preventive aspects of child health, including the care of the handicapped, and their new rôle should be recognised by the title child health practitioner.

5. In their clinical preventive work including immediate treatment where necessary, child health practitioners should be responsible for the children they see.

6. Each child health practitioner should be associated with one or two group practices, and have an independent personal professional status within the primary care field.

7. Some senior clinical medical officers should be regarded as eligible to become consultant community paediatricians on the basis of their training and experience in paediatrics, in the care of handicapped children and educational medicine.

8. Senior clinical medical officers who lack sufficient general paediatric training, should be given the opportunity to become eligible for appointment to consultant posts in community paediatrics after successful completion of short intensive training in paediatrics.

9. To take account of the position of senior clinical medical officers who

are not eligible or do not wish to become consultants there should during the period of transition be a specialist career grade in paediatrics, called clinical specialist in paediatrics, carrying responsibilities in both hospital and community that parallel those of consultants.

10. Appointments in the grade of clinical specialist in paediatrics should be "personal" to the doctors concerned and should be made by a special appointment committee.

11. AHAs should be formally asked to review the situation five years from the date of commencement of implementation of our proposals to discover whether additional measures or incentives are needed to accelerate progress.

CHAPTER 20

IMPLICATIONS FOR TRAINING

1. New programmes of training will be needed in many fields but the initial emphasis should be on supplementary training for those who are doing the work at present.

2. Courses for GPs and Clinical Medical Officers wishing to become GPPs should be integrated as far as possible and provided through general practice vocational training schemes.

3. Child health practitioners will need to attend concentrated or day-release courses in clinical paediatrics and preventive child health.

4. CHVs should be registered nurses who have completed a suitably designed post-registration course leading to a Higher Certificate in Health Visiting. Some paediatric nurse-training which would usually be obtained through modules in the training for basic certification and registration would also be required.

5. Health visitors at present in post would need to attend concentrated or day-release courses in paediatric nursing if they wish to become CHVs.

6. AHAs should be required to employ in the child health visiting service only those nurses accredited with post-registration health visitor training or health visitors already qualified.

7. Child health nurses should have obtained their Certificate in Nursing Practice, with experience in paediatric nursing, and taken an option or additional module of training in community nursing.

8. The Council for the Training and Education of Health Visitors (or any educational body who may carry this responsibility in future), in association with the appropriate Teacher Training Body, should be asked to design a course leading to a Higher Certificate in Educational Nursing and to indicate the necessary arrangements for implementing it.

9. Paediatrics should be represented on the Central Council for Postgraduate Medical Education.

10. University Departments of Child Health, working with Departments of Social Medicine, General Practice, Child Psychiatry, Education and Social Work, should initiate or expand post-graduate training programmes for doctors wishing to take up posts as consultant community paediatricians.

11. The Association of Clinical Professors and Heads of Paediatric Departments should be asked to estimate the increase in academic staff required to begin to develop the new pattern of consultant paediatrics and to pursue its implementation with the University Grants Committee.

12. The Specialist Advisory Committee of the Joint Committee on Higher Medical Training should examine with the Royal College of General Practitioners the implementation of their suggested four-year training programme leading to "specialist status", as a framework for GPP and specialist and consultant training, and for clinical specialists in paediatrics.

393

13. Area Nurses (Child Health) should be qualified RSCN and HV in present terms; ultimately, they should have obtained their Higher Certificates in Health Visiting and in Paediatric Nursing.

14. Social workers concerned with handicapped children and children in hospital should be trained first in the care of children and their families.

15. The Specialist Advisory Committee in Paediatrics of the Joint Committee on Higher Medical Training, together with the Women's Medical Federation, should examine the question of realistic part-time training schemes for women in paediatrics, and with the DHSS coordinate these with the development of posts.

16. The contribution of paediatrics to the training of SCM(CH)s should be the subject of joint consultation between the Faculty of Community Medicine, the Royal College of General Practitioners and the British Paediatric Association.

17. The Association of Clinical Professors and Heads of Paediatric Departments, the Specialist Advisory Committee in Paediatrics of the Joint Committee on Higher Medical Training, and the University Grants Committee, should be asked to work out a policy for providing and coordinating a range of training programmes for a variety of medical personnel, and the academic staff that will be required to implement it when the time is opportune.

CHAPTER 21

ADMINISTRATION

1. Joint Consultative Committees should consider how best to ensure that the particular needs of children receive due attention, and in this context they may wish to appoint a sub-committee of members of health and local authorities to advise on the development of services for children.

2. High priority should be given to the establishment of district planning teams for children's services; their remit should include services for mentally ill children and those who are mentally or physically handicapped.

3. The composition of District Planning Teams and Joint Care Planning Teams, when these are concerned with services for children, should always reflect the need to see the provision and operation of these services as a joint exercise involving health, education and social services at every level.

4. The SCM(CH) should be entitled to direct access to the Area Team of Officers on all matters relating to the child health services.

5. In England the SCM(CH) should be responsible for liaison with social services departments of local authorities in all matters relating to the health of children.

6. In Wales the responsibilities of the SCM (Child Health and Special Needs Groups) are too heavy and should be divided between an SCM (CH) and an SCM (Adult Social Services).

7. In multi-district health areas the SCM(CH) should establish a small paediatric advisory group with representation from the constituent districts, and in teaching areas from the Academic Department of Child Health.

8. Where a single division of child health is established within the Cogwheel system its membership should include representatives of other disciplines involved in the health care of children.

9. Child health practitioners who are attached to group practices should be represented on the Local Medical Committee.

10. The Area Nursing Officer's responsibility for providing comprehensive nursing services to local education authorities should be delegated to the Area Nurse (Child Health).

11. The Area Nurse (Child Health) should be entitled to direct access to the Area Team of Officers on all matters relating to nursing aspects of the child health services.

12. The Area Nurse (Child Health) should have delegated to her responsibility for liaison with the social services department of the local authority in nursing matters where social services for children are concerned.

13. With the introduction of a system of child health visitors, Nursing Officers should similarly have responsibility for health visiting services for children and families or for other groups.

14. In addition to their responsibilities for their own group of nurses, Nursing Officers (Child Health Visiting) should have a further responsibility for providing a link with hospital and community services, and for providing advice up the line for a specific feature of nursing services, eg handicapped children.

15. There should always be a senior nurse (of at least Grade 8 of the Salmon Scale) responsible that children's needs are met and understood wherever there are children under hospital care, and she should have the RSCN qualification.

16. The senior nurse (referred to in recommendation 15) should additionally have a responsibility for providing advice on the special needs of sick children to other nursing divisions within the district.

17. The membership of Community Health Councils should include mothers with young children and some younger persons.

18. Health authorities should be able not only to pay travel and subsistence allowances but also to reimburse non-working mothers for financial loss (eg cost of baby-sitters incurred through attendance at CHC meetings).

19. The terms of the Employment Protection Act 1976 should be extended to cover CHC membership.

20. A suitably constituted committee with representatives from the Advisory Committee on Hospital Medical Records, should be set up to consider the question of clinical records for children in hospital and in the community including those under the care of the local authority social services department.

21. The DHSS should consider the introduction and design of a health record book, similar to the Carnet de Santé.

22. The Children's Research Liaison Group should ask the MRC and SSRC to provide an annual statement of those parts of their research programme that are relevant to the needs of children so that there is nationally a comprehensive picture of the work being done in this field.

APPENDIX A

THE COMMITTEE'S METHOD OF WORKING

Appointment and Terms of Reference

On 13 July 1972, the Rt Hon Sir Keith Joseph Bt MP then Secretary of State for Social Services and the Rt Hon Margaret Thatcher MP then Secretary of State for Education and Science announced that, in conjunction with the Rt Hon Peter Thomas QC, MP, Secretary of State for Wales, they had decided to initiate a review of the child health services. In the following year a committee was established with the following terms of reference:—

"To review the provision made for the health services for children, up to and through school life; to study the use made of these services by children and their parents, and to make recommendations."

The membership of the Committee is given on page iii. The first meeting took place in September 1973 and it has met subsequently on 26 occasions including four 3-day residential meetings. On each occasion all or almost all members have been present.

Method of Working

The spirit of a committee is difficult to capture in words. We agreed that we would always try to record what was going well before measuring needs and seeking new remedies. The first three months were an extended introduction in which, through a series of discussion papers, members shared their experience and attitudes. The frankness and good temper of these conversations quickly changed a collection of individuals into a committee. We could then proceed to the next stage in which smaller groups made a detailed analysis of the subject. The natural divisions were seen as: fetal and perinatal health, child development and the advancement of health, children families and society, health for education, dental health, illness, physical and mental handicap, psychiatric disorders, consumer needs, and the organisation of services.

Evidence

At the same time, organisations and individuals were invited through the press to send us facts, observations and advice arising from their experience. In addition letters of invitation were sent to selected organisations. Altogether written evidence was received from 138 organisations and 123 individuals. Some produced reports so rich in information and so well presented that we hope they will be published in full. The Committee also invited representatives of organisations and particular individuals to come and discuss points of special interest in their submissions, together with other queries arising from these.

The written submissions were a useful starting point for the working parties, who went on to gather factual evidence and informed opinion from published sources and in conversation with experienced individuals and the representatives of relevant organisations. Each working party produced a formal report which, after discussion and revision by the Committee, collectively formed the basis of the final Report.

Visits

We did not remain confined to a committee room. Groups of members with the chairman visited group practices, health centres, day nurseries, schools, special schools, district hospitals and University centres in many parts of the country. The places and institutions visited are shown in Appendix C. On every visit we were able to meet, in large and small groups, men and women involved professionally or voluntarily in the care of children and some senior pupils at schools. Brief visits risk being superficial and discourteous, but due to excellent local planning and the provision of local data in advance, they were remarkably informative and left a feeling of wider personal contact and consultation. We record our thanks to the Area Medical Officers and Area Administrators and their staff, to all who showed us their work, and especially to the Specialists in Community Medicine (Child Health) who so often acted as guides and interpreters throughout the visit. They knew that we were looking for success more than failure, for excellence in an established service, or a promising experiment. We were deeply impressed by the many examples of initiative and achievement we found, often in the face of stubborn obstacles and frustrations.

APPENDIX B

ORGANISATIONS AND INDIVIDUALS WHO GAVE EVIDENCE

Organisations

Association for all Speech Impaired Children
Association for Research in Infant and Child Development
Association for Spina Bifida and Hydrocephalus
Association for the Improvement of Maternity Services
Association for the Study of Infectious Disease
Association for the Welfare of Children in Hospital
Association of British Adoption Agencies
Association of British Paediatric Nurses
Association of Child Psychiatrists
Association of Child Psychotherapists
Association of Directors of Social Services
Association of Educational Psychologists
Association of Hospital Management Committees
Association of Workers for Maladjusted Children

Booth Hall Children's Hospital
British Association for Early Childhood Education
British Association for the Study of Community Dentistry
British Association of Occupational Therapists
British Association of Orthodontists
British Association of Orthopaedic Nurses
British Association of Otolaryngologists
British Association of Paediatric Surgeons
British Association of Social Workers
British Dental Association
British Epilepsy Association
British Housewives League
British Medical Association
British Orthopaedic Association
British Orthoptic Society
British Paediatric Association
British Paedodontic Society
British Psychological Society
British Society for the Study of Orthodontics
British Society of Audiology

Camden Social Services Department
Central Council for the Education and Training of Health Visitors
Chartered Society of Physiotherapy
Cheshire Area Health Authority
Child and Family Guidance Clinic, Bristol
Child Guidance Clinic, London Borough of Sutton
Child Poverty Action Group
Childminding Research Unit
Children's Hospital, Birmingham

399

Coeliac Society
College of Speech Therapists
Community Development Project, Upper Afan Valley
Community Relations Commission
Consultant Orthodontists Group
Council for Children's Welfare
Cyd—Bwyllgor Addysg Cymru (Welsh Joint Education Committee)
Cystic Fibrosis Research Unit

Disabled Living Foundation

Employment Medical Advisory Service

Faculty of Dental Surgery, Royal College of Surgeons of England
Faculty of Ophthalmologists
Family Planning Association
Family Service Units
Foundation for the study of Infant Deaths

General Dental Council

Health Education Council
Health Visitors Association
Health Visitors '74
Health Visitors in Huddersfield
Hospital for Sick Children, Great Ormond Street

Inner London Education Authority
Invalid Children's Aid Association
IPC Magazines

Joint Board for Clinical Nursing Studies
Joint Committee of Ophthalmic Opticians
Joint Four

King Edward's Hospital Fund for London

League of Jewish Women
Liverpool Community Development Project

Maternity Infant Care Association
Medical Officers of Schools Association
Medical Sociology Research Centre, University College of Swansea
Medical Women's Federation
Mothers in Action
Mothers Union
Mudiad Ysgolion Meithrin (National Association of Welsh Medium Nursery
    Schools and Playgroups)
Muscular Dystrophy Group of Great Britain

National Association for Deaf, Blind and Rubella Children
National Association for Gifted Children
National Association for Maternal and Child Welfare
National Association for Mental Health
National Association for the Prevention of Cruelty to Children

National Association for the Welfare of Children in Hospital
National Association of Certificated Nursery Nurses
National Association of Chief and Principal Nursing Officers
National Association of Counsellors in Education
National Association of Head Teachers
National Association of Nursery Matrons
National Association of Probation Officers
National Association of School Masters
National Children's Bureau
National College of Teachers of the Deaf
National Council for the Divorced and Separated
National Council for Special Education
National Council of Women of Great Britain
National Deaf Children's Society
National Federation of Women's Institutes
National Housewives Register
National Marriage Guidance Council
National Union of School Students
National Union of Teachers
Northwick Park Hospital

One Parent Families Association

Paediatricians at the London Hospital
Paediatric Pathology Society
Patients Association
Portsmouth Community Child Health Services
Pre-school Playgroups Association

Royal College of General Practitioners
Royal College of Midwives
Royal College of Nursing
Royal College of Obstetricians and Gynaecologists
Royal College of Psychiatrists
Royal College of Physicians
Royal National Institute for the Blind
Royal National Throat, Nose and Ear Hospital
Royal Victoria Infirmary, Newcastle upon Tyne

Salvation Army
Scottish Home and Health Department
Society of Chief Nursing Officers (Public Health)
Society of Community Medicine
Soroptomist International
Spastics Society
Standing Conference of Representatives of Health Visitor Training Centres
Surrey Education Authority

Totnes Action Group for Handicapped Children

Undeb Cenedlaethol Athrawon Cymru (National Associaton of the Teachers of Wales)
University of Birmingham (Dept of Dental Health)

Wales Council for the Disabled
Westminster Childrens Hospital
Whittingham Hospital (Dept of Psychiatry for the Deaf)
Women's National Commission
Women's Royal Voluntary Service
Young People's Unit, East Cheshire HMC

Individuals

Mrs G Adamson
Mr R Astley
Dr C M Atkins
Professor C F Ballard
Dr F N Bamford
Dr M C Bax
Dr J Beale
Mr R Bettles
Dr J A Black
Miss A G Brenton
Dr F S W Brimblecombe
Dr A R Buchan
Professor N Butler
Mr C L Carmichael
Dr A Cartwright
Mr J Charlton
Dr I Chesham
Dr N J Cook
Dr J Corbett
Dr C M Cowan
Mr D Cruse
Mr H Colin Davis
Miss J Davis
Dr J A Davis
Dr K S Deas
Mrs P Dickinson
Mr G Dickson
Dr S Dische
Mr J Dixon
Mr T B Dowell
Mr M C Downer
Dr M Eastwood
Dr P R Evans
Mrs M la Frenais
Dr D Garrow
Professor P Graham
Dr R Graham
Dr D J Pereira Gray
Dr N Gordon
Mr A Green

Dr J Grubb
Dr I Hadfield
Miss D Harding
Dr D Harvey
Professor P M Higgins
Mr J H Hovell
Mr B M Howell
Dr A G Ironside
Dr F E James
Professor P M C James
Dr M J Jameson
Mrs A Jones
Rev Erastus Jones
Dr P Jones
Mrs M Kay
Dr C W Kesson
Professor E G Knox
Dr R Lansdown
Dr R K Levick
Dr A Little
Mr C MacFarlane
Dr R MacKeith
Dr R B McGucken
Dr D W McLean
Miss C McLoughlin
Dr J P Maher
Dr B K Mandal
Lady Marre
Mr P Mellor
Dr E Midwinter
Professor R G Mitchell
Dr G A Neligan
Dr E Newson
Dr A P Norman
Mr D H Norman
Dr C H Nourse
Mrs B O'Neill
Miss M Oswin
Mr J W Owen
Mrs J Page
Mr J D Palmer
Professor J Pemberton
Mrs P Phillips
Dr M Pollak
Miss J Pollitt
Mr L Power
Dr I Radford
Dr M Radford
Dr A S Raikes
Dr T A Ratcliffe

Dr B Ricks
Dr D M Ricks
Mr R Ritchie
Mr C D Roberts
Mrs A E Robinson
Dr L W Robinson
Miss P M Scarborough
Mr J E Scott
Dr B E Shortland
Dr M J Simkiss
Dr G Simon
Dr C Simpson Smith
Professor G L Slack
Professor M Stacey
Dr G D Starke
Dr G M Steiner
Dr H Steiner
Dr W J Stephen
Mr F H Stewart
Professor A Summerfield
Mr H Taylor
Professor I G Taylor
Dr F G Thorpe
Dr P Tiplady†
Mrs A Tomkins
Mr K G Tucker
Dr J Tudor-Hart
Professor W J Tulley
Mr G Turner
Mrs C M Valentine
Professor J H Walker
Dr R Walters
Dr E M Wallis
Dr A Heaton Ward
Dr T J Watson
Dr P G Whitfield
Dr L Wing
Professor G B Winter
Mr A Wynn
Mrs M Wynn
Dame Eileen Younghusband
Mr W Yule

† On behalf of a group of school doctors.

APPENDIX C

VISITS MADE BY THE COMMITTEE

BIRMINGHAM AREA HEALTH AUTHORITY (TEACHING)

Canterbury House Central School Health Clinic
Children's Hospital and Regional Child Assessment Centre
Paediatric Home Nursing Scheme

BRADFORD AREA HEALTH AUTHORITY

Bradford Children's Hospital Handicapped Assessment Unit
Green Lane Child Health Clinic
General Practice, Drs Quershi and Mir
Manor Row Central School Clinic
Odsal House School for the Deaf and Partially Hearing
Westwood Hospital School for the Mentally Handicapped

CAMDEN AND ISLINGTON AREA HEALTH AUTHORITY (TEACHING)

Accommodation for Homeless Families (Holloway Road)
University College Hospital, Neonatal Intensive Care Unit
Kentish Town Health Centre

DEVON AREA HEALTH AUTHORITY

Honeylands Short Term Day and Residential Unit for Handicapped Children
Paediatric Research Unit
Special Care Baby Unit
Royal Devon and Exeter Hospital

EALING, HAMMERSMITH AND HOUNSLOW AREA HEALTH AUTHORITY (TEACHING)

Heston Audiology Clinic
Martindale School for the Physically Handicapped
Child Development Research Project

GATESHEAD AREA HEALTH AUTHORITY

High Fell Special School for the Severely Mentally Handicapped
Percy Hedley School, Hostel and Sheltered Workshop
Queen Elizabeth Hospital, Children's Department
Rawling Road Day Nursery and Assessment Unit
Wickham General Practice Health Centre
Experimental Paediatric Home Nursing

HAMPSHIRE AREA HEALTH AUTHORITY (TEACHING)

Aldermoor Health Centre, University Teaching General Practice
Hamptun Youth Advisory and Self-Referral Centre
Heathfield Special School, Fareham
Miltonford School, Portsmouth
Moorhill Comprehensive Secondary School, Southampton
Regional Subnormality Unit

405

Southampton Children's Hospital (Bursledon Annexe) for Chronic Illness and Handicap
Southampton General Hospital Day Admission Ward
The Wessex Child Psychiatry Unit

HERTFORDSHIRE AREA HEALTH AUTHORITY
Harpenden Memorial Hospital
Leavesden Hospital

HUMBERSIDE AREA HEALTH AUTHORITY
Hessle Health Centre
Hull Child Guidance Centre
Royal Infirmary, Hull, Children's Department
School Dental Clinic
Maternity Hospital Special Care Baby Unit

LAMBETH, SOUTHWARK AND LEWISHAM AREA HEALTH AUTHORITY (TEACHING)
Angell Pre-school Playgroup
Kings College Hospital Neonatal Intensive Care Unit
Lilly Davis Special Playgroup for the Physically and Socially Handicapped
Loughborough Health Clinic—Centre for the Study of Local Needs, Experimental Service and Health Education in Brixton

NEWCASTLE-UPON-TYNE AREA HEALTH AUTHORITY (TEACHING)
The Mother and Babies' Hospital
Feversham Residential School for Maladjusted Children
Fleming Memorial Hospital, Paediatric Surgery Department
Nuffield Child Psychiatry Unit
Pendower Hall Special School for Physically Handicapped Children
Royal Victoria Infirmary
The Victoria School for the Blind

SHEFFIELD AREA HEALTH AUTHORITY (TEACHING)
Charles Clifford Dental Hospital, Children's Department
Chaucer Comprehensive School
Ecclesfield Health Centre
Jessop Hospital for Women, The Teaching Maternity Hospital
Northern General Hospital, Adolescent Paediatric Unit
Ryegate Assessment Centre for the Handicapped
Sheffield Children's Hospital, Wards and A and E Department
Shirle Hill Child Psychiatric Unit
St Joseph's Hospital for Mentally Handicapped Children

THE HOSPITAL FOR SICK CHILDREN, GT ORMOND STREET.
NEW CROSS SCHOOL FOR DENTAL AUXILIARIES
WALES
Dr Barnardo's Day Nursery, Ely, Cardiff
Erw'r Delyn School for the Physically Handicapped, Penarth
Fairwater Health Centre

406

Llandough Hospital, Children's Department
Llanedeyrn University Teaching Health Centre
Merthyr Hospital Children's Department
Penarth School for the Deaf
Preswylfa Child and Family Centre and Nursery School, Cardiff
University Hospital of Wales Children's Department

SCOTLAND
Craigshill Health Centre, Livingston
Royal Hospital for Sick Children, Yorkhill, Glasgow
Scottish Home and Health Department
Woodside Health Centre, Glasgow

APPENDIX D

THE WORK OF A LOCAL AUTHORITY'S CHILD
AND SCHOOL SERVICES

TABLE 1

Survey of the Work of Health Visitors in the Community Child Health Clinics of Newcastle upon Tyne during a Two-week Period in June 1973: Reasons Given by 1,093 Mothers for Visiting the Clinic

Reasons Given for Visiting the Clinic	Number of Children Age Group (months)					% of all 1,093 children
	0–6	7–12	13–24	24+	Total	
For weighing*	447	219	107	64	837	77
Feeding advice	162	54	13	7	236	22
For a birthday check	—	17	41	39	97	17†
For advice about a medical problem	83	44	28	21	176	16
For immunisation††	28	36	39	51	154	14
For advice about growth and/or development	38	16	20	22	96	9
To buy food or vitamins	9	3	—	3	15	1.4
For advice about a social problem	3	4	2	4	13	1
For advice about a maternal problem (eg anxiety, depression)	6	5	2	—	13	1
To play in playgroup	—	—	—	4	4	0.4
For advice about family planning	3	4	3	—	10	0.9
Miscellaneous	13	12	7	4	36	3

* This provides an opportunity for discussion about the child's growth and development, during which reassurance and advice is often given by the health visitor.

† Out of a total of 579 children aged over 6 months.

†† These children had for various reasons not been immunised at the regular monthly immunisation sessions held in the clinics.

Note. More than one reason was often given.

TABLE 2

Survey of the Work of Medical Officers in the Community Child Health Clinics of Newcastle upon Tyne during a Two-week Period in March 1973: Reasons Given by 343 Mothers for Consulting Clinic Doctor

Reasons Given for Consulting the Clinic Doctor	No of Children Age Group (months)					% of all 343 Children
	0–3	4–12	13–24	24+	Total	
Birthday check	—	23	31	28	82	41*
For a health check	70	11	—	—	81	24
Skin problem	21	18	7	6	52	15
Immunisation†	1	13	19	12	45	13
Respiratory infection	11	16	5	5	37	11
Feeding problem	16	12	3	1	32	9
Vomiting and/or diarrhoea	9	5	6	6	26	8
Eye problem	3	4	4	1	12	4
Orthopaedic problem	1	1	5	4	11	3
Behaviour problem	—	2	2	7	11	3
Developmental problem	—	3	2	1	6	2
Social problem	—	4		3	7	2
Maternal problem (eg anxiety, depression)	5	1	—	—	6	2
Speech problem	—	—	—	—	4	1
Miscellaneous	19	17	8	3	47	14

* Percentage of 200 children aged over 6 months.

† These children had not been immunised at the regular monthly sessions.

Note. More than one reason was often given.

Taken from: Steiner, H (1975). Paediatrics in hospital and community in Newcastle upon Tyne. In: *Bridging in Health,* ed: Brimblecombe, F S W *et al.* Oxford University Press for Nuffield Provincial Hospitals Trust.

TABLE 3

Fresh Defects Found at School Entry Examination in a Sample Study of 1,255 Children Born in Newcastle upon Tyne During 1960

Type of disorder	Total	Referred to hospital at 5 years	Total clinically significant	Clinically significant %
Nose, throat and otitis media	174	29	77	44.30
Vision and squint	56	3	52	92.86
Orthopaedic	79	11	41	51.90
Skin	56	1	17	30.36
Speech	48	0	39	81.25
Enuresis	44	2	12	27.27
Chests	37	2	13	35.14
Hearing	31	1	25	80.65
Undescended testis	33	1	24	72.73
Behaviour	23	0	5	21.74
Heart murmur	16	5	8	50.0
Fits and epilepsy	7	1	1	14.29
Others	70	2	25	35.71
Total	674	58	339	50.29

Taken from: Lowden, G M, and Walker, J H (1975). The School Health Service and the School Doctor. In: *Bridging in Health,* ed: Brimblecombe, F S W *et al.* Oxford University Press for Nuffield Provincial Hospitals Trust.

Tables reproduced by permission of the Oxford University Press.

APPENDIX E

THE SCOPE AND RESPONSIBILITIES OF THE
SCHOOL HEALTH SERVICE

1. The School Health Service, including the school nursing service, was first established in 1907. The early origins of the service, its changing pattern especially following the introduction of the National Health Service in 1948 and the implementation of the Education Act 1944, and the scope, organisation and structure of the service in the years just prior to the reorganisation of the NHS in 1974, have been described fully in three official publications of the Department of Education and Science (Plowden Report—1967 Appendix 2; the First Report of School Health Service sub-committee of the Working Party on Collaboration 1973; and The School Health Service 1908–1974, published in 1975).

2. In short the services provide:

regular tests of vision and hearing;

as often as necessary, medical examinations to supervise the health of pupils, especially in relation to:

their education in school

their need for free milk between the ages 7–12 years

their medical fitness to participate in work-experience schemes before leaving school

their medical fitness to undertake employment outside school hours or to take part in public entertainment performances;

as often as necessary, hygiene inspections combining health education and cleanliness inspections, and any consequent disinfestation;

a programme of immunisation and vaccination as necessary; advice to parents, teachers and LEAs on the nature and extent of any handicap on account of which a pupil might need special education or of any medical condition significant for the child's care in school;

supervision of the health care of such children, whether they attend ordinary or special schools;

participation of doctors and nurses in health education in school; medical examination of teachers, school meals and other staff on taking up posts in the education services;

and oversight of features of the school environment that may affect the health of pupils, eg standards of lighting, heating and hygiene of premises, especially school kitchens.

3. The NHS Re-organisation Act 1973 brought together responsibilities for Local Authority health services for the pre-school child, for the medical and dental inspection and treatment of school children and for the services for children provided by general medical and dental practitioners and hospital and specialist services, under the Area Health Authorities, with the object of establishing a comprehensive range of integrated health services for children.

4. The Act made Area Health Authorities responsible for providing staff and services needed by Education Authorities for their responsibilities for

    (a) Handicapped pupils under Sections 33 and 34 of the Education Act 1944.

    (b) Certain miscellaneous functions for which they require advice and/or action by a medical officer such as the powers to ensure cleanliness, medical advice on the employment of children, medical supervision of entrants to teacher training etc.

5. Area Health Authorities were made responsible for medical and dental inspections and treatment and Section 3 of the NHS Re-organisation Act 1973 states that "It shall be the duty of the Secretary of State to make provision for the medical and dental inspection at appropriate intervals of pupils in attendance at schools maintained by Local Education Authorities and for the medical and dental treatment of such pupils".

6. DHSS Circular HRC(74)5 sets out in Annexes 1 and 2 the miscellaneous functions of LEAs for which they require advice and/or action by a medical officer.

7. NHS Re-Organisation Circular HRC (74)5 on the child health services, including school health services, and DES Circular 1/74 stress the need for Area Health Authorities and matching Local Education Authorities to work closely together and Section 5 of the DHSS Circular described the medical, dental and nurse staffing arrangements needed to be made by the AHA in conjunction with its matching LEA for the child health services, including the school health services in order to provide for

    (a) Organisation and planning of all child health services for the AHA.

    (b) Advice to the LEA and executive responsibility for certain services.

    (c) Advice about child health services to the Joint Consultative Committee (composed of members of the AHA and the LEA and meeting regularly) and participation of the joint planning of Associated Services provided by the AHA and LEA.

These responsibilities were set out in detail in Annex 3 of the circular.

8. The staff at Area Health Headquarters required to discharge the responsibilities set out above included a Specialist in Community Medicine (Child Health), a Senior Dental Officer (who the circular thought would usually be the Area Dental Officer but might on occasions be one of the senior members of the staff) and a Senior Nurse. These appointments are made by the AHA in agreement with the matching LEA.

9. The Area Medical Officer carries responsibility for coordinating child health services including the school health services. The Specialist in Community Medicine (Child Health), is accountable through the Area Medical Officer to the AHA for the functions described in Annex 3A 1.1, his NHS responsibilities, but is directly accountable to the LEA for the functions in Annex 3A 1.2, his education responsibilities. It should be noted that this in-

cludes providing advice and having executive responsibility in relation to the LEA on the health aspects of its functions and that among other matters it is a duty of the Specialist in Community Medicine (Child Health) to ensure that the medical and other necessary health services staff are available for the LEA's functions under Sections 33 and 34 of the Education Act 1944.

10. The Circular HRC(74)5 states that the Area Nurse (Child Health) will have responsibility in consultation with the LEA for the nursing aspects of child health (including school health) and that in collaboration with the District Nursing Officers will have direct management control of nurses and nurse managers in the field of school health.

11. The Area Dental Officer is directly accountable to the AHA for the child dental services.

12. Where certain responsibilities or functions for child health services are allocated to a District Community Physician, the DHSS circular emphasises that he must for these functions accept accountability to the Specialist in Community Medicine (Child Health) at AHA headquarters.

APPENDIX F

AT RISK REGISTERS

Extract from the Report of The Working Group on Risk Registers
(chairman: Professor T. Oppé), Paragraphs 9-16.1

The Child at Risk

9. It is known that handicapping conditions do not occur at random through-out the child population, and that some children do have a greater risk of inheriting or acquiring a potentially handicapping condition. We will now review this general concept of the child "at risk" and in particular its application to registers maintained by health authorities.

10. Statistical associations, not necessarily of a causal nature, exist between the occurrence of defects giving rise to handicaps, and definable adverse events before, during and after birth. Some of these events such as maternal rubella have a specific relationship with a particular disability or group of defects, but most adverse factors have only an ill-defined association with a variety of defects.

11. Doctors, with great advantage, use significant, or supposedly significant factors in their patients' histories to assist in diagnosis, but it is only recently that such factors have been used predictively in selecting individuals or groups of individuals for deliberate follow-up. It is therefore reasonable to apply the term "at risk" to an individual or to groups who can be predicted, on present information, to be more likely to fall victim to a particular disease or injury. It is only in the last decade or so that attention has been paid to the organisation of administrative schemes to assist doctors and health visitors in providing surveillance for children thought to be most in need of it. It is our task to examine such administrative schemes, to assess the theoretical assumptions on which they are based and their operational effectiveness.

Brief Historical Review of Risk Registers

12. Lindon (1961) was the first to propose registration by local health authorities of children "at risk": he found that many children with defects were being diagnosed too late for treatment to be fully effective. He considered three possible methods of early detection – symptomatic, total population screening and screening of an "at risk" group. As the first method was proving inade-quate and the second depended on resources which were not available, Lindon concluded that a Risk Register would be an immediate and practical addition to the existing symptomatic method of detection. He emphasised that in the absence of total population screening at least 30% of handi-capping conditions were unlikely to be found by the remaining two methods. If resources were largely concentrated on 20% of the infant population, roughly 70% of defects could be detected early. Shortly afterwards, Sheridan's well-known article amplifying the principles and categories of risk factors was published in the Monthly Bulletin of the then Ministry of Health and the Public Health Laboratory Service (December 1962, Vol 21 Section 1). Before research studies or any operational evaluation had been

413

made, the majority of Medical Officers of Health had established schemes for the maintenance of Risk Registers, in the main basing their categories of risk upon Sheridan's guidelines.

13. The organisation and use of Risk Registers has proved difficult. Frequently mentioned problems have been the lack of precise definition for some of the risk factors, difficulty in obtaining complete obstetric information, neglect of social factors, the risk of ignoring children not on the Register and of causing unjustified anxiety among mothers of those who were on the Register. Furthermore, strict and uncritical application of risk factors, when combined with a high standard of reporting, led to large numbers of infants being included on Risk Registers. Overall, the proportion of handicapped children found to be already on Risk Registers was disappointingly small and a large number of handicapped children appeared from those who were not.

14. Hughes (1964) suggested revision of the commonly used risk factors, to eliminate the less reliable ones and so reduce the size of Registers and increase their effectiveness. Decreasing the number of risk factors did reduce the size of Registers, but also led to a greater proportion of handicapped children eventually being found in the not "at risk" category (Rogers 1967). Local health authorities tried to solve the various problems in their own ways. Discrepancies were revealed when Oppé (1967) sought information from 66 authorities: he found that some had abandoned the attempt to maintain a Register and the remainder were dealing with different "at risk" populations according to individual interpretations of "risk" and selection of infants. Few had succeeded in making satisfactory, systematic follow-up arrangements. It was disappointing that this study revealed no factual information about the effectiveness of Risk Registers in expediting the detection of handicapping disorders in the pre- or early symptomatic stage. That Risk Registers were not in practice fulfilling their aim was also shown by Hamilton *et al* (1968) and Knox and Mahon (1971).

15. Richards and Roberts (1967) criticised the theory of Risk Registers and concluded that the early detection of all handicapping conditions could be achieved only by examinations of all neonates, prescriptive screening for metabolic and auditory defects, and careful serial observation of every infant's developmental progress. Other studies (Rogers 1968, Thomas 1968), showed that it is not yet possible to achieve good discrimination between a small group among which nearly all defects and disabilities will occur and on which resources should be concentrated, and a larger one in which few, if any, handicaps will arise. Butler (1969) concluded from analysis of data from the National Child Development Study that the majority of individual pregnancy and labour risk factors, commonly used as items for entering an infant on the Risk Register were poor predictors. However, a small number of such factors appeared to be better predictors when combined with each other, or when used together with other factors – birth order and socio-economic background being important. Utilising the same data, Alberman and Goldstein (1970) produced statistical evidence that, given restricted resources, optimum detection would be achieved by their differential allocation to groups of high and low risk, and that the value of such an approach is greater in areas where the existing detection rate is low, and vice versa.

DHSS Survey of Risk Registers

16.1 A survey of practice with regard to Risk Registers was undertaken by the Department of Health and Social Security among 12 local health authorities in 1969–70, and the results confirmed the practical difficulties and theoretical objections previously mentioned.

Alberman, E D, and Goldstein, H (1970). *British Journal of Preventive and Social Medicine* 24, 129.
Butler, N (1969). *Concern,* No 3, 8.
Hamilton, F M W, *et al* (1968). *Medical Officer.* 119, 201.
Hughes, E (1964). *Practitioner.* 192, 534.
Knox, E G, and Mahon, D F (1970). *Archives of Disease in Childhood.* 45, 634.
Lindon, R L (1961). *Cerebral Palsy Bulletin.* 3, 481.
Oppé, T E (1967). *Developmental Medicine and Child Neurology.* 9, 13.
Richards, I D G, and Roberts, C J (1967). *Lancet.* ii, 711.
Rogers, M G H (1967). *Medical Officer.* 118, 253.
Rogers, M G H (1968). *Developmental Medicine and Child Neurology.* 10, 651.
Sheridan, M D (1962). *Monthly Bulletin of the Ministry of Health and the Public Health Laboratory Service.* 21, 238.
Thomas, G E (1968). *Medical Officer.* 120, 162, 177, 191, 208.

SURVEY OF FIFTH AND SIXTH FORM ATTITUDES

In the Autumn 1974, nine secondary schools in Cheshire and another nine in Devon, Surrey, Gloucestershire, Cambridge, Nottingham, Birmingham, Sheffield and Westmorland, were visited and enquiries made of samples of children in either Vth or VIth forms as to their knowledge of the health services and their views regarding changes in these, especially in the school health services.

The procedure was for the headteacher to be asked to invite a group of adolescents to meet the person carrying out the enquiry; in Cheshire this was a senior member of the education advisory staff and in the other schools it was a doctor from the Department of Education and Science. The purpose of the enquiry was explained, and the students then asked to fill in a short questionnaire. They were asked to put the name of their school at the top but no personal identification was required. A group discussion was then held for the remainder of the session, approximately 45 minutes, on themes arising from the questionnaire and their response to it.

The schools included secondary modern, grammar and comprehensive schools, in both rural and urban (inner city) areas.

The data has been set out in four tables showing: awareness of the names of their family doctor and school doctor, and whether they had been seen by either during the last 12 months; their experience of hospital services; whether they enjoy watching films or television programmes about doctors and nurses, and if so, whether such viewing makes their own hospital experience less worrying; and finally, their response to some suggestions about changes in the customary school health service procedures. The figures in the tables have been rounded to the nearest whole number; they are therefore approximate, and they have not been treated statistically for significance. 573 pupils completed a questionnaire and differences were looked for between the replies of boys and girls, Vth and VIth form pupils and pupils in urban and rural schools.

TABLE I

90% of the children knew the name of their family doctor; there were no marked differences between the two groups in each of the three sub-samples.

60% had actually visited their GP during the year (1974); girls were much more likely to have done so than boys, and pupils in urban schools rather more than those in rural schools.

In contrast, only 3% knew the name of their school doctor, although 10% of the girls knew this doctor. 2% had been seen by the school doctor for personal reasons and 3% had similarly been seen by the school nurse. Many others had been seen by the school doctor or nurse at routine age-specific inspections but no importance can be attached to differences between the sub-sample groups since such routine inspections randomly reflect the policy of the authority concerned and not the needs of the pupils personally.

TABLE II

Three out of every four children remember attending hospital at one time or another during their school years; some attended more than one department:

38% attended an accident and emergency department

41% attended an out-patient department

41% were admitted to the wards

Girls were much more likely than boys to have been admitted as an in-patient; nearly two-thirds of admissions were for operation, 20% were for the treatment of accidents and 17% for illnesses. Again, the sex differences were the most marked: 80% of the boys' admissions were for operation but only 5% were for illness, whilst accidents were less often a cause for the admission of a girl than a boy.

With regard to visiting, four out of five pupils who were in-patients were visited by some person, almost invariably their parents; if they were not visited this was usually because of a very short period of admission. Visiting was as often as three or more times a week as it was confined to visiting hours; girls more often reported being visited three or more times a week than boys, and so did pupils from VIth forms compared with those from Vth forms. A little over one-third were visited by friends, but boys less often saw their friends (one in five).

TABLE III

43% of the children enjoyed watching films and television programmes about doctors, nurses and hospitals, but just as many were indifferent to such viewing. There were some differences in respect of sex and age-group: girls and Vth form pupils enjoyed them more whereas boys and VIth formers were more inclined to be indifferent to such programmes or to frankly not enjoy them.

Of the 410 pupils who watch such programmes *and* remember having been to hospital for any reason (not necessarily as an in-patient), 41% did not think their viewing had made their hospital experiences less worrying and just as many were uncertain; only a minority (18%) found them helpful, and more of this group were boys than girls. 55% of girls did not find these films and TV programmes helpful in dealing with their hospital experience.

TABLE IV

Five suggested changes in the school health service were put to the pupils to comment on; they were asked if these sounded helpful or not. About one in five were not sure about any of the suggestions.

44% thought it would be helpful if the school doctor visited the schools more frequently, although boys and pupils in rural schools were least enthusiastic for this.

They were equally divided about more frequent visits from the school nurse, 38% thinking this might be helpful and the same proportion doubting this. Boys were again least enthusiastic about this suggestion.

Half (56%) of the pupils welcomed the suggestion that the doctor and nurse might take more part in teaching human biology and personal development; boys were the least interested in this but pupils in rural schools were very keen.

Three-quarters (72%) of the pupils would have liked the school doctor to hold a clinic in the school when health or personal problems could be discussed privately and in confidence but only half the boys and rural school pupils were in favour of this.

Two-thirds of the pupils did not want their GP to be the school doctor and girls, VIth formers and pupils in urban schools were even more emphatic about this (between 72–78% of each group answering "no" to this question).

TABLE I
Pupils who Knew Their GP and SMO, and Used Their Services

%	All Pupils N–573	Boys N–62	Girls N–63	V Form N–339	VI Form N–120	Urban N–112	Rural N–159
Q 1 Knew name of GP	90	85	93	90	89	90	90
Q 2 Visited GP this year	61	42	75	62	60	74	60
Q 6 Knew name of SMO	3	5	10	5	nil	5	5
Q 8b Seen by SMO for special problem	2						
Q 9b Seen by school nurse for special problem	3						

TABLE II
Experience of Hospital Services

%	All	Boys	Girls	V Form	VI Form	Urban	Rural
Q 3 Remember attending hospital N–410	73	74	74	69	78	73	60
Q 3c Remember being admitted to Ward	41	31	54	42	46	38	40
Of those admitted to Ward N–235:							
Q 5a for accident	20	20	12	18	20	16	18
for illness	17	5	21	13	22	14	18
for operation	63	80	66	67	59	72	60
Q 5c Visited more than three times per week	46	50	60	43	60	42	41
Visited by friends	35	20	30	35	44	42	36

Table III

Effect of Doctor/Nurse Films or Television Programmes on Hospital Experience

%	All	Boys	Girls	V Form	VI Form	Urban	Rural
Q 11 Enjoy such programmes	43	22	50	50	33	52	44
Don't enjoy such programmes	13	23	5	8	17	13	17
Indifferent to such programmes	43	55	45	42	50	35	43
Of those who watch such programmes AND remember attending hospital: N–410							
Q 12 Such programmes did make hospital less worrying	18	31	23	21	10	13	10
Such programmes did not make hospital less worrying	41	19	55	40	40	35	40
Not sure	41	50	22	39	50	52	60

Table IV

Suggested Changes in School Health Service

%		All	Boys	Girls	V Form	VI Form	Urban	Rural
Q 13a Want SMO to visit more frequently	Yes	44	30	40	43	32	45	28
	No	31	40	43	28	45	34	30
	Not sure	25	30	17	29	23	21	42
Q 13b Want SN to visit more frequently	Yes	38	19	44	40	30	43	28
	No	38	50	38	31	50	31	36
	Not sure	24	31	20	29	20	26	36
Q 13c Want more teaching from SMO and SN	Yes	56	34	63	57	50	54	70
	No	26	32	25	24	30	34	10
	Not sure	18	34	12	19	20	12	20
Q 13d Want SMO to hold personal clinic	Yes	72	54	72	75	72	74	50
	No	13	23	18	9	20	18	8
	Not sure	15	23	10	16	8	8	12
Q 13e Want GP to be the SMO	Yes	13	14	10	15	12	11	17
	No	67	62	72	67	75	78	56
	Not sure	20	24	18	18	13	11	27

419

Comment

The following broad conclusions emerge from this data and from the inspectors' and doctors' reports of their discussions in the schools:

1. *The curative health services have some meaning for almost all V- and VI-form pupils.* They usually know their family doctor and a majority of them have visited him during any year. Very many of them have attended hospital for one reason or another during their school years and recollect the experience. Their chief criticism of the service is of the long wait in surgeries and out-patients' departments of hospitals for what is eventually a very brief interview or examination by the doctor.

2. *The preventive school health service means very little if anything to them.* They rarely know the school doctor by name and they have only the vaguest idea of the purpose of the service. Infrequent visits and constant changes of doctor (at least seven school doctors visited one rural school during the last five years) certainly contributes to their not knowing the name of the school doctor but many of these pupils will have had an interview if not an examination by a doctor during their fourth year in the secondary school. A number of them, when asked, did not know how they would contact the school doctor if they had wanted to but they could not imagine why they should ever want to. It was exceedingly rare for any of them to have asked to see the doctor and clearly he was not regarded as a source of help or advice. VI-formers in one school recognised its usefulness in detecting visual or hearing defects; in another several pupils asked whether the service was concerned with anything other than "flat feet and eyes". At a third group discussion it was considered that only doctors of the poorest quality worked in the school health service.

3. *There was a general feeling that neither family doctors nor school doctors communicate effectively with them, and that neither have time to discuss health and personal problems in the depth they would like.* Family doctors "don't talk to you" or they "talk to your parents in front of you as though you didn't exist". As a consequence of the family doctor seeming to be so busy and the school doctor visiting so infrequently they generally attributed the lack of time to talk to them to overwork.

4. *A large proportion of the pupils were in favour of a doctor holding clinics to which they could go for personal health advice and counselling.* This is clear from their replies to Question 13d (table IV) but it was equally evident from the reports of the discussions. The data and discussions also showed they would welcome a more prominent medical contribution to health education in school, particularly in relation to sexual relationships, venereal disease and drug-taking. However, from the reports of the discussions there is some reason to suspect that this is but another reflection of their desire for more personal and confidential advice to be available; some pupils specifically said they would welcome this from professionals with a wider specialist knowledge than teachers could possibly have.

420

5. *There was less agreement as to which kind of doctor should attend such clinics and where they should be held.* Some of these adolescents would prefer that their family doctor should be more readily (and leisurely) available for health advice but others were worried that the GP would not fully respect their confidence because he was the family doctor and knew the parents. In fact, a majority did not see the GP staffing such clinics and taking part in health education in school; rather, they wanted an independent (school) doctor to do this, although some concern was expressed lest the school doctor be too closely associated with the teachers and school authorities. At several discussions the suggestion was made (usually from personal experience) that these difficulties could be overcome by such advisory clinics being provided off the school premises.

6. *In schools where a nurse had been established full-time, it was clear that she had met some, but by no means all, of the demand for a personal advisory service.* The school nurse was not always free from criticism: she was seen by some as a purveyor of aspirin (as one boy remarked "even if your head fell off, you'd still get an aspirin") and by others as a head-inspector. But in general she was welcomed not only to dispense aspirin but also to give confidential advice about medical and personal matters.

7. *There was a general call for more information – especially through the press and television – about the services that are available for health care.* Their greatest difficulty was in knowing what they could reasonably expect of the health services.

ENQUIRY OF VIth FORM STUDENTS School: ....

HEALTH SERVICES DURING THE
SCHOOL YEARS LEA: ....

Please put a circle round the answer that applies, unless a written answer is required.

1. What is the name of your family
   doctor? Dr ..../don't know

2. Have you visited him this year
   (1974)? Yes/No

3. Do you remember being a patient:
   (a) in a hospital accident or casualty department? Yes (Year 19......)/No
   (b) in an out-patient department? Yes (Year 19......)/No
   (c) admitted to a ward? Yes (Year 19......)/No

4. Nobody likes being in hospital but
   if you remember being in any
   department mentioned in Question
   3:
   (a) did the doctor explain what
   was going to happen and why? Yes/No/Don't remember
   (b) were the nurses friendly and
   helpful? Yes/No/Don't remember

5. If you remember being admitted to
   a ward?
   (a) was it for an– Accident/Illness/Operation
   (b) were you visited– on visiting days only
   or/ more than three times a week

   (c) were you visited:
   by your parents? Yes/No
   by your brothers and sisters? Yes/No
   by friends? Yes/No

6. What is the name of your school
   doctor? Dr ..../don't know

7. When did you last seem him (her)? Year 19....../don't remember

8. If you remember seeing him (her),
   was this:
   (a) as part of a general examination
   of all pupils in the form? Yes/No
   (b) for a special problem of your
   own? Yes/No

9. Have you been to the school nurse
   this year (1974)? Yes/No

10. If you have been to the school nurse
    this year, was this:
    (a) as part of a general inspection
        of all pupils in the form?   Yes/No
    (b) for a special problem of your
        own?   Yes/No

11. Do you enjoy films and/or TV
    programmes about doctors and
    hospitals?   Yes/No/Indifferent

12. If you do watch them AND you
    have been to hospital either as an
    in-patient or an out-patient, did
    they make either experience less
    worrying?   Yes/No/Not sure

LASTLY:

13. Do you think any of the following
    changes in the school health service
    would be helpful:
    (a) for the school doctor to visit
        more frequently?   Yes/No/Not sure
    (b) for the school nurse to visit
        more frequently?   Yes/No/Not sure
    (c) for the school doctor and
        school nurse to take more part
        in teaching human biology and
        personal development?   Yes/No/Not sure
    (d) for the school doctor to hold a
        clinic in the school for senior
        pupils where any health or
        personal problem could be
        discussed privately and in con-
        fidence?   Yes/No/Not sure
    (e) for your family doctor to be
        the school doctor?   Yes/No/Not sure

423

APPENDIX H

SURVEY OF CHILD AND ADOLESCENT PSYCHIATRIC UNITS

Questionnaire to Consultant Psychiatrists in Child and Adolescent Units (England). Analysis of 57 replies received to 58 questionnaires issued. One consultant was unable to answer questions 3–7 as he was new to his unit and no records had been kept by his predecessor.

1. HOW MANY BEDS ARE AVAILABLE IN YOUR UNIT FOR (a) PRE-ADOLESCENT CHILDREN (b) ADOLESCENTS OF SCHOOL AGE (c) OLDER ADOLESCENTS ABOVE SCHOOL AGE?

19 units had beds for more than one of the classes and did not specify how these were allocated between the classes. This was usually because the number of beds available to each class could be varied to allow for fluctuation in pressures between the various types of cases. Figures are included for all 58 units. Figures for beds:

Class a	458	29 units
Class b	257	15 units
Class c	5	2 units
Classes a and b mixed	107	6 units
Classes b and c mixed	191	11 units
Classes a, b and c mixed	10	2 units

TOTAL 1,088 beds

2. HOW MANY BEDS IN THESE CATEGORIES ARE ORDINARILY IN USE?

31 of the 57 units who replied to this question (54%) reported 100% bed occupancy. The overall average rate was 88% (956 beds). Only 3 units reported a rate below 70%, one of which was a new unit restricting admissions until the staff were fully trained, another had staffing difficulties.

3. HOW MANY PERSONS IN EACH CATEGORY ARE CURRENTLY ON THE WAITING LIST?

Of the 56 units who replied to this 16 did not have a waiting list. Of these 5 said this was a matter of policy and 8 did not need a waiting list at present.

Of the remaining 40 units, 8 grouped more than one of our classes together; the following figures emerge:

Class a	131
Class b	81
Class c	9
Class a and b mixed	77
Class b and c mixed	12
Class a, b and c mixed	30

TOTAL 340 on waiting list

424

This represented an average of 8.5 for the 40 units which have a list and an overall average of 6.0 per unit.

4. WHAT WOULD BE THE AVERAGE TIME ON THE WAITING LIST FOR EACH OF THESE CATEGORIES?

56 units supplied information varying from the very precise to the very vague. 7 units were so non-committal that no meaningful answers could be arrived at, and 13 had no waiting times. A reasonable average for the remaining 36 units would probably be about 10 weeks, representing an overall average of 6 weeks.

5. IN YOUR JUDGEMENT IS THE PRESSURE ON BEDS IN EACH OF THESE CATEGORIES INCREASING OR DECREASING IN THE AREA YOU SERVE?

Some units replied to this in respect of the classes with which they were involved, whilst others offered opinions on all 3 classes. Percentages are based on the number of answers received in each class:

	PRESSURE IN CLASS A	34 replies
	Increasing	13 (38.2%)
	Static	12 (35.3%)
	Decreasing	8 (23.5%)
	Don't know	1 (2.9%)

	PRESSURE IN CLASS B	34 replies
	Increasing	18 (52.9%)
	Static	10 (29.4%)
	Decreasing	5 (14.7%)
	Don't know	1 (2.9%)

	PRESSURE IN CLASS C	15 replies
	Increasing	8 (53.3%)
	Static	5 (33.3%)
	Decreasing	1 (6.7%)
	Don't know	1 (6.7%)

6. IF IT IS CHANGING, WHAT IN YOUR VIEW HAVE BEEN THE REASONS FOR CHANGE?

26 units (46.4%) felt that pressure was increasing and gave reasons for this. The most common factor (9 instances) was the increasing awareness of the local medical staff and the community at large of the unit's existence and of the service it provided. Next most common factor (8 instances) was the inability of the local Social Services Departments to cope with cases of disturbance, attributed by some to the lack of residential/hostel accommodation for this type of case. 6 units felt the increase in pressure was due to an actual increase in the incidence of disturbance. 3 units dealing with class b patients suggested that the increase in the school leaving age had caused an increase in pressure whilst one unit had experienced practical difficulties which had restricted the number of beds it could staff. Another felt that generally inadequate facilities in this field was the cause. 3 units did not know to what the increase could be attributed. 10 units (19.6%) said there had been a decrease in pressures due to improvements in other services: particularly day patient service increases, more

425

work in the community and also the opening of new units elsewhere in their region. A further 17 units (30.4%) felt that pressures were static and 2 (3.6%) could not say what the situation was.

7.   IN YOUR JUDGEMENT, ARE IN-PATIENT FACILITIES IN YOUR AREA FOR EACH OF THESE CATEGORIES ADEQUATE, INADEQUATE OR MORE THAN SUFFICIENT?

Here again some units offered answers relevant only to the classes with which they were actually involved, whilst others commented on all 3. Percentages are in terms of the number of replies in each classification rather than the overall number of replies.

CLASS A	44 replies
Adequate	18 (40.9%)
Inadequate	23 (52.3%)
More than sufficient	3 (6.7%)
CLASS B	50 replies
Adequate	13 (26.0%)
Inadequate	35 (70.0%)
More than sufficient	1 (2.0%)
Don't know	1 (2.0%)
CLASS C	42 replies
Adequate	6 (14.3%)
Inadequate	36 (85.7%)
More than sufficient	— —

An analysis of the replies to this question on a regional basis did not reveal any significant variations.

8.   OTHER COMMENTS

Many replies contained comments on the service's shortage of day unit places, and several noted the difficulties in providing day or in-patient care for children with their families. The lack of hostel accommodation was also mentioned and there was general agreement that there was a particular service shortage of long-term in-patient facilities for adolescents with severe chronic psychiatric handicaps and of facilities (social and psychiatric) for the care of severely disruptive adolescents.

APPENDIX I

PRESENT DISTRIBUTION AND DESIRABLE INCREASE IN PAEDIATRIC SPECIALTIES

See Chapter 18, paragraphs 18.10–22

Specialty	Existing Centres			Necessary Centres			Present Consultants			Needed Consultants			Specialist–Population Ratio Present/ Desirable per million total		Necessary Increase in Specialists Whole-Time Equivalents (whole numbers)
	PE	L	W	PE	L	W	PE	L	W	PE	L	W			
Perinatal Paediatrics	7	2	1	12	4	1	8	3	0.5	12	4	1	1:4	1:0.5	6
Complex Handicap	7	3	1	12	4	1	6.5	2.5	0.5	12	4	1	1:7	1:2.5	8
Neurology	4	2	0	12	4	1	5.5	3.5	0	12	4	1	1:4.5	1:2.5	8
Cardiology	7	7	1	5	2	0	8	4	0	15	6	0	1:4.1	1:2.3	9
Nephrology	4	2	0	6	2	1	2.5	2	0	9	3	1.5	1:10	1:3.5	9
Endocrinology	4	3	0	6	3	1	2	1.5	0	7	3	1.5	1:14	1:4.1	8
Gastro-Enterology	1	2	0	3	2	0	3.5	3	0.5	7.5	3	0.5	1:7	1:5.5	4
Haematology	5	1	0	12	4	1	6.5	2	0.5	12	4	1	1:5	1:2.8	8
Oncology	7	1	1	8	2	0	2.5	0.5	0.5	6.5	3	0.5	1:12	1:3.5	7

PE = Provincial England, L = London, W = Wales.
Consultant numbers are whole-time equivalents.

APPENDIX J

THE PAEDIATRIC TRAINING REQUIRED BY THE GENERAL PRACTITIONER
A REPORT BY A JOINT WORKING PARTY OF THE BRITISH PAEDIATRIC ASSOCIATION AND THE ROYAL COLLEGE OF GENERAL PRACTITIONERS

Aims

The working party was given the following remit by the Councils of the Association and the College: "To examine the content and methods of the paediatric training required by the general practitioner and to make recommendations".

SUMMARY. This report has been written because special programmes of training for general practice are being developed in many parts of the country and there are questions about the paediatric component of training which need to be discussed nationally.

An important part of this report is devoted to listing educational objectives which should be attained in paediatrics by the general practitioner at the end of his training.

Recommendations

(1) All vocational training schemes for general practice should include formal training in paediatrics.

(2) Training in paediatrics should normally take place in four learning situations ie in junior hospital posts, in the community health services, in teaching practices, and on day or half-day release courses.

(3) (a) Junior hospital training posts should last not less than four months. In most training schemes six months will prove to be the minimum, for practical reasons.

(b) They should usually be in acute non-specialised paediatric units and should include experience in neo-natal paediatrics.

(c) The support of the British Paediatric Association is sought in encouraging paediatricians to allow six monthly changes in the occupancy of most of their senior house officer posts (SHO posts), rather than a longer period, as the majority of their senior house physicians will become general practitioners.

(d) Even so, there will be a shortage of paediatric SHO posts for training purposes in some localities. The help of the Central Manpower Committee is sought in encouraging regional authorities to create a small number of additional posts where service need makes this justifiable.

(e) While in hospital, trainees should have experience of general paediatric surgery and those surgical sub-specialties which are particularly relevant to general practice, ie orthopaedics and ENT.

(4) There should be discussions within local training schemes between the paediatrician, the scheme organiser, and the general-practitioner teachers about

---

428

the objectives of training and their distribution between the four learning situations.

(5) Developmental paediatrics and the early detection of handicap are essential subjects for general practitioners. Since they must be taught partly in teaching practices, these could with advantage run special sessions for screening well-babies and toddlers. Alternatively, a local arrangement will need to be made with a child health clinic.

(6) It is important to teach about the impact of children's needs on practice organisation—especially the need for easy contact, quick appointments, and satisfactory emergency cover.

(7) Emotional disturbance in children needs to be considered at all stages of training. The subject lends itself to group discussion about particular patients and their problems.

Paediatricians, child psychiatrists, and general practitioners can contribute valuably to such discussions.

Child psychiatrists, who are too few in number, can spread their influence by teaching general practitioners to take increasing responsibility in this field. Selected child guidance clinics might contribute as learning situations on a day-release basis. More academic departments of child psychiatry are needed to produce such teachers.

Introduction

The main reason for this report being required and written at this time is the development of special programmes of training for general practice after registration ("vocational" or "professional" training). These have appeared in all parts of the United Kingdom and hitherto they have depended to a large extent on local initiative. Local organisers were at first free to devise their own training patterns, but during the last ten years there has been a growing consensus of opinion about aims, content, and teaching methods. But there are still some issues about which opinions vary.

In relation to paediatric training—apart from uncertainties about the pattern of paediatric care in the community—there are such questions as:

(1) What does the future general practitioner need to know and be able to do at the end of his special training?

(2) What should he have learned as an undergraduate and what as a vocational trainee or mature doctor?

(3) Is a junior paediatric hospital post a desirable learning experience for him? If so, how long should it last?

(4) Assuming that it is, what should be learned in hospital and what in the teaching practice?

(5) Does he need to learn developmental paediatrics? If so, who should teach it and where?

(6) Should he learn what is needed for work in the school health service?

(7) Are there enough junior hospital posts for the needs of both future paediatricians and future general practitioners?

(8) The MRCP, MRCGP, DCH and the D(Obst)RCOG examinations all include paediatrics in varying degrees. What, if any, is the place of each?

Although the special training of the general practitioner after registration is the main reason for this report, and its main focus, the working party realised very early in its discussion that it must consider undergraduate education in paediatrics. It decided also to take continuing education into account. Thus it follows the general contemporary trend of thinking of medical education as a continuous process from school to retirement.

The general practitioner's rôle in paediatrics

It seems to us essential, before discussing training, to say something about the general practitioner's rôle in the care of children, whether well or sick. We need to reveal any assumptions we have made about this, and point to topics of uncertainty, if they have a bearing on his training.

We assume that all general practitioners will undertake the care of children in their practice and that they will have responsibility, as doctors of first contact and continuing presence, for promotion of health, prevention of diseases, and the diagnosis and treatment of established disease. They will, of course, continue to refer some of their child patients and problems to consultant paediatricians who will usually be based in a hospital. Both will try, wherever possible, to keep and treat sick children at home.

We believe that there are bound to be some general practitioners who have a special interest in children and who will wish to increase their training and experience. We believe this desirable. It might take the form of hospital attachment or more detailed work in developmental assessment or work in the school health service and might particularly suit married women at some stages in their career.

We do not go beyond this and suggest, as some do in this country and many elsewhere, that some general practitioners should confine their practice to children. There are one or two experiments of this kind in this country, but they have not yet demonstrated the advantage of having a different doctor for children at the primary level and thereby losing the concept and reality of the family doctor. Our report is based on the predominant situation—the same general practitioner for adults and children, and ideally the same for all members of the family living in one household.

We believe that knowledge of human development is essential for any doctor dealing with children. We consequently do not think that the general practitioner can practise without some knowledge of developmental paediatrics.

We believe that some general practitioners will be required and will wish to work in the school health service. This is likely to deal in the future with medical conditions limiting a child's ability to take advantage of normal education or requiring special education. (Illnesses and injuries presenting at school are likely to be dealt with through the ordinary practice arrangements.) In so far as this work is different from the paediatric work done by every general practitioner in his own practice setting, they will need special training. This must be provided by paediatricians, child psychiatrists, psychologists, and general practitioners with appropriate training or clinicians at present working in the community service.

We do not feel able now to state the content of the additional training needed by doctors who wish to increase their skills in developmental assessment or to take part in the school health service, but they will obviously require to train in a comprehensive assessment centre.

The present state of vocational training for general practice

Although five years after registration is expected to be the eventual length of in-service training required for general practice, the effort now and in the foreseeable future is concentrated on providing three-year programmes for all future principals.

Approximately 1,200 individual three-year programmes are required to be available by the beginning of 1977, if this training is to be the normal requirement for all principals in 1980 (England, Wales, Scotland, and Northern Ireland). The usual pattern of learning experience is two years in junior hospital posts, one year in training practices and a variable length of time on day-release courses. These proportions may change in the near future.

Until recently it was assumed that all 1,200 programmes would need to be provided as "packages" ie a planned series of rotations in one locality. It is now clear that a proportion of trainees prefer to plan their own rotations within broad guide lines laid down by the Royal College of General Practitioners and approved by the regional Postgraduate Dean. They need guidance in their choice of post. All that is said in this report about the content and standards of training applies as much to them as to the others.

At the time of writing this report there are 450 programmes available annually in three-year planned rotations ("packages") and 199 doctors are choosing their own rotations. (Council for Postgraduate Education England and Wales (1974), personal communication).

Paediatrics is regarded as one of the four most important hospital appointments by most scheme organisers—with adult medicine, psychiatry, and obstetrics and gynaecology (although this last is not regarded as essential training for all entrants). A survey by post at the end of 1973 showed that in the Oxford region 90% and in the North of England (Newcastle) region 85% of individual programmes included a paediatric hospital appointment, but in Scotland the proportion was lower (Royal College of General Practitioners, 1974).

THE TRAINING OF GENERAL PRACTITIONERS—OBJECTIVES

The working party set out, as its first task, to decide what knowledge, skills, and attitudes should belong to the doctor as he finishes his three-year postgraduate training and starts as a principal in a general practice.

We are able to divide the educational aims into the five headings in *The Future General Practitioner—Learning and Teaching* (Royal College of General Practitioners, 1972) generally accepted as suitable in any consideration of the content of training for this branch of the profession. However, for children, it seemed appropriate to make one change in the usual order:

(1) Human development

(2) Health and diseases

(3) Human behaviour

(4) Society and medicine

(5) Practice organisation

(1) Human development

At the completion of his training the doctor should be able to demonstrate that:

(a) He has knowledge of the important norms of physical, intellectual, emotional, and social development at different ages.

(b) He can carry out the basic methods of assessment of these modes of development from birth up to, and including, adolescence.

(c) He can recognise common deviations from the normal.

(d) He understands the rôle of the health visitor in developmental assessment.

(e) He can recognise when there is a need for referral for more elaborate or specialised assessment.

(2) Health and diseases

A. Health

At the completion of his training the doctor should be able:

(a) Through his knowledge of the norms of development, physical, intellectual, emotional and social, to describe what characterises health in children.

(b) To describe the needs of children at different ages and the factors, whether hereditary or environmental, which favour their health and happiness (Appendix).

(c) To demonstrate that he recognises the value of health education, whether about parenthood in general, or about feeding and physical care of children; and the value of disease education ie the prevention of certain diseases, the recognition and home management of common disorders and the use of health and social services.

B. Diseases

He should be able always to recognise and in many instances to treat the following conditions:

(a) *Acute conditions threatening life*
In the newborn: infections, surgical conditions, some life-threatening congenital abnormalities, hypoglycaemia and hypothermia.
In infants: acute respiratory disorders, gastrointestinal infections, meningitis.
In older children: asthma, the "acute abdomen", accidents (including self-poisoning).
In adolescents: suicidal behaviour.

(b) *Conditions which, if not recognised early, can lead to disability or premature death.*
In the newborn: infections, jaundice, congenital malformations not immediately apparent, renal conditions, metabolic errors. The recognition of prematurity and dysmaturity.
In infants and older children: malignant disease, respiratory infections with complications, epilepsy, abnormal relations in a family, including battering.

432

(c) *Common conditions*
In the newborn: minor disorders, eg birth marks, feeding problems.
In infants: feeding and sleep problems, respiratory tract infections, parasitic infections, and eczema.
In older children: minor injuries, epilepsy, migraine, behaviour and sleep problems, enuresis and faecal incontinence.
In adolescents: behaviour problems, hypochondriasis, depression.

(d) *Handicaps and their supervision*
Asthma, congenital handicaps, including heart disease, diabetes, haemophilia, epilepsy, cerebral palsy, mental handicap, social disadvantage.

In relation to all these conditions listed in *B. Diseases* above, he should be able to demonstrate that he has been concerned with some aspects in particular:

1. Early diagnosis.
2. Prevention, where possible.
3. Management at home.
4. Psychological and social aspects, where important.
5. The sick child's individuality.
6. The indications for referral to a consultant or a social agency.
7. Education of parents about common disorders and about the use of health services.
8. Children who are especially vulnerable.

(3) Human behaviour

At the end of his training the doctor should be able to demonstrate his understanding:

(a) Of the ways in which the doctor's behaviour towards a child and/or his parents can influence the success or failure of a consultation and the solution of a problem.

(b) Of the ways in which the behaviour of a child, acutely or chronically ill, can influence the behaviour of the rest of the family.

(c) Of the ways in which the behaviour of the family, particularly the parents, can influence the health, happiness and social behaviour of a child (and the behaviour of a child that of his parents).

(d) Of the ways in which family relationships and attitudes, healthy and unhealthy, towards children may persist from one generation to another.

(e) Of the potential importance of the "milestones" or "normal crises" in a child's life (weaning, habit training, separation from mother, starting school, puberty, falling in love and early sexual experience, as causes of persisting difficulty and indicators of family stress).

(4) Medicine and society

At the end of his training the doctor should be able to demonstrate:

(a) That he understands the influence of culture and class on the incidence, presentation, and management of different illnesses.

433

(b) That he is aware of the prevalence of the different types of children's illnesses in his practice population.

(c) That he is aware of the contribution of epidemiology to understanding of the causes of some disorders of children.

(d) His knowledge of the rôles of health visitors, social workers, and other helping agencies in the care of children, whether well or ill.

(e) That he is aware of what is known about the incidence, cause and prevention of socio-medical problems such as smoking, alcoholism, drug addiction, pregnancy in girls still at school, and juvenile crime.

(f) That he understands the medical aspects of adoption.

(5) Practice organisation

At the end of his training the doctor should be able:

(a) To demonstrate his knowledge of the organisation of paediatric services in this country and compare them with contrasting systems in other countries.

(b) To describe how practice organisation must meet the special challenges of sick children—the need for easy contact, quick appointments, and satisfactory emergency cover; the need for time for dealing with parental anxiety, for communicating with health visitors and social workers, for home visits; the need for suitable accommodation and equipment in the practice building.

(c) To describe the organisation of a well-baby clinic (screening, records, immunisation).

THE CONTINUUM OF EDUCATION

In listing the objectives, we have stated what we believe that the doctor should be able to do at the end of his training and at the moment when he will take up practice as an independent principal. Nothing has been said about which parts should be learned as an undergraduate, which as a postgraduate, or about which parts should be learned by postgraduates in a paediatric hospital post or in a training practice.

Although the undergraduate period caters for all students whatever their future career and should be an education rather than a training, in practice the line between education and training is impossible to define. There will undoubtedly be an overlap between what is learned as an undergraduate and what is learned in a postgraduate training for general practice.

(1) Undergraduate education

By the time of qualification it can be expected that the student will have learned how history-taking, physical examination, the presentation and varieties of illness, and the general approach to management differ in childhood from what he has learned about adult medicine.

It is reasonable to expect the newly qualified and registered doctor to have:

(a) A general impression of the scope of hospital paediatric practice and the paediatricians' ways of seeing disease and treatment in the context of total growth.

434

(b) Mastery of the basic skills of paediatric history-taking and examination.

(c) A limited experience of practical preventive paediatrics, including immunisation and infant feeding.

(d) Basic knowledge of growth and development and the assessment thereof.

(e) Awareness of the principles of paediatric therapeutics as applied to acute illness and handicap.

(f) Awareness of the nature of the doctor/patient relationship—applied to third-party consultations.

Thus the undergraduate will have a thorough grounding in human development, diseases, and clinical method. He may have had some grounding in human behaviour and about medicine and society from pre-clinical courses on psychology and sociology. He will have learnt almost nothing about practice organisation.

But even in human development and diseases he will need to know more and he will need plenty of opportunity for practising his skill in clinical method. Thus all areas are open for further training after qualification.

Adequate experience of neonatal medicine is important.

The student will gain invaluable experience by spending time in the casualty department.

(2) Early postgraduate training

Since the objectives of training have been set out above, we need:

(a) To justify their distribution between three learning situations—junior hospital posts, teaching practices, and day-release courses.

(b) To indicate which objectives are best served by one of these learning situations rather than another.

Although some advocate a training programme which takes place entirely in the setting of the future work, ie the practice, we believe that the experience gained in junior hospital posts in paediatrics cannot be omitted without important loss.

These posts offer a concentration of experience of a wide range of disorders, including some rare ones, of opportunities to practice clinical method and to gain understanding and confidence in recognising the child who is ill and dealing with serious disorders. Hospital posts in a district general hospital may lend themselves better to the future general practitioner's needs than those of a teaching hospital, assuming that the standard of clinical teaching is equally high. Adequate neonatal experience, which is essential, is now difficult to obtain except in hospital. It is an advantage that children with general or orthopaedic surgical conditions are now usually nursed in paediatric wards.

We believe that a four-month resident appointment is the minimum requirement. The post must have a service commitment, include experience in the outpatient department, and allow time for day-release, for tutorials and for reading. In most training schemes six months will prove to be the minimum, for practical reasons.

A full-time hospital appointment creates a difficulty for some married women doctors. This might be resolved, as in the Oxford region, by the creation of one-year posts of shared tenure.

The hospital outpatient department can provide a setting for learning about common disorders, chronic ones and the assessment of development and handicaps. It also offers experience under supervision in counselling parents and in the emotional disorders of children, especially if the department of child psychiatry cooperates. Teaching about common orthopaedic conditions also takes place in outpatients.

A day-release course can offer theoretical knowledge whether by lecture or discussion. There are theoretical aspects in all five areas, but particularly in health, human behaviour, medicine and society, and practice organisation.

A great deal of overlap is possible and desirable between what is taught in hospital posts, teaching practices, and courses.

Learning in hospital posts should concentrate most on the skills of clinical method and on knowledge of diseases, particularly the more serious and less common ones which it is nevertheless important for the future general practitioner to see if he is to recognise them later in life. The more serious chronic disorders and handicaps will also be seen through outpatient experience. As much as possible, emotional disturbances of childhood should also be included and demonstrated. As nine out of ten babies are born in hospital, neonatal experience must be obtained there.

Learning in a teaching practice should be maximal about prevention, including well-baby clinics, normal development and immunisation, about the early diagnosis of all disorders, including the psychological and social assessment of the children presenting them, about home management and the counselling of parents, about the indications for referral and the results thereof, about working in the domiciliary health team, about the assessment and management of multiple problems, about making rapid decisions, about the sick child in the family, the influence of the family on the child's health and the effects of the various social agencies; about practice organisation and the demands made on it by the special needs of children and their parents.

Learning in day-release courses may be maximal about human development, health, human behaviour, society and medicine, and practice organisation.

We believe it to be important that a training scheme organiser, his trainers and the paediatrician involved in the training scheme should discuss together the objectives of training and the distribution of content, as a syllabus, between the three settings.

(3) Continuing education

The general principle of detecting areas of ignorance or uncertainty, either through self-discipline or through inviting the scrutiny of others, then proceeding to the appropriate learning, applies as much to paediatrics as to any other subject.

During the life-long period when continuing education is required, the doctor should be able to satisfy himself that he:

(a) Has kept in mind such acute conditions as intussusception, which occur very rarely, yet threaten life, or lead to irretrievable damage if not diagnosed early.

(b) Is aware of important new advances, particularly in diagnosis, treatment, and prevention.

436

DEPARTMENT OF HEALTH AND SOCIAL SECURITY

ALEXANDER FLEMING HOUSE

ELEPHANT AND CASTLE

LONDON S.E.1. 6BY

TELEPHONE: 01-407 5522   Ext 6033

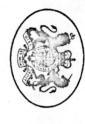

15 December 1976

To: Regional Administrators

Dear Administrator

REPORT OF THE COURT COMMITTEE ON CHILD HEALTH SERVICES

1.   The Secretaries of State for Social Services, for Education and Science and for Wales have today published the Report of the Committee on Child Health Services under the Chairmanship of Professor Court. (A copy of the Report is enclosed.)

2.   The Committee's recommendations, which call for far-reaching changes in the pattern of child health services and would have major implications for the professional staff concerned, would, in any circumstances, require widespread consultations before decisions are reached, and in a Statement in the House of Commons Mr Ennals said that the Government would be seeking the early comments of interested organisations and individuals on the Committee's recommendations. He went on to draw attention to the Committee's view that many of their recommendations would have very significant resource imp lications, particularly in respect of manpower and training and could be implemented only over a long period as the economic recovery of the nation proceeds. He also noted that there were a number of recommendations involving little or no additional resources.

3.   Ministers are anxious that careful consideration should be given now to the desirability of, and scope for, implementing at the appropriate time the Report's major recommendations. This of course must take place

e. the child guidance and child psychiatric services should be integrated as a single child and adolescent psychiatric service;

f. there is a need for a body at national level to look at the way children's needs are being met and to carry out the functions described in Chapter 16 of the Committee's report, which might be fulfilled by a joint committee of the Personal Social Services Council and the Central Health Services Council.

6. A number of the Committee's recommendations are in line with existing Departmental policy. Others clearly reflect innovations by individual authorities. We would welcome views, particularly from those who have been involved in any such developments, on which of the Court recommendations it would be both desirable and feasible to make some progress in the short-term given current resource constraints. Experience may have shown that rationalisation of some services in fact leads to savings.

7. We should be grateful if comments could be sent, no later than 30 June 1977, to Children''s Division (C), Room B1510, Alexander Fleming House, Department of Health and Social Security, Elephant & Castle, London SE1 6BY. 6 copies of this letter are enclosed for your RTO. Copies of the letter and a copy of the Report are being sent to Area Administrators, District Administrators and Family Practitioner Committees.

Further copies of the report can be obtained from HMSO.

Yours sincerely

P V FOSTER

From:

Children's Division (C)
Alexander Fleming House
Elephant and Castle
London SE1 6BY

Department will be attempting a more rigorous analysis of the human and financial resource implications of implementing the Report than was possible for the Committee.

4. Against this background the Department would like to have the views of your RTO on the Court Committee's recommendations, taking into account the views of Areas and districts in your region. (Community Health Councils are being consulted individually.)

5. With a wide ranging report of this kind there will clearly be many points on which you will wish to comment. It would however be of particular assistance to Ministers in considering what would be involved in reaching early decisions on the major issues of principle if your reply could specifically indicate your views on the following propositions underlying the Committee's key recommendations:

a. the long-term aim should be to provide pre-school and school health services through general practitioner paediatricians;

b. there should be a degree of specialisation in health visiting leading to the establishment of child health visitors;

c. there should be increased involvement of paediatricians in work in the community, including the establishment of posts for consultant community paediatricians;

d. there should be district handicap teams with responsibility for all handicapped, including mentally retarded, children;

1

(c) Can deal critically with the literature, particularly that provided by drug firms.

The many methods of postgraduate continuing education do not need to be listed. We would like to stress the value of short attachments to consultant paediatricians and particularly the domiciliary consultation where both doctors meet—the more so since neither are always easy to arrange; also the self-administered questionnaire as a simple means of detecting weak areas of knowledge and skill.

Experiments could with value be made whereby consultant paediatricians pay regular visits to practices. Large group practices or health centres would lend themselves most easily to this purpose. The paediatrician would see children as a consultant, with the child's doctor, and might also take part in group teaching sessions.

Examinations

We expect that undergraduates would always be examined in paediatrics as part of their final examination. General practitioners would be expected to examine.

Paediatrics forms part of the MRCGP examination which can be taken at the end of the three-year period of training. Trainees are encouraged to have their standards evaluated by this examination.

There is uncertainty at present about the purpose and value of the DCH examination, particularly as intending principals in general practice seem to have the paediatric component of their training covered in the MRCGP examination. We believe it would find a useful place for those general practitioners who wish to work part time in child health clinics or the school health service and that preparation for it might take place, in part, after the end of the three-year training period. If vocational or professional training eventually occupies five years, the DCH examination might be taken during the last two.

If the examination is reviewed, it would be an advantage if general practitioners as well as paediatricians were on the examining board.

Adequacy of present opportunities for training

(1) *Hospital posts*

Between 20 and 40 senior house officer posts are required annually for training paediatricians in England and Wales while about 450 posts are needed twice a year for training future general practitioners (Council for Postgraduate Education in England and Wales (1975) Personal communication), ie the same post needs to be occupied by a different trainee every six months. On paper there are enough posts for all needs; but in practice there are not, because the same doctor often occupies the post for a year or even longer, and this is obviously an advantage to the consultant concerned, since he has a more experienced senior house officer to support him. If senior house officer posts are to be correctly used for general professional or vocational training, the help of paediatricians must be sought in ensuring that appointments are for six months. The support of the British Paediatric Association is needed.

A number of these posts are in children's hospitals. Posts in district general hospitals provide as a rule the most suitable training for general practice.

Some posts might combine medical and surgical paediatrics. This might enable the number of SHO posts in a unit to be increased from two to three.

437

The cost of new posts should be set against the present cost of overtime pay and locums.

We do not think that the duration of the senior house officer post should be shortened to help married women doctors, but we support the idea of a post being shared by two women doctors, half-time each, during a year.

(2) *Paediatric consultants*

Most senior house officers will enter either general practice or some branch other than paediatrics itself. General practice and paediatrics would both gain if paediatricians based their aims in training on the likely future career requirements of their senior house officers. To achieve this, they should have been exposed to general practice.

In the training for consultant paediatricians it has been agreed by the British Paediatric Association that a six-month elective period in general practice would be appropriate. This would probably involve up to 20 doctors annually. Many general practitioners and paediatricians are beginning to feel that it should be mandatory.

General practice could be given the same weighting in consultant training as paediatrics is given in the training of the general practitioner.

(3) *Teaching practices*

There are at present a greater number of teachers than trainees looking for teachers. Further development needs to be in the direction of greater understanding of what should be taught about children in teaching practices and the best methods of teaching.

Addendum

The members of the working party were: Dr J. P. Horder, *O.B.E.* (Chairman), Dr J. P. Bound (Hon. Secretary), Professor J. A. Davis, and Drs W. Henderson, L. Hersov, C. G. W. Sykes, and C. Waine. Dr G. W. Hatcher later replaced Dr Henderson.

Acknowledgements

We wish to thank Miss Therese Searson for the considerable secretarial work involved in this report.

We also wish to thank all those members of the Academic Board of the British Paediatric Association (together with Dr Ronald McKeith) and the members of Faculties of the Royal College of General Practitioners who have read and commented on the final draft of this paper.

Appendix

The needs of children are well described in a paper written for this working party by Dr Lionel Hersov:

"Throughout a child's development the parents have to meet the infant's, child's, adolescent's needs for affection, praise and acceptance, security, and a sufficient degree of stimulation both cognitive and emotional. In addition, children need freedom for bodily activity, the opportunity for new experiences and increasing responsibility and above all a comfortable loving relationship in which recognition and praise as well as disapproval, when appropriate, are consistently provided."

Dr Hersov's paper discussed the ways in which parents fulfil or fail to fulfil these needs. It also stresses the effects of children on their parents—how for instance a more active baby can stimulate more demonstrations of affection from its mother so that there is a stronger and earlier attachment.

In general he points to the need to think and teach about the mutual interaction of two persons—mother and child (or father and child)—rather than concentrating too much on the child and his needs.

REFERENCE

Royal College of General Practitioners (1972). *The Future General Practitioner—Learning and Teaching,* London: British Medical Journal.

APPENDIX K

PRESENT ARRANGEMENTS FOR PAEDIATRIC NURSE TRAINING

1. Since 1972 nurse training has operated in an educational twilight. The signposts for the future have been erected, but the road ahead has not been made. While waiting expectantly we must keep the established road in reasonable repair. Nurses have more continuous and intimate contact with children and parents than doctors do. They must be equipped and ready to meet not only the needs of illness but the needs of children and parents for explanation and comfort, and they must be skilled at involving parents as fully as possible in the care of their children. If they are to become effective at this their training must include experience of normal children, and greater knowledge than in the past of child development, family relationships, psychiatric disorders and handicap and its effects on child and family. The 1969 syllabus for the RSCN certificate has been widened to include these subjects, and training can take place in the community, in nurseries, child health clinics and special schools as well as in hospital.

2. At present there are six ways in which to train for nursing sick children:
   (i) A combined course of three and a half years leading to the double qualification of SRN/RSCN. Over the past ten years the number of such courses has risen from 9 to 14.
   (ii) A post registration course of 13 months for nurses who are already SRN, leading to RSCN. The number of these courses has increased from 9 to 20.
   (iii) An experimental, post registration, combined scheme of 104 weeks at the Hospital for Sick Children, London, leading to RSCN and Diploma in Nursing Part A and Part B in Paediatrics.
   (iv) An experimental post registration course of 6 months at Sheffield for SRNs with not less than 2 years senior experience in a post of responsibility in children's nursing.
   (v) A 3 year course leading to the qualification of RSCN. Until 10 years ago this was the main method of entry to children's nursing, but this pattern of training is gradually being phased out and the number of schools offering training has fallen from 19 to 1.
   (vi) A 2 year course leading to the qualification of SEN, 18 months of which are given to sick children. There are 11 schools providing this experience.

3. In the view of the General Nursing Council for England and Wales the integrated course in its present form is a satisfactory substitute for the 3 years RSCN course. In 1963 there were 19 RSCN courses, 9 integrated courses and 9 post registration courses (total 37); the corresponding figures for 1974/75 were 3, 28 and 20 (total 51); and for 1975/76 they were 1, 14 and 20 (total 35). In 1968, 800 students were admitted to one or other of these courses; in 1974/75 the number was 970. There has therefore been a modest increase in the numbers of students entering courses leading to the RSCN qualification, although we have been given to understand that there have been some restrictions placed on the numbers accepted for training in certain schools during 1976. Furthermore

440

over the past 5 years the discontinuation rate has fallen from 57% in 1964/65 to 24.8% which is lower than the average discontinuation rate of 31.1% for all nursing students.

4. We see integrated and post registration courses continuing to be the main source of RSCNs in England and Wales. We hope the 6 month "experimental course" in Sheffield will continue and that it will soon be possible to decide whether similar courses should be introduced elsewhere. We would like to see a considerable increase in the number of paediatric SEN courses, the existence of which is still relatively unknown, even within nursing and medicine.

APPENDIX L

THE TRAINING OF WOMEN DOCTORS

1. Specialist training raises special issues for women doctors and their contribution to paediatrics can be more clearly seen if the general position is understood. In the last twenty years the proportion of women entering medical schools has steadily increased; it is already at 35% and may soon reach 50%. Ways of improving the professional opportunities of those who temporarily or permanently can work only part-time must be found; and part-time post-graduate and vocational training makes little sense without established part-time career posts afterwards. The previous Secretary of State indicated her belief that planning should prepare for a situation when half of all new medical graduates will be women. This is clearly relevant to our proposals, which call for an increase in doctors.

Part-time Career Grade Posts

2. Important contributions to the work of the Health Service can be made on a part-time basis. From time to time, general practices take in partners with a limited commitment to the practice work or part-time salaried assistants. The Medical Practices Committee does on occasion approve admission to the medical list in a restricted area of married women doctors whose choice of area is determined by their husband's work. The Community Health Services have long offered a range of opportunities in clinical and administrative work, and without the part-time contribution of women doctors the work of the child health and school health services could not be maintained. There is some evidence to suggest that this situation is in part due to domestic necessity rather than professional choice. Wider opportunities could therefore reduce the numbers available in this area of paediatrics unless the present isolation and lack of a satisfactory career structure are overcome.

3. On the hospital side the Department will consider applications for the establishment of new part-time consultant posts. It is also possible for the field of recruitment for established posts to be enlarged to include doctors who can work only part-time because of domestic commitments. Some Health Authorities have indicated when advertising whole-time or maximum part-time posts that they will also consider applications from doctors who because of domestic commitments are able to offer only 7 sessions, and the use of this formula has met with some success. The concept of an intermediate career grade between consultant and trainee has not so far found favour with the profession. Necessity however has compelled the creation of a limited number of "medical assistant" posts. These can be established with the Department's approval: and the criteria are that the post meets both a specific service need and the personal circumstances of a doctor who has completed two years of registrar training or its equivalent but cannot, for personal reasons, go on to higher training and a consultant post. We believe that for training purposes the "medical assistant" should be seen in the wider context of the "clinical specialist in paediatrics". There are a few "clinical assistants" providing sessional help to fill short or long term gaps in a particular specialist service. These posts are generally unsatis-

factory for the individual and the service; a more rational career structure should make them unnecessary and specific training is not indicated.

Postgraduate Training

4. The corollary of part-time appointments is part-time training. This is recognised by the Training Bodies, and their hopes have been feelingly expressed. "The Joint Committee recognises that there are special problems with the training of married women doctors who have domestic ties. It is very much hoped that they will make every effort to continue their postgraduate medical education even though they may have acquired family responsibilities. All employing authorities should be prepared to make facilities for general professional and specialist training flexible to meet their needs on a part-time basis and the Specialist Advisory Committees will cooperate in the approval of such programmes. The visiting team will enquire specifically about the provision of these facilities. It should be noted that in this context "part-time" is interpreted as meaning at least half time. Married women doctors should be prepared to do at least this number of sessions together with periods of on-call and emergency duties."[1]

5. At present both the hospital and the general practice components of vocational training schemes for general practice may be undertaken part-time with the twelve months training in general practice spread over a period of up to 2 years. Doctors wishing to return to medical practice as general practitioners may receive assistance with retraining. There are special arrangements to enable health authorities to establish part-time senior registrar, registrar and SHO posts for doctors with domestic commitments. The harsh fact is however that the implementation of these schemes falls far short of the intake of women students and the expectations of an increasing number of able graduates.

6. The "women doctors retainer scheme" can be a useful bridge. The object is to enable doctors with substantial domestic commitments to maintain contact with professional work by undertaking at least one session a month and at most two sessions a week in the NHS, including general practice. They are paid for these sessions, with an annual "retainer" to cover basic expenses. They also attend a minimum of seven educational sessions a year, agree to maintain registration with the General Medical Council and membership of a medical defence organisation, and to subscribe to a medical journal. This is a holding activity until return to a substantial professional commitment is again possible.

---

[1] Second Report of the Joint Committee on Higher Medical Training (1975). Royal College of Physicians.

APPENDIX M

THE REORGANISATION OF THE NATIONAL HEALTH
SERVICE AND THE CENTRAL DEPARTMENTS

Background to the Reorganisation

1. There were three main reasons for the introduction of the National Health Service in 1948. The first was that many people were experiencing great difficulty in finding the money to pay for medical treatment. Second, the hospital services were running into serious financial trouble. (This was not just a matter of too few beds and too many of these unsatisfactory, but also because there were two separate systems of administration—voluntary hospitals and local authority hospitals.) Third there was a need to remedy the uneven distribution of staff and other resources between different geographical areas and between different parts of the services.

2. To deal with these problems a unified service was needed and had been intended, but for political reasons and because health services had grown up that way, the NHS was saddled with a tri-partite structure. In one part were the hospital and specialist services. In another were the general practitioner services, administered by autonomous Local Executive Councils. In the third part were the local authority health services administered by the major local authorities. This division of responsibility led to lack of balance, overlap and deficiencies in the services, particularly in services for children, old people and people with mental illness, mental handicap or physical handicap. On the hospital side the services for these groups had failed to attract the financial and other resources they needed, while on the local authority side complementary domiciliary and community services had been slow to develop and were developing unevenly. For these and other reasons the framework of the NHS was re-designed and on 1 April 1974, a new administrative structure was introduced under the NHS Reorganisation Act (1973).

Outline of the reorganised administrative structure

3. The stated purposes of the change were to unify the local administration of health services under new Area Health Authorities; to base the day-to-day running of the services on Districts, each planned to provide comprehensive health services for a population of about a quarter of a million; to provide for collaboration between the NHS and certain related services for which local authorities still remained responsible; to give full weight to the views of the health professions in the planning and management of services; to correct disparities among regions and among specialties; and to provide a new means of representing the interests of the public in the health services at district level. The services brought together under Area Health Authorities were hospital and specialist services previously administered by Regional Hospital Boards, Hospital Management Committees and Boards of Governors of teaching hospitals; the personal health services previously administered by local authorities through their health committees (health visiting, home nursing, maternal and child health care, vaccination and immunisation, health centres etc.); and the school health services previously administered by local authorities through their educa-

tion committees. Details of the new structure are set out in "Management Arrangements for the Reorganised National Health Service", in "Management Arrangements for the Reorganised National Health Service in Wales" and in a wide range of DHSS and Welsh Office circulars. A summary of the arrangements is provided in what follows.

4. *Area Health Authorities.* These are the key authorities with boundaries drawn to correspond with matching local authorities. The chairman of the Authority is appointed by the Secretary of State, and the members by the matching Local Authority and by the Regional Health Authority (see below), after consultation with the professions and interested organisations. The AHA is responsible for planning and developing health services in its Area in relation to national policies and regionally determined strategies and in co-operation with the matching Local Authority. It allocates resources between districts and monitors the performance of the districts in relation to agreed plans. It is accountable to the RHA (in Wales there is no Regional Authority interposed between the AHA's and the Welsh Office—the central government department). The AHA is advised by an Area Team of Officers (Area Medical Officer, Nursing Officer, Treasurer and Administrator).

5. *Family Practitioner Committees.* The reorganisation has left unchanged the status of general medical and dental practitioners, ophthalmic medical practitioners, opticians and pharmacists. All continue to provide services as independent contractors under contracts administered by Family Practitioner Committees. AHAs have a statutory duty to set up FPCs. There is some cross-membership and a close working relationship is essential, but the FPC has sole responsibility for matters which relate to the administration of contracts with practitioners. The AHA is responsible for matters involving the planning of practice services, the development of health centres and arrangements for nurses (including health visitors) and other skilled staff employed by the AHA to work with general practitioners but the AHA will have the advice of the FPC. The AHA has to ensure that any plans affecting contractor services are acceptable to the FPC.

6. *District Management Teams.* Except in one-district Areas, the day-to-day running of the NHS is based on Districts. The District is not a separate tier of the administrative hierarchy but part of the Area administration so organised as to enable the AHA to meet community needs most effectively. The members of each District Management Team (District Community Physician, Nursing Officer, Finance Officer, Administrator and a consultant and general practitioner) are jointly responsible to the Area Health Authority (but are not accountable to the ATO, except in Wales) for most of the NHS services in their district. They assess existing services in the district, identify unmet needs, suggest priorities and draw up plans for the approval of the AHA. Within each district there is a *District Medical Committee* to represent all general medical practitioners and hospital specialist staff and to coordinate

445

medical aspects of the health services throughout the District. The views of the consumer of the district health services are represented by *Community Health Councils.*

7. *Joint Consultative Committees.* Four important health related services lie outside the NHS and are the responsibility of local government authorities: personal social services; educational services; housing; and environmental health services. Collaboration between the authorities responsible for these services and the health authorities is essential. To achieve this Joint Consultative Committees have been set up by Area Health Authorities and matching local authorities to advise on the planning and operation of services of common concern.

8. *Regional Health Authorities.* The principle rôle of the regional authorities is to develop strategic plans and priorities based on a review of the needs identified by the AHAs within its boundaries and on its judgement of the right balance between those areas' claims on its resources. In this rôle it is guided by national policies. It is also responsible for identification and provision, directly or through its AHAs, of services that need a regional approach such as arrangements for the less common specialties (eg neurosurgery, cardiac surgery, radiotherapy). Each RHA has at least one University Medical School within its boundaries and has a special responsibility for the service facilities needed to support undergraduate and postgraduate medical and dental education. In Wales there is no RHA.

9. *Dental Services.* The administrative structure of the Dental Services in the reorganised NHS follows a pattern intended to be comparable with that in medicine (ie the service is two-tiered with a tier at Regional and a tier at Area level and a central government department). It was originally proposed that there should be administrative Regional Dental Officers, Area Dental Officers and part-time District Dental Officers. In the event, no Regional Dental Officers and very few (only 45) District Dental Officers have been appointed but all Area Dental Officers are now in post. There is no comparable district dental committee: the interests of general dental practitioners are represented on the Area Dental Committee. Since reorganisation, the School Dental Service has been the responsibility of Area Health Authorities and the DHSS (the Welsh Office in Wales): prior to 1974, it was that of the local education authorities and the DES.

10. *Department of Health and Social Security.* The Secretary of State is responsible to Parliament for the administration of the NHS and in carrying out this task is assisted by the Department of Health and Social Security. That responsibility includes establishing national policies and priorities; agreeing with regions and areas on the objectives to be developed in the light of those policies and priorities; allocation of resources to enable regional authorities to put their plans into effect (family practitioner services are provided for separately and are not in-

cluded in regional and area budgets); development of the resources essential to the services (personnel, finance, property, supply); certain types of research; and the preparation of national statistics. Expert advice is available to the Department from a structure of advisory bodies.

The Welsh Office

11. The administrative structure of the health services in Wales differs from that in England in a number of respects. The most important of these is that there is no regional health authority. This means that the Welsh Office (the central government department) is itself responsible for strategic planning within the Principality and for monitoring the performances of the eight AHAs. The Secretary of State for Wales is directly responsible for all services for children and this includes the appropriate social services, primary and secondary education and housing as well as services within the National Health Service. Because there is no regional authority, substantially more planning and decision making responsibilities are delegated to the AHAs than in England. A special body, the Welsh Health and Technical Services Organisation, is responsible amongst other things for the design and execution of major capital works, the systematic evaluation of contracting arrangements for supplies, and for a computer-based management information service.

The Department of Health and Social Security

12. Although some of the health needs of children are met by elements of the NHS devoted exclusively to them—eg school health services and children's departments in general hospitals—many other needs are met by personnel and facilities shared with adults—eg ENT surgeons, GPs (medical and dental), diagnostic laboratory services and health centres. Children do not have a separate health service, they are clients of the NHS provided for the population at large. Similarly, local authority social service departments provide services for people of all ages, there is no separate management structure for their services for children. But both the NHS and social service departments provide specialised services and institutions for children and employ professional staff who specialise in the needs of children—eg community medical services for children, services for the residential care and fostering of children, consultant paediatricians and Specialists in Community Medicine (Child Health).

13. At the end of 1972 the headquarters of the Department of Health and Social Security was reorganised and a new Service Development Group was established. This group includes six divisions, three of which are concerned with the development of services on a "client group" basis, namely: Services for the Socially Handicapped, Services for Mental Health and Children's Division. The new organisation recognises that most of the Department's work requires several disciplines to act in partnership and provides professional groups alongside administrative divisions with related but direct responsibilities. Thus groups of medical, nursing and social work

447

service officers are associated with the Children's Division and are responsble between them for central oversight of NHS and PSS services provided exclusively for children. They do not take the lead in developing policy for the services which children share with adults. For these, the object is to provide advice to other divisions and groups on the special needs of children. For example mentally handicapped children in long-stay hospitals need specialised medical and caring services along with mentally handicapped adults. Yet as children they have other needs best met by child-oriented services. The two sets of needs are closely linked. When a problem arises for which particular expertise in mental handicap is required, the lead is taken by the Mental Health Division. The Children's Division takes the lead on those problems which arise directly from the fact that the patients are children (eg the provision of paediatric care and issues concerning such matters as play, recreation and parental visiting).

Printed in England for Her Majesty's Stationery Office by Williams Lea and Company Limited London
Dd 294753 K80 12/76